Masterclass in Neuroendocrinology

Volume 10

Series Editors

William E. Armstrong
Department of Anatomy and Neurobiology, The University of Tennessee Health
Science Center, Memphis, TN, USA

Mike Ludwig
Centre for Integrative Physiology, The University of Edinburgh, Edinburgh, UK

Masterclass in Neuroendocrinology is a co-publication of the INF (International Neuroendocrine Federation) that aims to illustrate the highest standards and promote the use of the latest technologies in basic and clinical research, while also providing inspiration for further exploration into the exciting field of neuroendocrinology. It is intended for established researchers, trainees and students alike.

Each book
- is edited by leading experts in the field
- is written by a team of internationally respected researchers
- includes assessments of different experimental approaches, both in vivo and in vitro, and of how the resulting data are interpreted.

Founding Series Co-Editors: William E. Armstrong and John A. Russell

More information about this series at http://www.springer.com/series/15770

Francis J. P. Ebling • Hugh D. Piggins
Editors

Neuroendocrine Clocks and Calendars

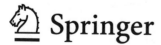 Springer

Editors
Francis J. P. Ebling
School of Life Sciences
University of Nottingham
Nottingham, United Kingdom

Hugh D. Piggins
School of Life Sciences
University of Bristol
Bristol, United Kingdom

ISSN 2662-2068   ISSN 2662-2076   (electronic)
Masterclass in Neuroendocrinology
ISBN 978-3-030-55645-7   ISBN 978-3-030-55643-3   (eBook)
https://doi.org/10.1007/978-3-030-55643-3

Cover illustration by deblik, based on an image from © Nablys/stock.adobe.com

This Springer imprint is published by the registered company Springer Nature Switzerland AG.
The registered company address is: Gewerbestrasse 11, 6330 Cham, Switzerland

*This book is dedicated to the memory of
Gerald Lincoln, who died after a short illness
on 15 July 2020 at the age of 75. Gerald was a
Fellow of the Royal Society of Edinburgh, and
lately Emeritus Professor of Biological
Timing at Edinburgh University.
He had completed the first chapter of this
book; this provides a historical overview of
how we have arrived at our current
understanding of seasonality,
photoperiodism, and circannual rhythmicity.
No person could have been better placed to do
this, as Gerald played a leading role in these
fields. He was an outstanding naturalist and
scientist, a deep thinker, and a vibrant and
engaging communicator. Gerald is best
known for studying the semi-domesticated
Soay sheep breed as a model to explore
seasonal cycles in neuroendocrine function,
but his broad interest in biology and
understanding of comparative studies
underpinned his approach to science. His
studies utilising surgical approaches to
remove sympathetic innervation of the pineal
gland in Soay rams and then the replacement*

of melatonin implants contributed hugely to our understanding of how photoperiodic information is transduced in mammals. Likewise, his studies in Soay sheep where the pituitary gland was surgically disconnected from the hypothalamus demonstrated the key role of the pars tuberalis *as a melatonin responsive tissue and as a locus for the generation of circannual rhythmicity. Gerald was passionate about his research, and his enthusiasm for understanding mechanisms and explaining the natural world stimulated and enthused everyone he came into contact with. The scientific community has lost an inspirational biologist and a wonderful person.*

Fran Ebling
22 September, 2020

Series Preface

This series began publication as a joint venture between the International Neuroendocrine Federation and Wiley-Blackwell and now is continuing with Springer Nature as publisher for the federation. The broad aim of the series is to provide established researchers, trainees and students with authoritative up-to-date accounts of the present state of knowledge and prospects for the future across a range of topics in the burgeoning field of neuroendocrinology. The series is aimed at a wide audience as neuroendocrinology integrates neuroscience and endocrinology. We define neuroendocrinology as the study of the control of endocrine function by the brain and the actions of hormones on the brain. It encompasses study of normal and abnormal function and the developmental origins of disease. It includes study of the neural networks in the brain that regulate and form neuroendocrine systems. It also includes study of behaviours and mental states that are influenced or regulated by hormones. It necessarily includes understanding and study of peripheral physiological systems that are regulated by neuroendocrine mechanisms. Clearly, neuroendocrinology embraces many current issues of concern to human health and well-being, but research on these issues necessitates reductionist animal models.

Contemporary research in neuroendocrinology involves the use of a wide range of techniques and technologies, from the subcellular to systems at the whole-organism level. A particular aim of the series is to provide expert advice and discussion about experimental or study protocols in research in neuroendocrinology and to further advance the field by giving information and advice about novel techniques, technologies and interdisciplinary approaches.

To achieve our aims, each book is on a particular theme in neuroendocrinology, and for each book, we have recruited a pair of editors, expert in the field, and they have engaged an international team of experts to contribute chapters in their individual areas of expertise. Their mission was to give an update of knowledge and recent discoveries, to discuss new approaches, 'gold-standard' protocols, translational possibilities and future prospects. Authors were asked to write for a wide audience, to minimise references and to consider use of video clips and explanatory text boxes; each chapter is peer-reviewed and has a glossary and a detailed Index. We have been guided by an Advisory Editorial Board.

The Masterclass Series is open-ended; books in the series published to date are *Neurophysiology of Neuroendocrine Neurons* (2014, ed. WE Armstrong & JG

Tasker), *Neuroendocrinology of Stress* (2015, ed. JA Russell & MJ Shipston), *Molecular Neuroendocrinology: From Genome to Physiology* (2016, ed. D Murphy & H Gainer), *Computational Neuroendocrinology* (2016, ed. DJ Macgregor & G Leng), *Neuroendocrinology of Appetite* (2016; ed. SL Dickson & JG Mercer), *The GnRH Neuron and its Control* (2018; ed. AE Herbison & TM Plant) and *Model Animals in Neuroendocrinology* (2019, ed. M Ludwig and G Levkowitz). The first two books of the series published by Springer Nature are *Neurosecretion: Secretory Mechanisms* (ed. J Lemos & G Dayanithi) and *Developmental Neuroendocrinology* (ed. S Wray & S Blackshaw). Books in preparation include *Glial-Neuronal Signaling in Neuroendocrine Systems* and *Neuroanatomy of Neuroendocrine Systems*.

Feedback and suggestions are welcome.

International Neuroendocrine Federation—http://neuroendonow.com/

University of Edinburgh,   Mike Ludwig
Edinburgh, UK
The University of Tennessee Health Science Center,   William E. Armstrong
Memphis, TN, USA

Volume Preface

Life on planet Earth has evolved in a rhythmic world, surviving in environments that change with completely predictable timescales, most notably the day–night cycle, but also in tidal and seasonal cycles. Intrinsic biological timing mechanisms, 'clocks' and 'calendars', improved the fitness of organisms as they allowed them to anticipate these regular changes in the environment. Their importance in ensuring metabolic efficiency and survival is evident from the almost ubiquitous existence of timing mechanisms across all life forms. We are not exempt; our lives are governed by our daily (circadian) rhythmicity and, perhaps to an extent that we underestimate, by our seasonal cycles. Every time our alarm clock wakes us from our slumber, or when we toil through the night on a shift-work rota, we are fighting our natural circadian biology. Only now are we starting to recognise the impact of circadian misalignment on our physical and mental health.

Circadian rhythms have an ancient evolutionary heritage, so are a feature of unicellular organisms, reflecting both transcription/translation feedback loop mechanisms, but also metabolic cycles based on oxidation–reduction cycles of peroxiredoxin proteins. Cell-based oscillations were conserved in the evolution of multicellular organisms, but in vertebrates the input of environmental information to synchronise rhythms with the external world and the communication of timing information to peripheral metabolic and physiological systems is very much the realm of hypothalamic function and neuroendocrinology.

The objectives of this volume are to provide a comprehensive account of the pathways and mechanisms underlying circadian and circannual rhythmicity, and to shine a light on the substantive and in many cases unexpected advances that have been made in this area of neuroendocrinology in the last few decades. These include a sophisticated understanding of how interconnected translational-transcriptional feedback loops can generate circadian rhythmicity within cells. The identification of novel retinal photoreceptors utilising melanopsin that convey information about the external light–dark cycle to the hypothalamus. The discovery that astrocytes in the master hypothalamic clock, the suprachiasmatic nucleus, have as much functional importance as neurons in generating co-ordinated circadian function. The realisation that the *pars tuberalis* in the pituitary gland stalk is a pivotal structure in generating circannual rhythmicity and in relaying hormonal signals about photoperiod to the hypothalamus. And finally, the recognition that another group of glial cells, namely hypothalamic tanycytes, are a major integrator of photoperiodic information that directs changes in hypothalamic and neuroendocrine structure and function.

Although the focus of this volume is on mammalian systems including man, there are chapters specifically devoted to timing systems in fish and birds; these outline the similarities and differences between the major vertebrate groups. Throughout, the value of interdisciplinary and varied experimental approaches is stressed, as is the importance of different animal models. For example, intensive breeding has resulted in seasonal traits being lost from most laboratory strains of mice and rats, so comparative studies have been essential to develop our understanding of mechanisms underlying photoperiodism and circannual rhythmicity. We hope that this book will also appeal to a wide range of readers, from undergraduates to senior researchers, who seek to understand how innate rhythmicity affects the neuroendocrine and hypothalamic systems that underlie so many aspects of physiology and behaviour.

Nottingham, UK   Francis J. P. Ebling
Bristol, UK   Hugh D. Piggins

Contents

Photoperiodism and Circannual Timing: Introduction and Historical Perspective

Gerald A. Lincoln and Francis J. P. Ebling

Abstract

Almost all vertebrates display some form of seasonality across their life cycle that requires profound cyclical adaptations in behaviour, physiology and morphology. These are fundamentally controlled by neuroendocrine processes, since it is the brain that senses the environment and co-ordinates seasonality through endocrine and autonomic outputs. This chapter briefly considers how seasonality may impact upon our own species, then provides an introduction to these seasonal processes, considering landmark discoveries and advances in understanding from a historical perspective. It discusses how much of the initial focus was on the direct effects of changing photoperiod on seasonal timing, but how more recent long-term experimental studies have identified innate circannual timers. Seasonal rhythms arise from the interaction of direct photoperiodic effects and circannual rhythms, and timing can also be modified by proximate environmental and social cues; the relative contribution of these processes reflecting the lifespan and environmental ecology of each species.

Keywords

Season · Cycle · Reproduction · Neuroendocrine · Body weight

G. A. Lincoln
Centre for Reproductive Health, University of Edinburgh, Edinburgh, UK

F. J. P. Ebling (✉)
School of Life Sciences, University of Nottingham, Nottingham, UK
e-mail: fran.ebling@nottingham.ac.uk

F. J. P. Ebling, H. D. Piggins (eds.), *Neuroendocrine Clocks and Calendars*,
Masterclass in Neuroendocrinology 10, https://doi.org/10.1007/978-3-030-55643-3_1

1.1   Introduction

Most environments on our planet are highly seasonal in that the climate fluctuates in a predictable manner over the course of a year. This has major implications for the evolution and survival of organisms, whether the seasonality is the changing ambient temperature of cool and polar regions, or predominantly changes in rainfall in sub-tropical and tropical regions. The constraints of surviving in a seasonal environment have shaped human evolution and migration, have shaped our societies and cultures, and continue to influence our everyday lives, health and wellbeing. Identifying the mechanisms whereby seasonal rhythmicity is generated and regulates physiology and behaviour is not only important for understanding the natural world and relevant to animal production, it also offers many insights into the human condition. This chapter will provide an introduction to the biology and neuroendocrine mechanisms that underpin seasonal rhythmicity, adopting a historical perspective to allow readers to place the subsequent mechanistic chapters in context.

Box 1.1 Why There Are Seasons on Earth

It is a common misconception that our seasons arise from the fact that the Earth's orbit around the sun is not perfectly circular, so winter reflects the point at which our planet is most distant from the sun. This cannot be true, as when winter arrives in the northern hemisphere, so summer arrives in the southern hemisphere. The seasons actually arise because of the profound tilt in the Earth's axis relative to its plane of rotation around the sun (Fig. 1.1a). This 23.5° of tilt results in the sun's irradiance being spread over a far greater area in winter than in summer. At the summer solstice in the northern hemisphere, the sun appears directly overhead at the tropic of Cancer, an imaginary line of latitude at 23.5° north of the equator, so a given unit of irradiance is concentrated in the least possible area (Fig. 1.1b). However, at this time, the angle of the sun relative to the surface of the earth at the tropic of Capricorn in the southern hemisphere will be at its lowest point across the year (Fig. 1.1c). The same given unit of solar irradiance is therefore spread across a far greater area, so the heating of the Earth's atmosphere and surface is correspondingly reduced. Additionally, the tilt of the axis means that the duration of sunlight is far greater in the summer than winter, so at 55°N day length would be over 16 h at the summer solstice, but just under 8 h at the winter solstice (Fig. 1.1d). The effect of changing intensity of radiation across the annual cycle is markedly amplified by the duration of sunlight affecting all photosynthetic processes and primary food production.

1.1.1   Seasonality, Human Evolution and Culture

Jared Diamond offers many fascinating explanations for why the evolution and migration of man resulted in a very unequal distribution of agricultural and

Fig. 1.1 Seasons arise from the tilt in the Earth's axis relative to its plane of orbit around the sun (**a**), resulting in solar radiation being concentrated in a smaller area in summer (**b**) compared to winter (**c**) and in the sun being visible above the horizon for longer in summer than winter (**d**). See text Box 1.1 for details

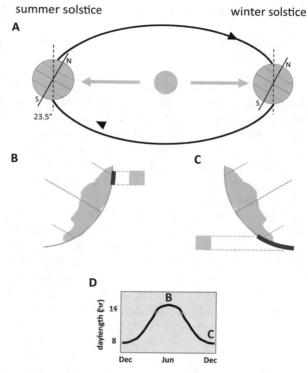

technological advancements across the planet (Diamond 1997). His core argument is that it is the environments that different human populations evolved in, rather than any innate genetic differences, that shaped mankind's destiny. Seasonality plays a key part in this environmental argument. After the last ice age 10 K years ago, a number of populations started to domesticate crops and animals, and adopt settled lifestyles rather than surviving as hunter-gatherers. This transition resulted in increased efficiency of food production supporting hierarchical societies and the development of cultural, military and other technologies. Developing societies were able to migrate from east to west through Eurasia because the animals they domesticated (sheep, goats, horses) and crop systems they relied on were highly seasonal, but could thrive as populations moved along the lines of latitude. In contrast, post ice age populations in continents that have a north-south axis (America, Africa) suffered from the biological constraints of seasonality that limited the propagation of agriculture across latitudes. Long before the establishment of the major religions, man observed and celebrated the passage of the seasons with festivals. Recent evidence has emerged that Mesolithic societies built earthworks that would allow them to track the phases of the moon and predict the lunar months (Gaffney et al. 2013). Remarkably these preceded by 5000 years the elaborate bronze age stone works such as Stonehenge that tracked solar cycles and identified the solstices!

1.1.2   Seasonality in Human Health and Disease

It is chiefly the changes of the seasons which produce diseases. Hippocrates (fifth century BC)

Those of us that live in temperate latitudes are by our very nature phenologists, we note the passing of the seasons as we observe the arrival of migrant birds in spring, lambs in the fields and the blossoming into leaf of deciduous trees and flowers emerging around us. What we commonly fail to realize is the seasonal rhythmicity within our own bodies. Shaving a patch of skin repeatedly over the course of a year will confirm that our hair growth is seasonal (Randall and Ebling 1991), but perhaps the most important aspect of human seasonality are changes in our susceptibility to disease and infection. Whilst we are familiar with regular epidemics of influenza in winter, Micaela Martinez has collated epidemiological data for over 60 communicable diseases around the world, and shown that all show seasonal cycles of prevalence (Martinez 2018). As she notes, 'To every pathogen there is a season', and the timing of peak prevalence differs for each infection (Fig. 1.2). The mechanisms underlying this seasonal cyclicity are numerous, complex, and different for each disease, for example relating to seasonality of vectors, and/or of annual differences in human contact rates. However, one factor is likely to relate to our innate cycle in immune function. As an example, the incidence of chicken pox, a common childhood disease that results from infection with the *varicella* zoster virus, peaks in the spring in both the northern and southern hemispheres (Fig. 1.2). This seasonal pattern may reflect changes in seasonal behaviour and exposure (Martinez 2018), but is likely to have a physiological cause. The *varicella* virus can lie dormant in neural tissue for several decades before reactivating to produce shingles in adulthood. This reactivation is a reflection of weakened innate immunity occurring most likely in spring, evidence for an innate

Fig. 1.2 Maximum prevalence of major infectious diseases in USA populations, adapted from Martinez (2018)

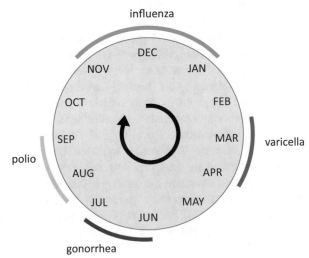

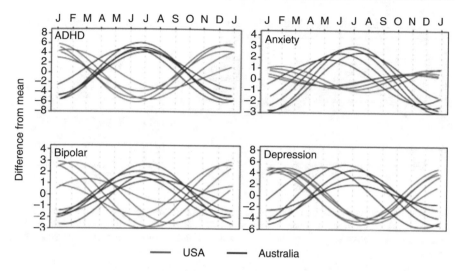

Fig. 1.3 Seasonal variation in Google search term records in the USA (blue) and Australia (red) over the course of 5 years. *ADHD* attention deficit hyperactivity disorder. Note the inverse relationship between cycles in the northern and southern hemispheres. Data from Ayers et al. (2013)

endogenous seasonal rhythm in immune function in man, as experimentally demonstrated in many other mammalian species (Weil et al. 2015).

A second area where seasonality impacts greatly upon us is in relation to mood and mental health. An increased occurrence of dysphoric mood and depression in autumn and winter has long been recognized, and the greater prevalence at more northerly latitudes supports the view that these phenomena are related to our seasonal environment. The diagnostic and statistical manual of the American Psychiatric Association (DSM V) specifically classifies seasonal affective disorder (SAD) as a major depressive disorder that only occurs at a specific time of year (usually winter) with spontaneously remission, but returns on an annual basis. SAD is just one of many conditions that shows seasonality in its prevalence. Large data sets mined from the Google search engine provide a fascinating insight into this, as analyses of search terms for conditions related to mental health show significant seasonal variation (Ayers et al. 2013). The seasonal trends of winter peaks and summer troughs for terms such as 'bipolar', 'anxiety', 'depression' and 'attention deficit hyperactivity disorder' (ADHD) are remarkably robust across years, and confirm that these trends exist in the southern hemisphere (Australia) just as in the northern hemisphere (USA), but are out of phase by 6 months (Fig. 1.3). As with seasonal cycles in the incidence of infectious diseases, the challenge is now to identify the underlying mechanisms, and in particular to establish the relative contribution of different environmental and social factors, as compared to the intrinsic annual rhythmicity that reflects our evolutionary history. Experimental studies in animal models have provided huge insights (see below).

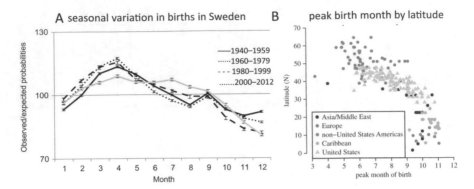

Fig. 1.4 Historical records from Sweden revealing a clear seasonal cycle in the probability of births occurring (**a**). Records from countries at different latitudes in the northern hemisphere indicate that the peak month for births occurs earlier at higher latitudes (**b**). See text Box 1.2 for details

---

Box 1.2 Seasonal Variation in Reproduction in Man
The systematic recording of the time and date of births over the past two centuries provides vast datasets from which further evidence of human seasonality can be gained. In almost all locations there is an annual rhythm in births (Fig. 1.4a; Dahlberg and Andersson 2018), the peak birth rate being around the summer solstice in North European populations (Roenneberg and Aschoff 1990). Clearly cultural, socioeconomic and biological factors contribute to these seasonal patterns, and it is notable that the amplitude of these rhythms has decreased in most locations in recent decades (Fig. 1.4a). That timing of peak births is closely linked to latitude (Fig. 1.4b; Martinez-Bakker et al. 2014) may point towards photoperiod as an important proximate time cue.

1.2   Seasonality Is the Norm for Vertebrates

Almost all vertebrates display some form of seasonality across their life cycle. Extraordinary examples exist, for example migration from river to sea and back of salmon, or arctic to antarctic migration of arctic terns, and the hibernation of reptiles and amphibians and some mammals in temperate and polar regions. These require profound cyclical adaptations in behaviour, physiology and morphology, but are fundamentally controlled by neuroendocrine processes, since it is the brain that senses the environment and co-ordinates seasonality through endocrine and autonomic outputs. Overt seasonal cycles reflect three underlying mechanistic processes: (a) innate long-term timing in neuroendocrine tissues, (b) responsiveness to change in daylength across the year, and (c) the modifying effects of nutrition, social factors

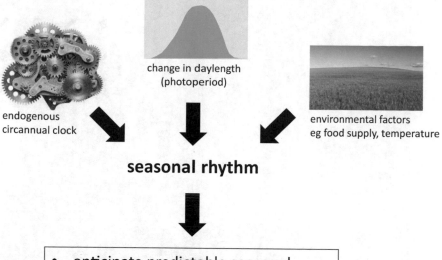

change in daylength
(photoperiod)

endogenous
circannual clock

environmental factors
eg food supply, temperature

seasonal rhythm

- anticipate predictable seasonal changes in environment
- optimise energy storage and usage
- optimise survival of the offspring

Fig. 1.5 Seasonal rhythms in physiology and behaviours such as food intake, reproduction and hibernation reflect three underlying processes: the influence of endogenous circannual oscillators, perhaps located in the *pars tuberalis* of the pituitary gland, the synchronising influence of the annual change in daylength, and the modifying effects of other local environmental factors

and other acute changes in the environment (Fig. 1.5). The critically important feature is that these mechanisms allow organisms to *anticipate* seasonal environmental change, and ultimately to *optimize* reproduction and survival of the offspring. Reproduction is an energetically costly process for both sexes, whether for egg production or supporting pregnancy, lactation and maternal care in females, or in males supporting intraspecific competition for territory and mates. As a consequence, seasonal control of energy balance and reproduction are tightly linked, as are the seasonal changes in morphology (for example, muscle growth, horns, antlers, fat deposition) and behaviour that are integral to reproductive success.

Our knowledge of these seasonal mechanisms depends mainly on a select few species that are amenable to experimental analysis often in laboratory settings (Ludwig and Levkowitz 2018). Ferrets, hamsters (Box 1.3), voles and sheep have been important mammalian model organisms, and studies in birds have relied heavily on Japanese quail and a few passerine species. Although this is a limited range of model organisms, there seems to be substantive variation in the relative importance of the three basic control mechanisms. Historically much of the focus has

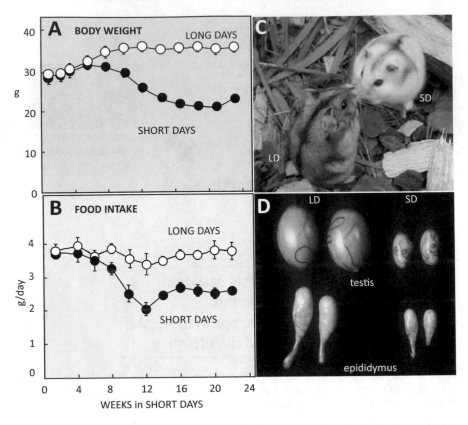

Fig. 1.6 Siberian hamsters (*Phodopus sungorus*) display seasonal cycles in body weight (**a**), voluntary food intake (**b**), coat colour (**c**) and reproductive function (**d**). In this study adult male hamsters were maintained in long days (LD) of 16 h light: 8 h dark, or transferred to short days (SD) of 8 h light: 16 h dark. See text Box 1.3 for further details

been on photoperiodism (Sect. 1.3), but almost certainly this reflects the fact that this phenomenon is most readily investigated in the laboratory.

Box 1.3 Seasonal Cycles in the Siberian Hamster, a Widely Studied Animal Model

The Siberian hamster (*Phodopus sungorus*) is a tractable rodent model that can be housed in conventional animal facilities but displays profound seasonal changes in behaviour and physiology when maintained in prolonged periods of alternating long-day photoperiod (16 h light:8 h darkness, LD 16:8) and short-day photoperiod (LD 8:16) (Fig. 1.6). Colonies were first established in Germany in the 1970s from founder animals captured from the wild in Djungaria in central Asia, and later exported to the UK and USA. Whereas

(continued)

Box 1.3 (continued)

body weight is maintained at around 30–40 g in males in long photoperiod, over the course of many weeks it declines by about a third in hamsters exposed to short photoperiod (Fig. 1.6a). This weight loss mainly reflects catabolism of intra-abdominal fat stores, and is driven by a reduction in voluntary food intake (Fig. 1.6b). By 12–16 weeks under short days the brown summer coat has been shed and replaced with a white winter pelage (Fig. 1.6c), and whereas spermatogenesis/fertility is maintained in hamsters in long days, testicular involution occurs in males in short days (Fig. 1.6d). These endpoints all reflect major changes in hypothalamic and neuroendocrine function, so the loss of spermatogenesis directly reflects decreased LH and FSH secretion from the anterior pituitary resulting from reduced GnRH output from the hypothalamus. Likewise, the moult to a white winter coat is predominantly a reflection of decreased prolactin secretion. These experimentally induced transitions provide a powerful approach for understanding control of neuroendocrine axes. Most strains of laboratory mice and rats are unusual in that photoperiodic responses and seasonality have been bred out of them by many decades of intense selection for fecundity, so relying on these species can give a very narrow view of neuroendocrine mechanisms. Understanding the natural decrease in motivation to eat and increased mobilization of fat depots in seasonal species like hamsters provides an opportunity to identify novel control mechanisms that might lead to therapeutic strategies for weight loss in man.

1.3 Photoperiodism

Observations that under laboratory conditions many species respond to changes in day-length by altering their physiology and behaviour have led to the simple view that seasonal biology is a passive response to the external light environment. This is a basic misunderstanding. We now recognize that photoperiod time measurement (PTM) is an innate highly complex neuroendocrine decoding mechanism, with interesting differences between species. It takes photoreceptors, circadian clocks and cellular transducers, to regulate long-term cycles in physiology. After decades of research, we are still unravelling the cellular and molecular basis of PTM.

1.3.1 Early Studies (1900–1950)

The striking precision in the timing of the many seasonal events in nature has long encouraged speculation that seasonal timing must be innate: evolved to anticipate environmental change. Each species' seasonal adaptations differ according to the organisms' size, longevity and ecology, and an array of ancestral characteristics. The first careful scientific approach was the analysis of the breeding times of long-distance migratory birds (Schafer 1907). Despite traversing continents to avoid cold winters, many birds appear to use increasing daylight length to synchronize egg laying to springtime. A Canadian biologist William Rowan was perhaps the first to demonstrate photoperiodic effects (Rowan 1925). He captured juncos migrating south in September and housed them over winter in aviaries. The addition of artificial light to simulate spring was shown to be very effective at promoting testicular regrowth and activating courtship singing (Rowan 1925).

Francis Marshall working in the 1930s was particularly instrumental in characterizing the effects of external factors on seasonal periodicity, notably based on the way animals realign their seasonal rhythms following transference across the equator. This included the observation on the effect of the translocations of red deer between the UK and New Zealand; the stags adjusted their antler cycles rapidly, while the hinds took at least 2 years to fully realign their breeding cycles (Marshall 1937). By the time the classic textbook, *Marshall's Physiology of Reproduction* was published in 1960, a full chapter could be devoted to the way environmental factors affect sexual periodicity. The distinction between 'ultimate factors' that directly affect reproductive success, and 'proximate factors' that act as seasonal time cues was already well recognized.

Box 1.4 Photorefractoriness as Part of Innate Circannual Rhythmicity
Although early experimentation demonstrated the potency of changing daylength as a proximate cue, it rapidly became clear that cycle generation is a dynamic process. Thus, the initial physiological response to a change in photoperiod often spontaneously reverses under prolonged exposure to the same photoperiod; a phenomenon termed 'photorefractoriness'. For example, in the Siberian hamster, exposure to long days (LD) induces testicular growth due to the activation of gonadotrophin secretion, and exposure to short days (SD) reverses this process. However, prolonged exposure to SD beyond 12 weeks results in spontaneous testicular recrudescence (Fig. 1.7a). There are parallel changes in the pelage cycle driven by prolactin. This refractoriness to winter photoperiod allows the hamster to emerge from hibernation in spring with an already developing summer physiology. In Soay sheep, the dynamics are somewhat different since initial exposure to LD is inhibitory to gonadal activity, but switching between LD, SD and LD drives the reproductive cycle. In this species prolonged exposure to LD results in spontaneous reactivation of the gonadal activity (Fig. 1.7b), and again photoperiod-induced cyclicity in prolactin secretion governs the pelage moult cycle. While the gonadotrophin regulation is different, the prolactin regulation is similar in sheep and hamster, indicating separate neuroendocrine control of these two basic physiological systems. Overall, the dynamic changes under constant photoperiod reveal that season rhythms are not simply a direct response to changing photoperiod, but result from underlying innate long-term interval timers (see Sect. 1.4).

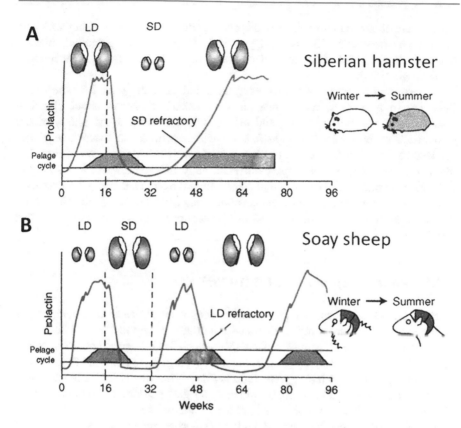

Fig. 1.7 Maintaining Siberian hamsters (**a**) or Soay sheep (**b**) in constant photoperiod for a prolonged period reveals innate endogenous timing processes, often referred to as 'photorefractoriness' as the physiological response is the opposite of the initial response to a change in photoperiod. Under prolonged short days (SD), the testes regrow in Siberian hamsters and prolactin secretion increases to initiate a moult to the summer pelage (**a**), whereas in Soay sheep, under prolonged long days prolactin secretion eventually decreases and testis growth restarts (**b**). See Text Box 1.4 for further details

1.3.2   Photoperiodism and Circadian Oscillators (1960s)

One of the first fundamental discoveries in this field occurred more than 50 years ago with the demonstration that PTM is dependent upon an organism's endogenous circadian rhythm–generating system. This work was pioneered over decades by the botanist Erwin Bunning. His experimental approach was to systematically expose individual bean seedlings to different lighting paradigms, including night interruption and non-24h cycles of light and dark, and record which seasonal response occurred, vegetative growth or flowering. This revealed that it is seldom the *duration* of daily light exposure that governs the seasonal response, but it is the *phasing* relative to an underlying endogenous circadian oscillator. Subsequently, similar results were obtained in organisms as disparate as insects, birds and mammals. Colin Pittendrigh extended the 'Bunning's Hypothesis' to propose two potentially interactive models for PTM: (1) 'external coincidence' and (2) 'internal coincidence' (Pittendrigh 1972).

The external coincidence model recognizes that the daily periodic exposure to light acts in two ways; on the one hand, to *entrain* the endogenous circadian clockwork in the cell/organism, and on the other, to *induce* the photoperiodic response. This only occurs if light falls coincident with a 'photosensitive phase' produced by the circadian oscillation, hence the concept of external coincidence. The internal coincidence model proposes that the daily light-dark cycle acts solely to determine the phase of multiple components within the circadian oscillator system— producing a different phase relationships under long days compared with short days. This is supported by experimental evidence for separate 'dawn' and 'dusk' circadian oscillators.

1.3.3 Photoreceptors for PTM (1970s)

Michael Menaker was another pioneer who recognized the value of a comparative biology approach using reptiles, birds and mammals to help understand the evolution of the vertebrate PTM mechanisms (Menaker 1971). In one ingenious experiment, 24-h locomotor activity profiles (perch hopping) were recorded in groups of sparrows exposed to 14 h *dim-green* light per day. This was effective at entraining the circadian behavioural rhythm, but did not alter the long-term reproductive status. He then added a short pulse of *white* light for 75 min per day at either the beginning or end of the 14-h green light period. Only the sparrows receiving the bright light at the end of the dim green light treatment showed activation of reproductive activity. Both groups received the same amount of light—thus circadian phasing is critical, used as evidence to support the external coincidence model for PTM.

In a second classical experiment carried out by Menaker's group, the site of the photoreceptors involved in PTM was investigated in different vertebrates. In one study, the injection of opaque Indian ink under the skin of the scalp in house sparrows was shown to block the gonadal response to long days, while unexpectedly blindfolds over the eyes were ineffective. Moreover, implantation of light-emitting particles into the cerebral ventricles and basal hypothalamus of sparrows activated the reproductive responses. These studies provided the first definitive evidence that daylight, penetrating the skull, can act through deep-brain photosensitive cells to drive seasonal timing in birds. In addition, the pineal gland was shown to be photosensitive—rhythmically secreting melatonin with an inverse pattern relative to the daily light cycle. Pineal cells from some vertebrates are light-responsive and express daily rhythms in tissue culture. This introduced the pineal gland into the complexity of photoperiodism.

In birds, melatonin is intimately involved in circadian rhythm generation, but has little effect on seasonal biology. This contrasts with the situation in mammals, where photoreceptors in the retina of the eyes are solely involved in PTM (Fig. 1.8). Here,

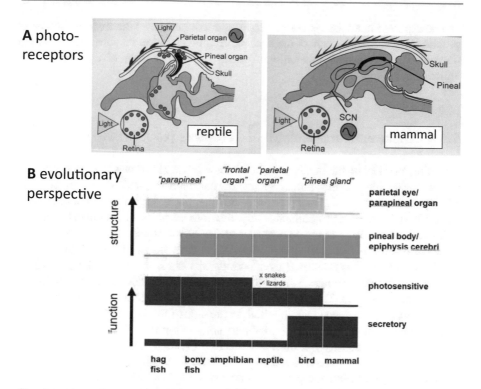

Fig. 1.8 Photoperiod sensing in mammals: (**a**) Schematic summary of the localization of photoreceptors (orange circles) in the reptile (left panel) and mammal (right panel) brain illustrating how in the ancestral vertebrate light acts through multiple sites (retina, parietal/pineal complex and deep-brain sites) to affect the photoperiodic control of seasonal cycles, while in mammals only the retina is involved. In this most derived system, light signals are conveyed from the retina to the suprachiasmatic nuclei (SCN, circadian clock), and to the pineal gland that secretes melatonin during the night, and the photoperiod induced changes in the 24-h melatonin pattern induces the seasonal response. (**b**) Evolutionary perspective across vertebrate groups of the relative importance of the different photosensitive and secretory tissues in the pineal gland/parapineal complex in regulating seasonal physiology

daily light signals from the eyes act to entrain the central suprachiasmatic nucleus (SCN) pacemaker system in the anterior hypothalamus that in turn governs the daily rhythm in melatonin production by the pineal gland. It is the changing characteristics of the daily melatonin signal that drives seasonal rhythmicity. The 'simplified' mammalian relay, with a single photoreceptor system in the eyes, is seen as the most derived vertebrate PTM light-sensing system—possibly related to a nocturnal bottleneck in mammalian evolution at the time of the dinosaurs that resulted in the loss of deep-brain photoreception. The comparison of form and function across vertebrate groups demonstrates an evolutionary progression in brain light-sensing systems (Fig. 1.8).

Taking a more global perspective, photoreceptor mechanisms undoubtedly first developed early in eukaryote cell evolution, and thus cell autonomous light sensing can be expected in all tissues in small transparent organisms. Moreover, melatonin is predicted to be there as part of the ancestral light-adaptation response based on the universal expression of melatonin in extant organisms from diverse taxa, both animals and plants.

1.3.4 Melatonin and Melatonin Receptors (1980–1990s)

Focusing on PTM in mammals, a major advance in the 1980s was the discovery that surgical excision of the pineal gland in the hamster and sheep blocks the photoperiodic control of gonadal activity and other physiological responses (Bittman et al. 1983). Moreover, programmed daily infusions of melatonin in pinealectomized animals, that precisely replicate normal patterns of melatonin in the blood, restore seasonal responses (Bartness et al. 1993). Short daily bouts of melatonin infusion (typically 6 h per day) repeated over periods of weeks, as seen under long days, activate a summer response, while long (>10 h) daily melatonin bouts produce a winter state (Fig. 1.9). This unequivocally demonstrates that it is melatonin *signal duration* that acts to decode photoperiod. In the case of the Siberian hamster (a long-day breeder), short daily signals activate gonadotrophin secretion and gonadal activity, while in the sheep (a short-day breeder) the reverse occurs. This illustrates how the seasonal reproductive phenotype is determined by differences in central neuroendocrine transduction pathways and not at the level of melatonin signalling. The same applies for the development of 'photorefractoriness' within an individual,

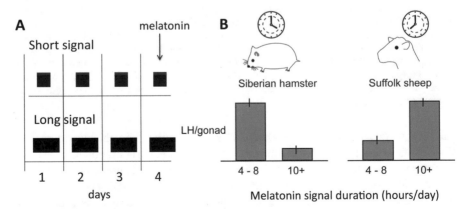

Fig. 1.9 Melatonin signal duration decodes photoperiod. (**a**) Short nocturnal melatonin signals that occur under long days (LD) produce a summer response, while long signals produced under short days (SD) produce a winter response. (**b**) Summary of the reproductive (LH/gonad, arbitrary units) effects of programmed daily infusions of melatonin delivered as short (4–8 h) or long (10 h+) bouts for many weeks in the Siberian hamster and Suffolk sheep. In the small species (long day breeder), short melatonin signals result in gonadal activation, while in the sheep (short-day breeder) short melatonin signals are inhibitory to reproductive function (after Bittman et al. 1983; Bartness et al. 1993)

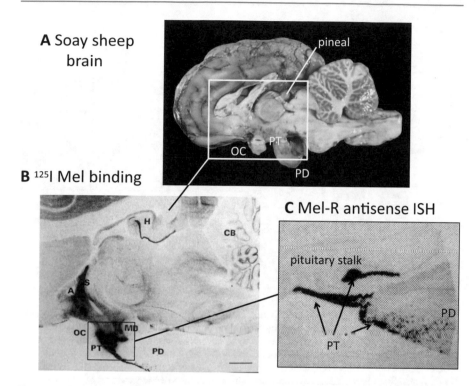

Fig. 1.10 Location of melatonin receptor expression in the sheep brain and pituitary. (a) Photograph of a sagittal section of the Soay sheep brain showing the optic chiasm (OC), pineal gland, *pars tuberalis* (PT) and *pars distalis* (PD). (b) Autoradiograph of iodinated melatonin (^{125}I-Mel) binding in the brain and pituitary gland. Abbreviations: medial basal hypothalamus (MB), hippocampus (H) and cerebellum (CB). (c) In situ hybridization (ISH) micrograph of localized area (black box, see autoradiograph) using an antisense Mt1 melatonin receptor riboprobe—note the specific Mt1 receptor expression in the PT of the pituitary stalk and associated with the blood vessels leading to the PD (seen as variable dots)

where the spontaneous physiology cycle proceeds under constant photoperiod (Box 1.4; Fig. 1.9), while the melatonin signal remains unchanged.

A second major advance in resolving the photoperiod decoding mechanism came with the sequencing of three melatonin receptors, and the demonstration that it is the high affinity mt1 sub-type receptor (Mel-R) that relays the effects of melatonin for mammalian seasonal timing (Reppert 1997). Using specific RNA probes for the receptor, the site of action of melatonin for PTM was then explored. Unexpectedly, hybridization of the melatonin-receptor probe was not in the medial basal hypothalamus (MBH) as predicted, but principally in the pituitary gland stalk within the *pars tuberalis* (PT), immediately adjacent to the MBH (e.g. sheep, Fig. 1.10). The PT has the highest density of Mel-R expression of any tissue, and the PT lights up as a *somatic cell–based* melatonin target tissue in all photoperiodic mammals studied to date (Fig. 1.10). Parallel in vivo studies investigated the local effectiveness of melatonin implants placed in different sites in the sheep brain (Fig. 1.11; Lincoln

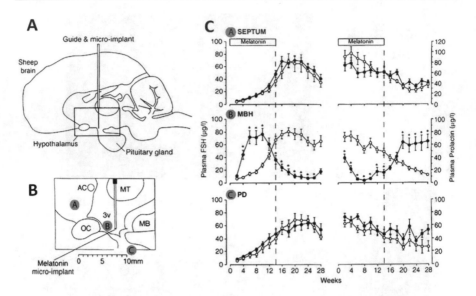

Fig. 1.11 Endocrine effects of local administration of melatonin in the Soay sheep brain using microimplants. (**a**) Sagittal section of sheep brain showing the needle implant with melatonin at the tip, placed by stereotaxic and Xray guidance. (**b**) Three brain areas targeted with melatonin microimplants: A: septum, B: mediobasal hypothalamus/PT (MBH) and C: pituitary *pars distalis* (PD). Abbreviations: optic chiasm (OC), third ventricle (3v), anterior commissure (AC), medial thalamus (MT), mammillary body (MB). (**c**) Long-term changes in blood concentrations of FSH (left) and prolactin (right) in groups of Soay rams ($n = 6$–8) treated with melatonin implants (filled circle, experimental) or empty implants (open circle, control) placed in the 3 target sites for 14 weeks (see horizontal bar) while the sheep were exposed to long photoperiod (LD 16:8). Note that melatonin delivery in the MBH but not in other sites blocked the effects of LD, so activated FSH secretion and testicular activity (not shown), and suppressed prolactin secretion and the pelage moult (not shown). (After Lincoln 1994)

1994). Melatonin placed in the mediobasal hypothalamus adjacent to the third ventricle, or in the PT, blocked the effect of long days and generated a short-day physiological state for the control of both gonadotrophin and prolactin axes (Fig. 1.11). Implants placed in other sites elicited no effect (Fig. 1.11). This is consistent with the view that melatonin acts via the high-affinity Mel-R expressed in the PT to regulate multiple photoperiodic rhythms.

1.3.5 Circadian Clock Gene Expression in the PT (2000–Present)

The full characterization of canonical circadian clock genes and their protein-protein interactions in the 1990s opened the way to dissect the circadian-basis of PTM at the level of the PT. The seasonal sheep model was particularly useful because of the large size of the animal, compared with small laboratory species, providing bulk samples of PT and other tissues from individual animals. Groups of sheep could be sampled at regular clock times across 24 h, repeated at different phases of photo-induction, and multiple tissue sections probed by in situ hybridization to measure local changes in the expression of clock genes, transcription factor genes and potential output genes in the PT. This was first performed in long- and short-day-acclimatized Soay sheep, comparing 24-h patterns of clock gene expression in the PT and SCN (Lincoln et al. 2002). The study revealed a photoperiod-regulated circadian profile of clock gene expression in the PT (*bmal1*, *clock*, *per1*, *per2* and *cry1*) that was distinct from the SCN. The PT was presented as a defined melatonin-decoding tissue, and the SCN as the central circadian pacemaker. Of special note was the rapid activation of *cry1* gene expression at the onset of darkness in the PT, but not in the SCN, under both long and short photoperiod. This was later shown to be a 'dusk-onset' signal acutely activated by melatonin at the beginning of the night (Hazlerigg et al. 2004). There was a corresponding peak in *per1* expression at the beginning of the day representing a 'dawn onset' signal. Changing photoperiod between long and short days thus produces a marked change in the *relative phasing* of the *cry* and *per* oscillations. This was proposed as the basis of an internal coincidence mechanism that decodes melatonin signal *duration* in the PT for PTM (Lincoln et al. 2002).

The PT cells that respond to melatonin are tissue-specific thyrotrophs that secrete TSH as the primary product (Hanon et al. 2008). Detailed analysis of the promoter region of the *TSHβ* gene has identified Tef1 as a key transcription activator that is potentiated by the ubiquitous gene-regulatory protein Eyes absent 3 (Eya3) (Dardente et al. 2010). This regulatory role for Eya3 is consistent with data from the Japanese quail where Eya3 and TSHβ were in the 'first wave' of gene activation induced by long photoperiods—a very rapid response system in birds, and also consistent with a comprehensive genomic analysis of photoperiod-induced TSH regulatory genes in a melatonin-proficient mouse strain (Masumoto et al. 2010).

In 2013, Oliver Ebenhöh and David Hazlerigg used the available evidence on circadian rhythmic gene expression in the PT to propose a modern coincidence model for PTM in mammals (Ebenhöh and Hazlerigg 2013). This highlighted the importance of the change in the relative phasing between peak Cry1 expression induced by the onset of melatonin secretion (dusk signal—acting as a suppressor) and peak Eya3 expression varying with photoperiod. Under short days, Eya3 expression occurs in the *night* and is inhibitory to TSH release producing a winter phenotype, whereas under long days, Eya3 peaks in the *day* and is stimulatory driving a summer phenotype (Fig. 1.12). The model predicts that Eya3 protein acts via a positive feedback loop, enhancing its own transcription, to generate a *bi-stability state* where a switch in photoperiod generates two very different stable end-states, a winter versus a summer physiology (Ebenhöh and Hazlerigg 2013). Similar dynamics in Eya3 activation governs organogenesis during embryonic development, for example, the regulation of eye formation and body segmentation. Thus the gene-based, long-term, cyclical PTM program governing seasonal transitions may well share regulatory domains with the overall life history program.

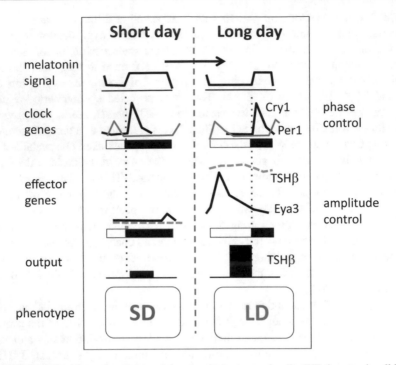

Fig. 1.12 Decoding the melatonin signal duration in the *pars tuberalis* (PT) thyrotroph cell in the short-day (SD) vs. long-day (LD) state. Parameters from top to bottom (arbitrary units): 24-h melatonin signal duration, phase control of Cry1 and Per1 clock gene expression in the PT cell, amplitude control of βTSH and Eya3 effector gene expression in the PT cell, and TSH output. The difference in TSH production, acting via its retrograde pathway (TSH-DIO2-TH), controls tanycyte activity in the hypothalamus and hence the local availability of biologically active thyroid hormone. This dictates the photoperiod phenotype (modified from Dardente et al. 2010)

1.4   Circannual Timing

While photoperiodism allows organisms to synchronize their seasonal physiology to the time of year, it is the innate circannual timing system that primarily governs the *long latency* of seasonal cycles. This is based on an extensive literature demonstrating that long-term rhythms in many different physiological traits persist even when photoperiod and temperature are held constant. Coelenterates, annelid worms, insects, molluscs, fish, reptiles, birds and mammals (primates included) all utilize endogenous circannual clockwork to control seasonal transitions in biology. Moreover, unicellular organisms (e.g. marine algae) and primitive plants have a circannual biology supporting the idea of an early evolution of innate circannual timing.

This presents a paradox that even small organisms utilize a circannual clock even though each individual may only live few weeks (Lincoln 2019). The explanation for this is that circannual timing can be trans-generational influencing the 'alternation of generations strategy' switching between summer vegetative replication and winter dormancy as part of the species life history. Circannual timing may control only one phase of the organism's life cycle, as for eclosion in insects, or operate in a short-lived mammals like the Siberian hamster to govern the process of photorefractoriness as discussed earlier (Box 1.4). Circannual timing is a universal trait, the consequence of natural selection in a profoundly periodic world.

1.4.1 Discovery of Circannual Timing (1950–1970s)

The first formal demonstration that mammals express innate circannual rhythms involved studies of hibernating golden-mantled ground squirrels (*Citellus lateralis*) (Pengelley and Fisher 1957; Pengelley et al. 1976). In one of Pengelley's early experiments, two ground squirrels were maintained under constant photoperiod (12 h light and 12 h darkness; LD 12:12) and constant temperature for more than 2 years. Both animals continued to hibernate about once a year, and each hibernating period was preceded by a dramatic increase in food consumption and body weight. Timing and coordination were similar to the natural summer-active/winter-rest seasonal cycle observed in squirrels living outdoors.

These studies were confirmed and extended by co-workers, and by other researchers using a range of seasonal species. In a more robust investigation, multiple groups of squirrels were kept for 47 months in constant darkness (DD), constant light (LL) or constant equatorial light (LD 12:12) (Pengelley et al. 1976). Some animals were blind and some were normally sighted (Fig. 1.13). The hibernation rhythms continued throughout the prolonged experiment in all individuals. The free-running period (*tau*) was consistently shorter than a year at 10–11 months, irrespective of whether the animals were blind or sighted (Fig. 1.13). In many studies, the normal phasing between the different physiological cycles of food intake, body weight, hibernation behaviour and gonadal activity has been shown to be maintained in the circannual free-running state.

In 1986, Ebo Gwinner working in Germany published a synthesis of the extant literature on circannual rhythms based on some 60 publications that each provided strong evidence for innate circannual rhythmicity. These covered diverse organisms from plants to mammals, alongside his remarkable scientific contribution from laboratory and field studies of migratory warblers, European starlings and stonechats. His book was entitled 'Circannual Rhythms: Endogenous Annual Clocks in the Organization of Seasonal Processes' (Gwinner 1986). This was the turning point for the discipline: from then on circannual timing mechanisms were recognized as of fundamental importance. In one much-quoted study, a male stonechat was caged in the lab under constant photoperiod (LD 12:12) and food supply for 12 years (Gwinner 1996). The stonechat is a common passerine bird species with both migratory and resident genetic variants. Testis size and feather moult were recorded regularly (Fig. 1.14). Impressively, circannual reproductive and feather moult cycles persisted throughout the bird's full life span, and there was no reduction in the

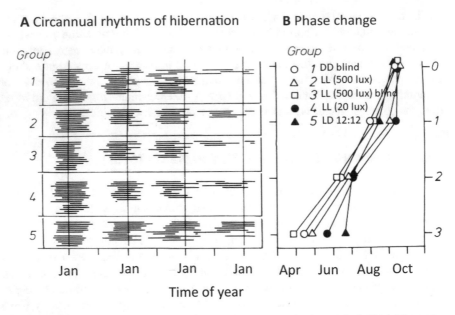

Fig. 1.13 Circannual rhythms in golden-mantled ground squirrels. (a) Individual hibernation rhythms (black bars arranged in horizontal rows) in groups of ground squirrels kept for 47 months at 3 °C under different constant photoperiods: Group 1, constant darkness (DD), animals surgically blinded, Group 2, constant light (LL, 500 lux), Group 3 constant light (LL, 500 lux), animals surgically blinded, Group 4, constant dim light (LL, 20 lux), Group 5, constant equatorial lighting (LD 12:12, 200:0 lux). (b) Symbols connected by lines indicate mean dates at which the animals of the various groups entered hibernation in successive cycles under the free-running conditions. (After Pengelley et al. 1976)

amplitude of these cycles with age. *Tau* was approximately 10.5 months, so during its 12-year life time in captivity the animal's concept of seasonal time advanced by more than a year relative to Earth orbital time. Studies across the full life history have been conducted in other passerine birds such as the blackcap and garden warbler with very similar results; feather moult following gonadal regression every circannual cycle. To establish whether this timing is truly innate, eggs from aviary-bred stonechats have been incubated artificially and the hatchlings reared by hand; at no stage was there contact with parent birds or the outside environment. Again, the birds continued to express robust circannual rhythms. The overall conclusion is that circannual timing in vertebrates is a component of the life-history programme.

1.4.2 Interaction with the Circadian System

With PTM dependent on the circadian timing system, and with both circannual and circadian rhythms showing similar formal properties such as specific periodicity, innateness, and a capacity to be entrained, it has been proposed that the period of a

African stonechat (passerine bird) caged under constant equatorial photoperiod (LD 12:12) throughout life

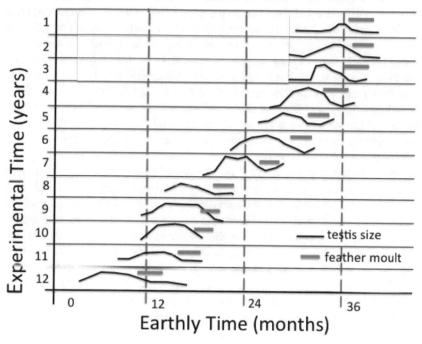

Fig. 1.14 Circannual rhythms sustained across the 12-year life span of a single male African stonechat that was caged in the laboratory under constant equatorial photoperiod (LD 12:12). Circannual cycles in testis size and feather moult persisted with a free-running period (tau) of ~10.5 months; peaks in gonadal size and sexual behaviour became progressively earlier in real time advancing by a complete cycle into old age. The post-breeding pelage moult remained phase locked to the innate reproductive cycle. Parallel studies were conducted where eggs were hatched in an incubator and the offspring were reared in a constant environment with no parental contact; the circannual periodicity still persisted indicating that cycle generation is part of the genetic life-history programme. (after Gwinner 1996)

circannual rhythm may be determined by the period of the circadian rhythm. This concept is called frequency demultiplication; the analogy is with an electronic clock that transforms the frequency of 50–60 cycles per second of the national electricity current into a 1-cycle per day frequency providing information about time of day. The prediction is that there will be a positive correlation between *tau* for the two endogenous timing systems, albeit perhaps rather weak considering the 1:365 ratio.

The frequency demultiplication hypothesis has been experimentally investigated in fish, birds, mammals and insects. One paradigm has been to expose groups of animals to different daily light-dark cycles of 22 h, 24 h and 26 h with equal lengths of day and night ('T-cycles'). These light-dark cycles have been maintained constantly for 2–4 years to allow the period of the circannual oscillations to be recorded.

Measurement of circadian perch-hopping rhythms of the birds has revealed that locomotor activity patterns are entrained to the different T-cycles; thus, the animals have true differences in their internal temporal organization. However, the observed small differences in period of the circannual rhythms (testicular size and moult) were not consistent with the frequency demultiplication prediction. There are technical difficulties in the design of these experiments, since minor differences in photoperiod-length may engage the photoperiodic system, but overall there has been no robust support for the frequency demultiplication hypothesis. A second approach has been to suppress or ablate circadian rhythmicity and look for a corresponding effect on circannual timing. Pinealectomy in many species of birds and lesions of the suprachiasmatic nuclei in mammals severely disrupt circadian locomotor activity rhythms, but in a wide range of experiments normal circannual rhythms have been shown to persist.

Despite this lack of support for the frequency demultiplication concept, there is an extensive literature describing a close association between changes in the phasing and intensity of circadian locomotor activity rhythms and the progression of the circannual cycle. This includes the observation that periods of migratory restlessness (*zugunruhe*) occur at specific phases of the circannual cycle in body weight and reproductive function in migratory birds, and changes in the phase-angle of entrainment (ψ) of locomotor activity patterns are very tightly linked to the 'circannual sensitive windows' characterized in the European hamster (Monecke et al. 2009). It still remains to be established whether these circadian phenomena are truly *causal* in the generation of circannual rhythmicity, or rather, the *consequence* of the underlying circannual pacemaker mechanism.

1.4.3 Entrainment of Circannual Rhythms

To achieve the optimal timing of seasonal biology, circannual rhythms need to be entrained by external cues, notably photoperiod, nutrition and/or social factors (Paul et al. 2008). In the case of photoperiodic entrainment, this involves the induction of phase advances or phase delays in the innate rhythm to synchronize with the 12-month environment. Because many free-running circannual rhythms have a *tau* value shorter than a year (<10 months), stable entrainment requires the induction of an overall phase-delay (lengthening) in the endogenous cycle by some 2 months, annually. The magnitude of this re-setting response has been determined by exposing experimental animals to a 'pulse' of inductive photoperiod (e.g. 4-week-long photoperiod under prolonged constant conditions). This has been repeated in different groups across the circannual cycle to produce a phase-response curve (PRC), representing the magnitude and direction of the phase shift. This is a routine procedure in circadian rhythm research, but a logistic nightmare for the circannual researcher.

A phase-response curve for the circannual system has been published for trout (Duston and Bromage 1988), European hamster (Monecke et al. 2009), and in most detail for the carpet beetle (Miyazaki et al. 2006). The results demonstrate that a long-day stimulus applied early in the subjective circannual year can cause a phase-delay of approximately 2 months. This predicts that animals will utilize the long days of summer for entrainment of their innate rhythmicity to a specific season. The suggestion that only part of the annual cycle in daylength is required for normal entrainment of the circannual clock has been elegantly confirmed by Fred Karsch and colleagues studying the annual reproductive cycle of Suffolk sheep (Woodfill et al. 1994). In their key experiment, groups of adult pinealectomized ewes housed outdoors were treated with a programmed infusion of melatonin to mimic either a long-day photoperiod (LD; short bouts 6 h/day) or short-day photoperiod (SD; long bouts 12 h/day) delivered for 90 days, once each year for 4 years (Fig. 1.15). The animals were also ovariectomized and given a slow-release implant of estradiol to standardize the reproductive status. Long-term changes in blood concentrations of LH were measured as an index of the circannual reproductive rhythm. The untreated pinealectomized sheep showed variable, asynchronous cyclical patterns in LH, while the animals given melatonin to mimic long photoperiod for 90 days given once per year (LD group), showed highly synchronized annual gonadotrophin cycles. Con-trastingly, the SD melatonin group remained asynchronous. The responsive LD animals showed a tightly regulated onset and offset of the annual reproductive rhythm, with a consistent *phasing* (3 month delay) relative to the end of the melatonin treatment (Fig. 1.15). The overall pattern was very similar to normal, pineal-intact animals living outdoors. These results illustrate that both period and phase control are mediated through LD melatonin signalling. Only a relatively short cue lasting just 3 months can interact with the innate clock mechanisms to produce the annual phenotype; this nicely demonstrates that most of the temporal control of long-term cycles in physiology is innate. It is interesting that in sheep, a 'short-day breeder', summer photoperiod provides the primary seasonal entrainment cue, while in the European hamster, a 'long-day breeder', it is winter photoperiod that synchronizes reproductive timing (Saboureau et al. 1999).

1.4.4   Circannual Chronotypes

In species adapted to temperate and cold climates, individuals are generally well synchronized in the timing of their seasonal rhythms, as seen for red deer living in the wild in Scotland (Fig. 1.16a). Within a population, however, there is notable variation between individuals independent of the effect of age (Lincoln et al. 1970); note the 'front-runner' called Broken Brow (Fig. 1.16a). This animal cast his antlers 6 weeks ahead of most of the adult stags and always left early for the rut over a 4-year period of observations. This illustrates how animals have an individual circannual *chronotype*, analogous to the 'larks' and 'owls' of the circadian domain. Rutting early is an evolutionary gamble targeting a few prime-breeding hinds, and is a genetic trait since hybrids between early and late phenotypes produce an interme-diate timing. The survival advantage of date of birth varies from year to year, which may explain how polymorphism in innate seasonal timing mechanisms can be maintained in a wild population.

Karsch pinealectomised sheep model

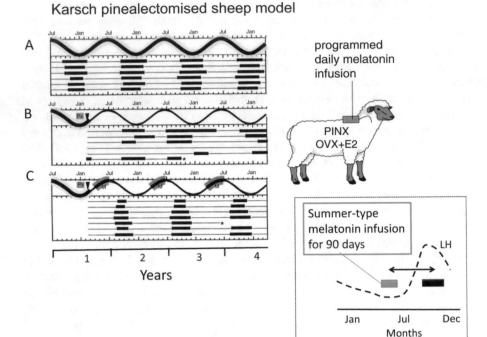

Fig. 1.15 Entrainment of circannual rhythms by once-yearly melatonin treatment in Suffolk sheep living outdoors. The sheep were initially pinealectomized to remove endogenous melatonin, and ovariectomized and given constant-release implants of estradiol (OVX + E2) to standardize the reproductive status (see diagram). The protocol was to treat the ewes with a programmed daily infusion melatonin replicating either a long day (LD, 6-h daily pulse) or a short-day (SD, 12-h daily pulse) photoperiod signal. This was delivered for 90 days (orange symbols) once annually over a 4-year study (see Box for predicted effect on circannual LH secretion). (**a**–**c**) Summary of individual reproductive cycles assessed from plasma LH concentrations where black bars indicate increased activity: (**a**) control ewes with no treatment; (**b**) pinealectomized ewes (operation see arrow) but no melatonin treatment; (**c**) experimental treatment with 3-month blocks of LD melatonin treatment (for timing see M). Note, the periodic LD melatonin group showed full re-entrainment of the annual LH cycle in all animals, with the onset of increased reproductive activity occurring some 3 months after the end of each melatonin phase, conceptually equivalent to an autumn breeding season. The periodic SD group failed to entrain (data omitted for brevity). (After Woodfill et al. 1994)

A most extreme case of variability occurs in Indian Chital deer adapted to living near the equator where individual males show asynchronous cyclicity (Fig. 1.16b). This occurs both in their natural habitat in India and Sri Lanka and in captivity at the London Whipsnade Zoo, where they have been living outdoors for more than 120 years (Loudon and Curlewis 1988). The period of the antler cycle rhythm is 10–12 months, as if the rhythm is free-running independent of daylength. The asynchrony between group members beautifully illustrates autonomous timing, since there is no geophysical feature that can explain the individual chronotypes. Equally impressive are the asynchronous musth cycles in male African elephants,

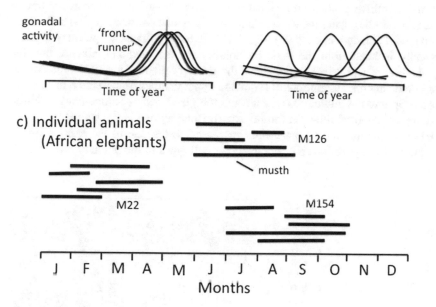

a) Synchronous (red deer)   **b) Asynchronous (Indian chital deer)**

gonadal
activity   'front runner'

Time of year   Time of year

**c) Individual animals
(African elephants)**   M126

musth

M22   M154

J F M A M J J A S O N D
Months

Fig. 1.16 Intraspecific variation in the phasing of the circannual rhythm: (**a**) *Synchronous* seasonal testicular cycles in a population based on wild red deer stags living in Scotland (Lincoln et al. 1970); (**b**) *Asynchronous* as observed in tropical Indian chital deer living in Sri Lanka or in the London Zoo (Loudon and Curlewis 1988); (**c**) *Asynchronous with marked variation between individuals*: musth behavioural cycles in bull African elephants living in the Amboseli National Park in Kenya (Poole 1987)

musth being a period of aggressive behaviour in males associated with elevated circulating testosterone concentrations (Fig. 1.16c). Here, once males are sexually mature at 15–20 years old, each bull comes into musth at a specific time of year: each animal adopts its preferred rutting time repeated for many years (Poole 1987). When dominant bulls have been killed by poachers, subordinates may take over the breeding slot, indicative of social inhibition and entrainment of the innate circannual cycle under natural conditions.

The occurrence of circannual chronotypes may also apply to man. People who experience severe symptoms of seasonal affective disorder (SAD) show striking individual differences in the onset, offset and severity of the clinical condition. SAD may be in part a natural adaptation to winter, where a change in appetite and increased body weight in autumn, and the development of social withdrawal behaviour in winter, was once an advantage to our hunter-gatherer ancestors (Levitan 2007; Wirz-Justice 2017).

1.4.5   Circannual Pacemakers 2000–Present

The first definitive evidence for a localized pacemaker system for circannual timing came from studies using the hypothalamo-pituitary disconnected (HPD) male Soay sheep model (Lincoln et al. 2006) (Fig. 1.17). In these animals the pituitary gland is surgically isolated from the brain by ablation of the median eminence and the implantation of a physical barrier above the pituitary gland. This blocks the normal anterograde neuroendocrine control from the hypothalamus. Importantly, the normal blood supply to the pituitary is retained and the gland retains autonomous viability, and support a normal life-span for the experimental animal in the laboratory.

HPD Soay rams have permanently regressed testes due to the loss of GnRH regulation of the gonadotrophs, but the other cell types in the pituitary *pars distalis*

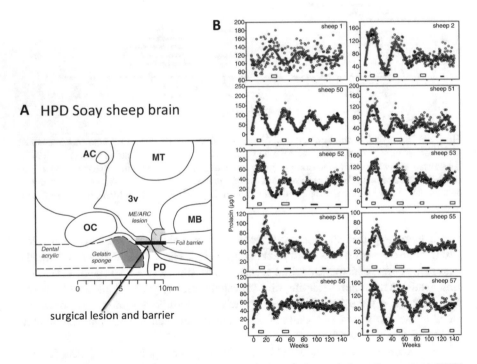

Fig. 1.17 Localization of a circannual pacemaker in hypothalamo-pituitary disconnected (HPD) Soay sheep. (**a**) Schematic sagittal section of the sheep basal hypothalamus illustrating the surgical procedure to visualize the pituitary stalk from the nasal area (dotted line—site later sealed), to ablate the median eminence and to place a permanent foil barrier (black bar) between the hypothalamus and pituitary gland. Abbreviations: optic chiasm (OC), third ventricle (3v), anterior commissure (AC), medial thalamus (MT), mammillary body (MB), *pars distalis* (PD), median eminence/arcuate nucleus (ME/ARC lesion); (**b**) Blood plasma prolactin concentrations in individual HPD Soay rams under constant long days (LD 16:8), across the 148-week study. Note, the persistence of circannual rhythmicity in prolactin release and a correlated pelage moult cycle (open boxes) throughout, with individual variation and the development of asynchrony in the group, consistent with innate regulation. Adapted from Lincoln et al. (2006)

(lactotrophs, thyrotrophs and corticotrophs) show varying degrees of secretory activity. Remarkably, HPD sheep still express normal, robust photoperiod-induced cycles in prolactin secretion, and a reoccurring circannual rhythm in prolactin under constant long photoperiod for at least four cycles. The prolactin-regulated wool growth cycle runs in parallel (Fig. 1.17). In this pivotal experiment conducted under constant long photoperiod (LD), each animal was found to have a unique cyclical prolactin profile, and the animals gradually lost synchrony within the group, indicative of innate control. The mean *tau* value was close to 10.5 months as for many circannual rhythms.

More recently, the pituitary pacemaker has been localized to the melatonin-responsive thyrotrophs in the *pars tuberalis* (PT) of the pituitary stalk (Wood et al., 2015), see Chap. 2. For this, groups of seasonal Blackface rams that had been castrated to standardize the reproductive axis were exposed to an abrupt switch from short photoperiod (SD) to a prolonged period of long days (LD) and killed at different times of day and at selected weekly/monthly intervals. Changes in the thyrotrophs in the PT were measured by immunohistochemistry and in situ hybridization on tissue sections through the pituitary gland. This revealed a progressive cycle in PT cell secretory activity over months; however, individual thyrotrophs cells were found only in one of two states: TSH secretory active 'summer like' (early in the study) or TSH secretory inactive 'winter like' (later in the study). This indicated that individual thyrotrophs 'flip' from one state to the other and gradually a *wave* of change pervades the tissue; the population effect explains the smooth profile of the circannual rhythm (Wood et al. 2015).

These observations are of fundamental importance because they indicate that circannual timing is potentially a cell autonomous process operating within each PT cell, and some form of long-term intrinsic timing and cell-cell coordination dictates the period of the cycle, as predicted for a pacemaker. These studies have shown that the retrograde PT TSH-Dio2-TH brain relay remains potentially functional, but it is the *switching off* of the PT thyrotrophs that inactivates the axis to produce the initial photorefractory response (Sáenz de Miera et al. 2014; Wood et al. 2015). The full circannual cycle of activation, regression and reactivation has so far not been characterized, and the fundamental mechanism that 'flips' the thyrotroph between on and off is unresolved.

In addition to the PT, there is increasing evidence for a parallel circannual pacemaker in the brain of certain mammalian species that is melatonin independent, but entrained by photoperiod and other seasonal cues (Fig. 1.18). This is supported by a detailed analysis of circannual regulation of gonadal activity, body weight and hibernation cycles in the European hamster (Sáenz de Miera et al. 2014). In this species, pinealectomy has a minimal disruptive effect on the expression of circannual rhythms, and the rhythmicity retains some degree of photoperiod responsiveness. Seasonal cycles with near-normal timing have also been observed in a diverse range of mammal that have been pinealectomized or had their superior cervical ganglion removed to ablate sympathetic innervation of the pineal gland (SCGx). This includes golden-mantled ground squirrel, mink, wolf, edible dormouse, Soay sheep, red deer and horse. Notably, this occurs in animals under natural

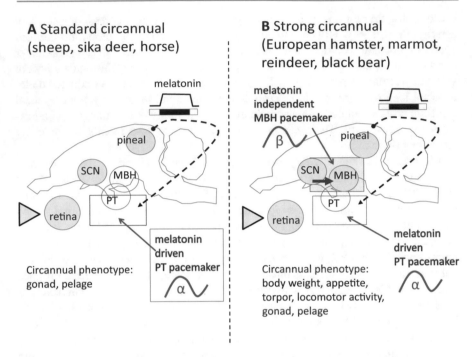

Fig. 1.18 Two models for circannual timing in mammals. (**a**) Standard circannual model—as seen in many temperate climate species (e.g. sheep, sika deer, horse) where photoperiod acts through the retinal-pineal-melatonin relay to entrain the *pars tuberalis* (PT) circannual pacemaker system (oscillator α) to time cycles in reproduction and moult. (**b**) Strong circannual model—as proposed for hibernators and arctic species (e.g. European hamster, marmot, reindeer, black bear) where photoperiod acts, in addition to well-documented relay, via a more direct melatonin independent SCN-hypothalamic pathway, to time a broader spectrum of seasonal behavioural and physiological traits. The prediction is for an associated central circannual pacemaker mechanism (oscillator β), possibly located within the tanycyte cell population lining the third cerebral ventricle. Abbreviations: suprachiasmatic nucleus (SCN), mediobasal hypothalamus (MBH)

conditions outdoors where other environmental variables may synchronize endogenous rhythmicity. Studies in the European hamster also point to the PT as a likely locus of a circannual pacemaker, as key genes involved in PTM continue to show circannual rhythms in expression in this tissue in hamsters housed under constant conditions (Sáenz de Miera et al. 2014), and can be photoperiodically regulated in the PT of pinealectomized hamsters (Sáenz de Miera et al. 2018). These observations raise an intriguing question, are there some mammals where photoperiodic information can be communicated from the SCN directly to the PT and/or hypothalamus? In this scenario, entrainment by photoperiod could arise either via the well-established pineal melatonin-pituitary PT-TSH-Dio2-TH pathway, and/or via the less well-characterized, retinal-SCN-hypothalamic tanycyte pathway (Fig. 1.18). In both cases, the focal pacemaker cell (PT thyrotroph and/or hypothalamic tanycyte) is from a basic somatic cell lineage. This ontogenetic feature may reflect the ancient origins of circannual timing systems.

References

Ayers JW, Althouse BM, Allem JP, Rosenquist JN, Ford DE (2013) Seasonality in seeking mental health information on Google. Am J Prev Med 44:520–525

Bartness TJ, Powers JB, Hastings MH, Bittman EL, Goldman BD (1993) The timed infusion paradigm for melatonin delivery: what has it taught us about the melatonin signal, its reception and the photoperiodic control of seasonal responses. J Pineal Res 15:161–190

Bittman EL, Dempsey RJ, Karsch FJ (1983) Pineal melatonin secretion drives the reproductive response to daylength in the ewe. Endocrinology 113:2276–2283

Dahlberg J, Andersson G (2018) Changing seasonal variation in births by sociodemographic factors: a population-based register study. Hum Reprod Open 4:29. https://doi.org/10.1093/hropen/hoy0151

Dardente H, Wyse CA, Birnie MJ, Dupre SM, Loudon ASI, Lincoln GA, Hazlerigg DG (2010) A molecular switch for photoperiod responsiveness in mammals. Curr Biol 20:2193–2198

Diamond J (1997) Guns, germs, and steel: the fates of human societies. Vintage, New York. isbn:9780099302780

Duston J, Bromage N (1988) The entrainment and gating of the endogenous circannual rhythm of reproduction in the female rainbow trout (Salmo gairdneri). J Comp Physiol A 164:259–268

Ebenhöh O, Hazlerigg D (2013) Modelling a molecular calendar: the seasonal photoperiodic response in mammals. Chaos Solitons Fractals 50:39–47

Gaffney V, Fitch S, Ramsey E, Yorston R, Ch'ng E (2013) Time and a place: a luni-solar 'time-reckoner' from 8th millennium BC Scotland. Int Archaeol 34. https://doi.org/10.11141/ia.34.1

Gwinner E (1986) Circannual rhythms. endogenous annual clocks in the organization of seasonal processes. Springer, Berlin

Gwinner E (1996) Circannual clocks in avian reproduction and migration. Ibis 138:47–63

Hanon EA, Lincoln GA, Fustin JM, Dardente H, Masson-Pevet M, Morgan PJ, Hazlerigg DG (2008) Ancestral TSH mechanism signals summer in a photoperiodic mammal. Curr Biol 18:1147–1152

Hazlerigg DG, Andersson H, Johnston JD, Lincoln GA (2004) Molecular characterisation of the long-day response in the soay sheep, a seasonal mammal. Curr Biol 14:1–20

Levitan RD (2007) The chronobiology and neurobiology of winter seasonal affective disorder. Dialogues Clin Neurosci 9:315–324

Lincoln GA (1994) Effects of placing micro-implants of melatonin in the pars tuberalis, pars distalis and the lateral septum of the forebrain on the secretion of FSH and prolactin, and testicular size in rams. J Endocrinol 142:267–276

Lincoln GA, Youngson RW, Short RV (1970) The social and sexual behaviour of the red deer stag. J Reprod Fertil Suppl 11:71–103

Lincoln GA, Messager S, Andersson H, Hazlerigg DG (2002) Temporal expression of seven clock genes in the suprachiasmatic nucleus and the pars tuberalis of the sheep: evidence for an internal coincidence timer. Proc Natl Acad Sci USA 99:13890–13895

Lincoln GA, Clarke IJ, Hut RA, Hazlerigg DG (2006) Characterizing a mammalian circannual pacemaker. Science 314:1941

Loudon ASI, Curlewis JD (1988) Cycles of antler and testicular growth in an aseasonal tropical deer (Axis axis). J Reprod Fertil 83:729–738

Ludwig M, Levkowitz G (2018) Model animals in neuroendocrinology: from worm to mouse to man. Wiley, Hoboken, NJ

Marshall FHA (1937) On the change over in the oestrous cycle in animals after transference across the equator, with further observations on the incidence of the breeding seasons and the factors controlling sexual periodicity. Proc R Soc Lond B 122:413–428

Martinez ME (2018) The calendar of epidemics: seasonal cycles of infectious diseases. PLoS Pathog 14(11):e1007327. https://doi.org/10.1371/journal.ppat.1007327

Martinez-Bakker M, Bakker KM, King AA, Rohani P (2014) Human birth seasonality: latitudinal gradient and interplay with childhood disease dynamics. Proc R Soc B 281(1783):20132438. https://doi.org/10.1098/rspb.2013.2438

Masumoto KH, Ukai-Tadenuma M, Kasukawa T, Nagano M, Uno KD, Tsujino K, Horikaw AK, Shigeyoshi Y, Ueda HR (2010) Acute induction of Eya3 by late-night light stimulation triggers TSHβ expression in photoperiodism. Curr Biol 20:2199–2206

Menaker M (1971) Rhythms, reproduction, and photoperiodism. Biol Reprod 4:295–308

Miyazaki Y, Nisimura T, Numata H (2006) Phase responses in the circannual rhythm of the varied carpet beetle, Anthrenus verbasci, under naturally changing day length. Zool Sci 23:1031–1037

Monecke S, Saboureau M, Malan A, Bonn D, Masson-Pévet M, Pévet P (2009) Circannual phase response curves to short and long photoperiod in the European hamster. J Biol Rhythm 24:413–426

Paul MJ, Zucker I, Schwartz WJ (2008) Tracking the seasons: the internal calendars of vertebrates. Philos Trans R Soc B 363:341–361

Pengelley ET, Fisher KC (1957) Onset and cessation of hibernation under constant temperature and light in the golden-mantled ground squirrel *Citellus lateralis*. Nature 180:1371–1372

Pengelley ET, Asmundson SJ, Barnes B, Aloia RC (1976) Relationship of light intensity and photoperiod to circannual rhythmicity in the hibernating ground squirrel, Citellus lateralis. Comp Biochem Physiol A Physiol 53:273–277

Pittendrigh CS (1972) Circadian surfaces and the diversity of possible roles of circadian organization in photoperiodic induction. Proc Natl Acad Sci 69:2734–2737

Poole JH (1987) Rutting behaviour in African elephants: the phenomenon of musth. Behaviour 102:283–316

Randall VA, Ebling FJ (1991) Seasonal changes in human hair growth. Br J Dermatol 124:146–151

Reppert SM (1997) Melatonin receptors: molecular biology of a new family of G protein-coupled receptors. J Biol Rhythm 12:528–531

Roenneberg T, Aschoff J (1990) Annual rhythm of human reproduction: I. Biology, sociology, or both? J Biol Rhythm 5:195–215

Rowan W (1925) Relation of light to bird migration and developmental changes. Nature 115:494–495

Saboureau M, Masson-Pévet M, Canguilhem B, Pévet P, Sassone-Corsi P (1999) Circannual reproductive rhythm in the European hamster (Cricetus cricetus): demonstration of the existence of an annual phase of sensitivity to short photoperiod. J Pineal Res 26:9–16

Sáenz De Miera C, Monecke S, Bartzen-Sprauer J, Laran-Chich MP, Pevet P, Hazlerigg DG, Simonneaux V (2014) A circannual clock drives expression of genes central for seasonal reproduction. Curr Biol 24:1500–1506

Sáenz De Miera C, Sage-Ciocca D, Simonneaux V, Pévet P, Monecke S (2018) Melatonin-independent photoperiodic entrainment of the circannual TSH rhythm in the pars tuberalis of the European hamster. J Biol Rhythm 33:302–317

Schafer EA (1907) On the incidence of daylight as a determining factor in bird migration. Nature 77:159–163

Weil ZM, Borniger JC, Cisse YM, Abi Salloum BA, Nelson RJ (2015) Neuroendocrine control of photoperiodic changes in immune function. Front Neuroendocrinol 37:108–118. https://doi.org/10.1016/j.yfrne.2014.10.001

Wirz-Justice A (2017) Seasonality in affective disorders. Gen Comp Endocrinol 258:244–249

Wood SH, Christian HC, Miedzinska K, Saer BR, Johnson M, Paton B, Yu L, Mcneilly J, Davis JR, Mcneilly AS, Burt DW, Loudon AS (2015) Binary switching of calendar cells in the pituitary defines the phase of the circannual cycle in mammals. Curr Biol 25:2651–2662

Woodfill CJI, Wayne NL, Moenter SM, Karsch FJ (1994) Photoperiodic synchronization of a circannual reproductive rhythm in sheep: identification of season-specific time cues. Biol Reprod 50:965–976

Further Recommended Reading

Bartness TJ, Powers JB, Hastings MH, Bittman EL, Goldman BD (1993) The timed infusion paradigm for melatonin delivery: what has it taught us about the melatonin signal, its reception and the photoperiodic control of seasonal responses. J Pineal Res 15:161–190. Review of studies on how melatonin conveys timing information to the neuroendocrine system.

Hanon EA, Lincoln GA, Fustin JM, Dardente H, Masson-Pevet M, Morgan PJ, Hazlerigg DG (2008) Ancestral TSH mechanism signals summer in a photoperiodic mammal. Curr Biol 18:1147–1152. Outstanding research paper demonstrating the importance in seasonal timing of signalling via the *pars tuberalis* to hypothalamic tanycytes.

Hazlerigg DG, Lincoln GA (2011) Hypothesis: cyclical histogenesis is the basis of circannual timing. J Biol Rhythm 26:471–485. Review that considers how circannual rhythmicity might arise from cellular changes in the *pars tuberalis*.

Lincoln G (2019) A brief history of circannual time. J Neuroendocrinol 31(3):e12694. https://doi.org/10.1111/jne.12694. Very recent review discussing the nature of circannual rhythms and their underlying mechanistic basis.

The *Pars Tuberalis* and Seasonal Timing

2

Shona H. Wood

Abstract

The *pars tuberalis* is part of the pituitary stalk that sits at the interface between the median eminence of the hypothalamus and the anterior pituitary gland (*pars distalis*). It primarily comprises thyrotrophs that produce βTSH, and folliculostellate cells. In all mammals studied to date it expresses a high density of melatonin receptors, so it is the key interface between the circulation and the hypothalamus for transduction of nocturnal melatonin signals that convey photoperiodic information. This chapter explores the mechanisms by which the changing duration of nocturnal melatonin regulates circadian 'clock genes', including cry1 and a 'developmental' gene EYA3 in the *pars tuberalis*, resulting in differential production of βTSH and 'tuberalins' to regulate hypothalamic and anterior pituitary function, respectively.

Keywords

Pars tuberalis · Seasonal · Circannual · Thyroid hormone · Melatonin

2.1   Introduction

The movement of the earth as it travels around the sun creates daily and seasonal cycles in local environments on its surface (Fig. 2.1a). The regularity of these cycles imposes a fundamental temporal framework upon which biological systems have

S. H. Wood (✉)
Arctic Chronobiology and Physiology Research Group, Department of Arctic and Marine Biology, UiT—The Arctic University of Norway, Tromsø, Norway
e-mail: shona.wood@uit.no

© The Editor(s) (if applicable) and The Author(s), under exclusive license to   33
Springer Nature Switzerland AG 2020
F. J. P. Ebling, H. D. Piggins (eds.), *Neuroendocrine Clocks and Calendars*,
Masterclass in Neuroendocrinology 10, https://doi.org/10.1007/978-3-030-55643-3_2

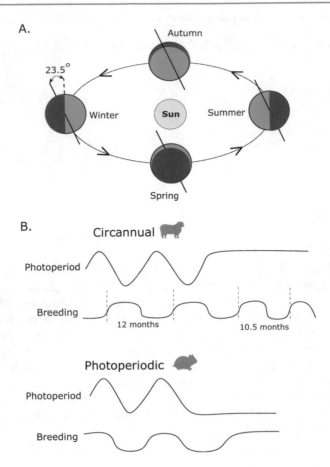

Fig. 2.1 (**a**) The earth as depicted from above the orbital plane is tilted on its axis by around 23.5°. The earth moves around the sun changing the relative day-length with the time of year depending on whether the axis is pointing, towards (summer solstice), away (winter solstice) or orthogonal to (equinoxes) the plane of solar radiation. (**b**) In mammals, the environmental photoperiod is inversely represented by rhythmic secretion of melatonin. Vertebrates use the annual change in photoperiod to entrain cycles in seasonal physiology, but if photoperiod is fixed then such cycles persist reflecting endogenous rhythmicity. While the photoperiod varies naturally or through stepwise changes in long (LP) and short photoperiods (SP), breeding is synchronised to short days in sheep and long days in hamsters. This difference is accounted for by relative gestation times to synchronise birth of offspring to the spring and the period of greatest food availability. If sheep are placed into constant LP the animal becomes refractory to the prevailing photoperiod and reactivates reproduction but then continues to show cycles of reproductive activation and inactivation, albeit with a shorter period of 10.5 months. This is a common feature of long-lived circannual species. Hamsters placed into constant SP will inhibit but then reactivate their reproductive circuits and subsequently remain in a reproductively active state, so only display one endogenously timed cycle

evolved. At high latitudes, the contrast in environment between winter and summer is particularly dramatic, and biological systems have developed remarkable adaptations to overcome the associated selection pressures. Migration, hibernation, aestivation, diapause, pelage/moult colour and quality, reproductive status and changing behaviour are all essential strategies necessary for life to exploit such challenging temporospatial niches. Each of these strategies needs to develop at the appropriate time of year to allow the individual to survive and successfully reproduce. Furthermore, major physiological change can take many weeks to complete; thus, the organism must intrinsically monitor the time of year and anticipate upcoming changes. Annual changes in day length (photoperiod) are a highly predictive signal that can be reliably used to activate a seasonal adaptive programme. Animals have evolved to use photoperiod in concert with endogenous long-term timers ('seasonal clock'). This allows them to keep track of seasonal time at tropical overwintering localities with constant day length, during migration through zones of rapidly changing day length, during polar summers with constant light, and in winter hibernacula or during polar winters with constant darkness. The fundamental biological basis of these seasonal clocks is not completely understood; however, the photoperiodic pathways and the anatomical structures involved in regulating the seasonal clockwork are becoming clearer. This chapter will focus on the *pars tuberalis* of the pituitary, which acts as a seasonal clock, and provides a lynchpin between the photoperiodic relay and the downstream seasonal physiological changes.

2.2 Photoperiodic and Circannual Species

Clocks must be able to be synchronised to external time signals (*zeitgeibers*), but also persist in the absence of such signals (endogenous rhythms). The suprachiasmatic nucleus (SCN) is the circadian master clock in the mammalian hypothalamus and robustly displays these properties on a daily basis, whereas the *pars tuberalis*, part of the pituitary stalk, appears to display clock-like properties on a yearly basis. There is however variation in the nature and persistence of the seasonal endogenous rhythm in different species based on differences in life history and longevity (Fig. 2.1b).

Using seasonal reproduction as an example, small short-lived seasonal species such as hamsters are programmed to breed in a single breeding season and seldom survive a second winter. In these species, the activation of reproduction in the spring will normally occur in response to increased photoperiod, but will also take place if hamsters are maintained on a fixed winter short photoperiod (SP). However, once these animals have entered a reproductively active state, they do not undergo any further changes in physiological state. This "photorefractory" mechanism is an almost universal feature of such species (Wood and Loudon 2014), and represents an ideal mechanism to drive onset of breeding for short-lived fossorial rodents (Fig. 2.1b).

In contrast, species that breed over two or more years will undergo persistent cycles when maintained on fixed photoperiods (i.e. SP, long photoperiod (LP) or

12:12), though the specific photoperiod will depend on the species (Gwinner 1986). Initially, this occurs as a consequence of refractoriness to the prevailing photoperiod, and then continues to cycle endogenously through the seasonal physiology (Fig. 2.1b). The eastern chipmunk has been shown to continue with these endogenous cycles for up to 6.5 years (Richter 1978). Birds, however, have some of the most impressive circannual cycles, the blackcap for example was shown to cycle through moulting for their entire lifespan (8 years) in constant conditions (Gwinner 1986). These refractory mechanisms, and therefore endogenously timed seasonal cycles, are common in mammals, marsupials (Brinklow and Loudon 1993), birds (Dawson 2015) and teleosts (Duston and Bromage 1991; Frantzen et al. 2004). It has been suggested that the different responses (circannual or refractory) are simply 'variations on a theme rather than fundamentally different models' (Follett and Nicholls 1985; Butler et al. 2010; Dardente et al. 2014).

What is clear from these responses is that there is an initial response to photoperiod that entrains the endogenous cycle, which, depending on life history, will continue to cycle in constant conditions for one or multiple cycles. The majority of the research has focused on the photoperiodic response and therefore the light-input pathways, encoding of photoperiod in the brain and the relay to the endocrine axis to initiate the changes in seasonal physiology.

2.3 Melatonin, the Photoperiodic Response and Circannual Rhythms

In mammals, light is received via the eye; this is the only photoreceptive organ and removal ablates the photoperiodic response (Reiter 1980; Nelson and Zucker 1981; Meijer et al. 1999). The photic input pathway from the retina to the SCN drives rhythmic melatonin production from the pineal gland (Fig. 2.2). Light inhibits the production of melatonin; therefore, there is an internal representation of the external photoperiod by the duration of melatonin production. This is the photoneuroendocrine system. Removal of the pineal gland (pinealectomy) blocks photoperiodic responses in mammals (Hoffman and Reiter 1965; Reiter 1980). Use of artificial patterns of timed melatonin infusion in pinealectomised individuals demonstrates that repeated daily exposure to melatonin is critical in the photoperiodic control of seasonal reproductive and metabolic responses (Bartness et al. 1993) (Bittman et al. 1983; Carter and Goldman 1983; Goldman 2001). Therefore, in most mammals, the nocturnal production of melatonin by the pineal gland provides a crucial step in the photoperiodic relay.

A rhythmic melatonin signal is also required for the generation of circannual rhythms (Zucker 1985; Woodfill et al. 1994). Pinealectomy of sheep and melatonin replacement by timed daily infusions led Fred Karsch's research group in the University of Michigan to make the striking observation that only 90 days of continuous exposure to the melatonin signal is required to entrain the annual cycle, with most effective responses being 90-day exposure to summer-like melatonin patterns, administered once a year (Woodfill et al. 1994). The capacity of arctic

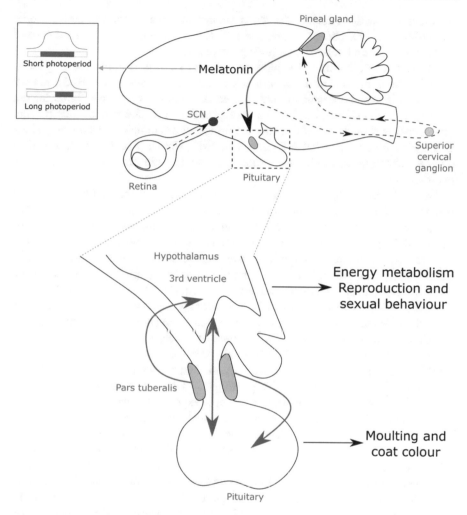

Fig. 2.2 In mammals, the photic input pathway from the retina to the SCN drives rhythmic melatonin production from the pineal gland, and this melatonin signal is sculpted by photoperiod to provide an internal endocrine representation for external photoperiod. Short photoperiods are represented by increased nocturnal duration of melatonin and long photoperiods by short duration melatonin. The only conserved site of melatonin binding in mammals is a region of pituitary stalk called the *pars tuberalis*, this ideally placed between the hypothalamus and pituitary to impinge on the hypothalamo-pituitary axis and appears to signal in a retrograde and anterograde manner to drive energy metabolism, reproduction and moulting. Adapted from Wood and Loudon (2017)

species (reindeer, ptarmigan, arctic charr), to maintain synchronisation of circannual rhythms, despite a breakdown of rhythmic melatonin secretion for long periods around the winter and summer solstices (Stokkan et al. 1994, 2007; Reierth et al. 1999; Strand et al. 2008), is also suggestive that only narrow windows of photoperiodic information are required to synchronise a circannual rhythm. It is important to note that circannual rhythms can persist in mammals after pinealectomy (Woodfill et al. 1994; Sáenz de Miera et al. 2014), but these are no longer entrained to the solar year and depend on a prior photoperiodic history.

The role for melatonin in the photoperiodic response in mammals is very clear, what is less clear is how melatonin contributes to the endogenous (circannual) rhythm. It is also important to note that unlike mammals, fish and birds have a directly photosensitive pineal gland and pinealectomy alone does not prevent photoperiodic responses, but can alter the timing of reproductive responses (Falcón et al. 2010; Migaud et al. 2010; Tsutsui et al. 2013; Ubuka et al. 2013). Birds and all other vertebrate groups additionally receive photoperiod information via deep-brain photoreceptors.

Given the importance of melatonin in the seasonal response, mapping where melatonin binds in the brain was the emphasis in early studies using auto-radiographic techniques to visualise binging of radiolabelled melatonin. This identified the *pars tuberalis* as the only consistent site of melatonin binding across a wide range of seasonally breeding mammalian species (Morgan et al. 1994). Subsequently, two subtypes of high-affinity G-protein-coupled (GPCR) melatonin receptors have been identified, termed MT1 (MNTR1A) and MT2 (MNTR1b) (Reppert 1997), one of which (MNTR1A) is strongly expressed in the *pars tuberalis*. A third GPCR melatonin receptor subtype, Mel1c (or MTNR1C), has been identified in fish, amphibians and birds, the orthologue of which in mammals is GPR50, but this does not bind melatonin (Reppert et al. 1996a, b). Interestingly, expression of GPR50 is not in the pituitary, but in hypothalamic ependymal cells in Siberian hamsters, where it is regulated by photoperiod (Barrett et al. 2006). It is also involved in hypothalamic control of energy expenditure and feeding (Ivanova et al. 2008), and knock-out studies in mice reveal a role in adaptive thermogenesis (Bechtold et al. 2012). Mel1c has evolved rapidly and under different selection pressures in fishes, birds and mammals (Dufourny et al. 2008), and the divergence of this receptor may represent changes in the photoperiodic organisation across vertebrates. Intriguingly, the Mel1c receptor is expressed in the chicken *pars tuberalis* (Kameda et al. 2002). In mammals, the MT1 receptor co-localises to the *pars tuberalis*, and is considered to be critical for photoperiodic signal transduction (Reppert 1997). Additionally the OPN5-positive neurons, the deep-brain photoreceptors of the paraventricular organ of the quail, are thought to be essential in relaying the photoperiodic signal to the *pars tuberalis* in birds (Nakane and Yoshimura 2010, 2014; Nakane et al. 2010; Yoshimura 2010, 2013). Therefore, current research points towards the *pars tuberalis* of the pituitary as the site receiving the photoperiodic readout and integrating this to the endocrine system to orchestrate downstream changes in seasonal physiology (Fig. 2.2) (Lincoln 2006; Sáenz de Miera et al. 2014; Wood and Loudon 2014, 2017; Wood et al. 2015; West and Wood 2018).

2.4   Anatomy of the *Pars Tuberalis*

The *pars tuberalis* sits at the interface between the median eminence and the main *pars distalis* (PD) regions of the anterior pituitary. Developmentally, it emerges from the rostral tip region of Rathke's pouch, and contains a mixture of *pars tuberalis*-specific thyrotrophs and folliculostellate (FS) cells. FS cells share a number of immunological markers with brain glial cells, including GFAP and S100 protein (Inoue et al. 1999). Gonadotrophs (LHβ protein) have been previously reported in the *pars tuberalis* (Gross 1984; Pelletier et al. 1992, 1995); however, expression is localised to the caudal-ventral region, where the border between the *pars tuberalis/ pars distalis* becomes ill defined. In sheep, rats and hamsters in the *pars tuberalis* the only detectable endocrine cell was the *pars tuberalis*-specific thyrotroph (Klosen et al. 2002; Dardente et al. 2003; Wood et al. 2015). The *pars tuberalis*-specific thyrotrophs contain the MT1 receptors (Klosen et al. 2002; Dardente et al. 2003; Johnston et al. 2006).

All glycoprotein hormones comprise a common α subunit (αGSU) and a specific β subunit, (βFSH/βLH/βTSH). In embryological development, αGSU is the first subunit gene expressed in the pituitary (Stoeckel et al. 1993; Akimoto et al. 2010; Inoue et al. 2013). In the main pituitary upon differentiation to specific endocrine cell types, expression of the β subunit is gained in adult endocrine cells. In this context, adult *pars tuberalis*-specific thyrotrophs are unique since they persist as αGSU+ precursors, and only mature into αGSU/TSHβ-expressing thyrotrophs that secrete TSH, when exposed to LP (Hanon et al. 2008; Nakao et al. 2008). The *pars tuberalis*-specific thyrotrophs lack receptors for the hypothalamic thyrotropin-releasing hormone (TRH) (Bockmann et al. 1997), and thus do not respond to conventional hypothalamic outputs. Anatomically, the long portal vessels linking the capillary bed of the median eminence to the *pars tuberalis* run through the parenchyma of the *pars tuberalis*. A sub-set of ventral hypothalamic tanycytes send projections to the *pars tuberalis* (Rodríguez et al. 2005). The *pars tuberalis* is ideally placed both as an integrator of the photoperiodic information for relaying signals to the hypothalamo-pituitary axis, to understand how it does this we need to look at the other hormones involved in the seasonal response, namely thyroid hormone and prolactin.

2.5   Thyroid Hormone and Seasonal Rhythms

Thyroid hormones (TH) are crucial for the expression of seasonal rhythms in multiple vertebrate species, and their role has been extensively reviewed (Hazlerigg and Loudon 2008; Yoshimura 2013; Dardente et al. 2014; Wood and Loudon 2014). This ancient signalling molecule originated before the divergence of the vertebrates from other deuterostome lineages, and has been linked to the control of breeding activity in echinoderms and the primitive chordate *amphioxus* (lancelet) (Heyland et al. 2005). Thyroid hormone comes in two forms, the biological active tri-iodothyronine (T3), and the less active precursor thyroxine (T4).

Thyroidectomy (TX) in starlings (Benoit 1936; Woitkewitsch 1940), Japanese quail (Follett and Nicholls 1985), sheep (Nicholls et al. 1988; Webster et al. 1991a, b), and red deer (Anderson and Barrell 1998) either blocks or dramatically alters the seasonal response of gonads, which in most cases is restored on T4 administration (Billings et al. 2002; Anderson et al. 2003). In rams, thyroidectomy during the nonbreeding season almost immediately reactivates the gonadotropic axis (Parkinson and Follett 1994). Therefore, TH appeared to transmit the message of long photoperiods. Microimplants releasing small amount of TH were then surgically placed within the brain of the ewe (Viguie 1999; Anderson et al. 2003), which revealed that TH acts centrally, and most likely within the medio-basal hypothalamus (MBH), to impact seasonal reproduction. Studies in Siberian hamsters using T3 microimplants showed that other seasonal axes are also controlled by central actions of T3. Infused T3 overrides the SP-induced inactivation of the gonadotropic axis (Barrett et al. 2007), seasonal inappetence, weight loss, and expression of torpor (Murphy et al. 2012). Similar outcomes are found when T3 is provided by daily subcutaneous injections to SP-exposed hamsters (Freeman et al. 2007). In contrast to these effects on reproduction and energy metabolism, T3 implants do not impact the lactotrophic axis (Duncan et al. 1985; Maywood and Hastings 1995). The moult cycle is dependent on the lactotrophic axis, which through anterograde signalling is coordinated via the *pars tuberalis*, but not TH (see prolactin and seasonal rhythms section and Figs. 2.2 and 2.3). Therefore, TH integrates and coordinates some but not all seasonal physiological changes.

Despite the clear importance of TH on the seasonal response, consistent changes in serum or CSF have not been identified [reviewed in Dardente (2012)]. TH metabolism is however precisely and locally regulated in the hypothalamus by the opposing actions of two deiodinase enzymes (Lechan and Fekete 2005). DIO2 converts the inactive T4 to active T3, while DIO3 inactivates T4 by converting to reduced T3 and degrading T3 to T2, with the opposing actions of these enzymes allowing for fine control over the local TH environment (Lechan and Fekete 2005). A key study in quail demonstrated photoperiodic control of the deiodinase enzymes within the tanycytes of the mediobasal hypothalamus (MBH) (Yoshimura et al. 2003). Under LP conditions, DIO2 is strongly expressed leading to a local increase in T3 (Yoshimura et al. 2003). In contrast, on SP, DIO3 is expressed and DIO2 repressed—leading to a reduced drive for conversion of T4 to T3, and greater catabolism of T3. Subsequent studies have revealed photoperiod-dependent regulation of one or both of these deiodinase enzymes in the hypothalamus of sparrows (Watanabe et al. 2007), Siberian hamsters (Watanabe et al. 2004), Syrian hamsters (Revel et al. 2006), sheep (Hanon et al. 2008), European hamster (Hanon et al. 2010), the common vole (Król et al. 2012), Fisher 344 rats (Ross et al. 2011), masu salmon (Nakane et al. 2013) and in the melatonin-proficient non-photoperiodic CBA/N mouse (Nakao et al. 2008). Therefore, local hypothalamic control of the availability of TH is a key regulator of seasonal metabolic and reproductive responses.

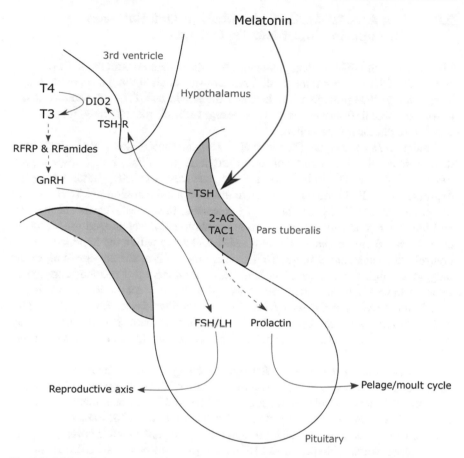

Fig. 2.3 Melatonin is sensed at the *pars tuberalis* via MT1 receptors on the *pars tuberalis* specific thyrotrophs. Under LP, the short-duration nocturnal melatonin signal activates βTSH. *Pars tuberalis*-derived βTSH is translocated back to the hypothalamus where it binds to TSH receptors (TSHR) expressed in tanycyte cells lining the third ventricle. Ligand binding of TSHR regulates the expression of deiodinase seleno-enzymes (Dio2 and Dio3), which, in turn, controls the local metabolism of thyroid hormone. RF-related peptides such KISS-1 serve as neuroendocrine intermediates in the regulation of reproduction across taxa, and their regulation is altered in response to photoperiod. RFRP subsequently acts either directly on GnRH neurons or indirectly via kisspeptin neurons or other interneurons in the arcuate nucleus (ARC) to synchronise reproduction with season in a species-dependent manner. Anterograde action is believed to control seasonal prolactin secretion from lactotrophic cells in the *pars distalis* , which, (PD) in turn, drives the pelage/moult cycle. The pathway is stimulated through secretion of low-molecular-weight molecules ('tuberalins') produced in the *pars tuberalis* and transported to the *pars distalis* through the portal blood system. Several tuberalin candidates have been proposed, including tachykinins (TAC1) and endocannabinoids (2-AG). Adapted from West and Wood (2018)

2.6   The *Pars Tuberalis* as the Missing Link Between Photoperiod Input and TH Output

The induction of DIO2 by long photoperiods is dependent on both the MT1 receptor and on the TSH receptor (Ono et al. 2008; Unfried et al. 2009; Yasuo et al. 2009). These studies thus provide a link between melatonin and TH, and, indicate that a retrograde signal from the MT1 expressing cells of the PT may mediate the deiodinase photoperiodic switch.

Studies in Japanese quail (Nakao et al. 2008) and sheep (Hanon et al. 2008) have demonstrated the importance of the retrograde signalling link between *pars tuberalis*-TSH and TH. In both species, the *pars tuberalis*-TSHβ subunit is highly expressed on LP. Using intracerebroventricular administration of TSH, it was demonstrated that TSH promotes Dio2 expression, in a cAMP-dependent manner, and initiates reproductive activation in short-photoperiod-suppressed birds (Nakao et al. 2008). Therefore, *pars tuberalis*-TSH acts locally within the hypothalamus to control DIO transcription through TSH-receptor-cAMP-mediated signalling in the tanycytes lining the 3rd ventricle (Fig. 2.3). Photoperiod-dependent changes in hypothalamic TH metabolism drive seasonal changes in physiology, and this in turn is regulated from the *pars tuberalis* through altered secretion of TSH. This TSH/DIO *pars tuberalis* /hypothalamic switch is now recognised as being highly conserved between birds, mammals and masu salmon (Nakane and Yoshimura 2014).

To summarise, *pars tuberalis*-TSH signals to hypothalamic tanycytes, which, in turn, modulate the seasonal biological availability of thyroid hormone (T3). Hypothalamic T3 status controls central structures involved in seasonal metabolic physiology and reproduction (Murphy et al. 2012; Klosen et al. 2013; Bank et al. 2017). Reproductive effects are mediated through alterations in the GnRH pulse generator, potentially involving kisspeptin and RFamides (Simonneaux et al. 2013; Hazlerigg and Simonneaux 2015; Beymer et al. 2016) (Fig. 2.3). Regardless of the animals breeding season LP has the same effects on TH; therefore, the mechanisms downstream of altered TH are likely to be where the reproductive switch occurs.

Collectively, these studies provide a model for the seasonal regulation of deiodinase enzyme expression, involving a 'retrograde' action of TSH from the *pars tuberalis* on receptor fields in the ependymal tanycytes, driving local TH metabolism in the hypothalamus (Fig. 2.3). However, this does not provide an explanation of how the melatonin signal effects TSH expression.

2.7   Circadian Circuits Driving the Response to Melatonin in the *Pars Tuberalis*

The photoperiodic response implies that an organism has the capacity to discriminate either the length of light or nocturnal phase, or both. Classical ground-breaking studies by Bünning (Bünning 1936) developed the concept that photoperiodic species might use the endogenous timing system of the daily circadian clockwork.

Here, both a light-requiring phase (photophil) of approximately 12 h, and a dark-requiring phase (scotophil) of approximately 12 h combine to a 24-h period (Bünning 1936). If light is experienced in the scotophil, then an LP response is triggered (external co-incidence). A variant of this hypothesis was proposed by Pittendrigh and colleagues (the internal co-incident timing model), in which light's only role is to entrain a multi-oscillator circadian system, with the phase of the dawn and dusk oscillators set by the length of the photoperiod (Pittendrigh and Minis 1964). Each of the oscillators will behave in a different manner, depending on the light–dark cycle and assume different phase-relationships with the entraining cycle. Changes in the 'internal' co-incidence of these oscillators would then determine the photoperiodic response. The Bünning external co-incidence hypothesis and the later model of Pittendrigh are now widely accepted as the basis for photoperiodic time measurement in birds and mammals (reviewed in: Wood and Loudon 2014).

The current model of photoperiodic entrainment focuses on the TH axis, and emphasises that changes in melatonin signal are transduced by a circadian-based 'coincidence timer' in the *pars tuberalis*. It is now known that the photoperiodic control of TSH production depends on up-regulation of TSHβ subunit expression by the transcriptional co-activator, EYA3 on long photoperiods (Dardente et al. 2010; Masumoto et al. 2010). It is proposed that the 'coincidence timer' uses the duration of melatonin signal to dictate the amplitude of expression of EYA3, which co-activates TSHβ (Dardente et al. 2010) (Fig. 2.4a). Short melatonin signals (in long photoperiods) generate large-amplitude EYA3 signals in the *pars tuberalis*, whereas long melatonin signals (in short photoperiods) suppress EYA3 oscillations. In both cases, the oscillation of EYA3 occurs approximately 12 h after dark-onset, which on LP is co-incident with light, but on SP coincides with the dark phase, and continued melatonin secretion.

EYA3 has been proposed as a key up-stream circadian-regulated component driving seasonal responses (Dardente et al. 2010; Dardente 2012). Promoter analysis and promoter-driven expression plasmids for ovine EYA3 demonstrated that the circadian transcription factors CLOCK and BMAL1 activate EYA3 transcription through E-box binding (Dardente et al. 2010). Thus, it is proposed that melatonin drives a local *pars tuberalis* slave oscillator by activating CRY1, which is phased to the dark onset/melatonin rise, allowing a CLOCK/BMAL1 drive approximately 12 h later (Dardente et al. 2010, 2014) (Fig. 2.4b). However, under SP conditions, persistent melatonin secretion of 12 or more hours in duration is proposed to repress target genes such as EYA3, through E-box or cAMP suppression. In contrast, on LPs, short-duration melatonin signals result in a de-inhibition of the suppressive effects of melatonin, which may be mediated by an LP-specific rise in cAMP at dawn (Hazlerigg and Loudon 2008) and subsequent CREB site activation. Several features of this model remain to be tested. For instance, although a role for melatonin inhibition of cAMP and CREB site activation has been demonstrated in vitro in *pars tuberalis*-thyrotrophs (Hazlerigg et al. 1993), a specific effect on EYA3 remains to be demonstrated, and it remains unclear what mechanisms may be involved in suppressing E-box activation in the dark phase in SP conditions; to date, no candidates or mechanisms have been identified. Also, studies on reindeer challenge

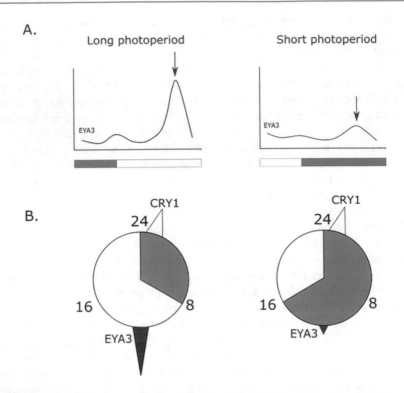

Fig. 2.4 (**a**) Representative schematics of the induction of EYA3 on transfer to LP. Sheep were acclimated to 8 h light/day and transferred to 16 h light/day (LP) by acutely delaying lights off. Tissue was collected at 4-h intervals throughout 24 h on SP and LP. The black horizontal bar in each graph indicates when lights were off during each sampling period. The red arrow indicates the time-point 12 h after dark onset. Adapted from West and Wood (2018). (**b**) Schematic representation of EYA3 transcription and the phase-relationship relative to Cry1 expression (a melatonin-induced circadian gene). This exemplifies clock control and inhibition by melatonin as the key factors in controlling the co-incidence of EYA3 with light. Black region represents darkness. Adapted from Dardente et al. (2014)

the assumption that circadian rhythmicity is important for seasonal rhythms because exposure to both constant illumination and constant darkness blocks circadian activity in reindeer, but they still progress through their seasonal life history (Hazlerigg, Blix and Stokkan 2017). Furthermore, circannual rhythms are seen in EYA3 (as well as TSH and DIO) (Sáenz de Miera et al. 2013, 2014; Wood et al. 2015), but not at the level of the circadian clock, which in the *pars tuberalis* continues to reflect the prevailing photoperiod (Lincoln et al. 2002, 2005). Understanding the role of the circadian clock in seasonal rhythms is not straightforward when considering endogenous rhythms and arctic species. It has been suggested that the 'generation of long-term cycles depends on the interaction between a circadian-based, melatonin-dependent timer that drives the initial photoperiodic response and a non-circadian-based timer that drives circannual rhythmicity in long-lived species'

(Lincoln et al. 2005), disentangling the photoperiodic response from a circannual process is the major challenge to overcome in the field.

2.8   Prolactin and Seasonal Rhythms

There is a TH-independent anterograde pathway from the *pars tuberalis* to the anterior pituitary gland (*pars distalis*: PD) controlling seasonal changes in pelage (coat colour and moult) (Lincoln and Clarke 1994; Dardente et al. 2014). The first clear demonstration of this anterograde pathway came from studies of the effects of surgical disconnection of the pituitary from the hypothalamus (hypothalamic-pituitary disconnection: HPD) in sheep. This removes the hypothalamic drive from GnRH neurons to gonadotrophs, thus inducing a hypogonadal state (Lincoln and Clarke 1994). However, seasonal rhythms in prolactin secretion that control seasonal changes in pelage in birds and mammals (Curlewis 1992) remain photoperiodic in animals where the pituitary has been surgically disconnected (Lincoln and Clarke 1994). Moreover, HPD sheep continue to exhibit circannual rhythmicity in prolactin secretion (Lincoln et al. 2006). Co-culture experiments of *pars tuberalis* cells and *pars distalis* lactotrophs from sheep revealed that the presence of *pars tuberalis* cells stimulated the production of prolactin from lactotrophs, suggesting that *pars tuberalis* cells produced an unknown prolactin-releasing factor that was then named 'tuberalin' (Morgan and Williams 1996; Morgan et al. 1996), an observation later confirmed in hamsters (Stirland et al. 2001). A hypothetical model was then proposed for tuberalin regulation of prolactin production via melatonin (Morgan and Williams 1996), based on the observed inhibitory effects of melatonin on cAMP production in pituitary cell cultures stimulated by forskolin treatment (Hazlerigg et al. 1993). Melatonin is proposed to inhibit cAMP production, which, in turn, reduces gene activation via CREB response elements (CREs) in the *pars tuberalis*. For this model to be relevant in vivo, it requires an endogenous stimulator of cAMP to be identified, which the authors termed "stim X" (Morgan and Williams 1996). Therefore, the balance between melatonin-mediated inhibition and 'stim x' activation was proposed to control tuberalin expression and subsequently prolactin secretion.

The cell-signalling mechanisms used to interpret the change in seasonal melatonin signal duration are still unclear. Melatonin onset not only acts as an inhibitor but also stimulates the expression of a range of genes in the *pars tuberalis*, which further complicates the model (Dupré et al. 2008; Fustin et al. 2009; Unfried et al. 2009; West et al. 2013). The identity of 'stim x' is still unknown, it is assumed it must be a stimulator of cAMP, and must be expressed in the PT, where the melatonin signal is received.

The identity of the secreted factor 'tuberalin', hypothesised to be regulated by 'stim x' and melatonin, has been sought by a number of groups. In sheep, the tachykinin 1 (TAC1) and neurokinin A (NKA) peptides emerged as candidates (Dupré et al. 2010), while other researchers have identified endocannabinoids (Yasuo and Korf 2011; Korf 2018) (Fig. 2.3). Specifically, 2-arachidonoylglycerol

(2-AG) emerged as a component of the endocannabinoid system produced in the PT that has the potential to increase prolactin release in the presence of adenosine or forskolin in Syrian hamsters (Yasuo et al. 2014). A striking feature of both NKA and 2-AG is that they are likely to act on folliculostellate (FS) cells in the pituitary gland. FS cells express the appropriate receptors (Dupré et al. 2010; Yasuo and Korf 2011), so may act as important neuroendocrine transducers in seasonal control (Wood and Loudon 2017). Since there are over 30 factors that can stimulate prolactin secretion (Freeman et al. 2000), the identification of specific factors from the *pars tuberalis* regulating prolactin secretion remains a challenge.

2.9   Evolutionary Conservation in the Photoperiodic Response and Anatomical Structures

The *pars tuberalis* is the regulatory hub for seasonal reproduction in birds and mammals and the TSH/DIO switch is highly conserved amongst vertebrates (Nakane and Yoshimura 2014; West and Wood 2018). However, the input systems vary, and in birds and fish can be melatonin independent (Fig. 2.5). The *pars tuberalis* is a common feature of all tetrapods, evidenced in stem-tetrapod fossils (Lu et al. 2012), but to date the role of the hypothalamic-pituitary-thyroid axis in photoperiodic control of reproduction in reptiles or amphibians in unknown. Fish have no *pars tuberalis*; however, LP induction of Dio2 has been observed in the *saccus vasculosus* (SV) of the masu salmon (Nakane et al. 2013). The SV is a highly vascularised fish-specific organ located on the floor of the hypothalamus and posterior to the pituitary gland (Maeda et al. 2015). Specialised coronet cells of the SV co-express Dio2, TSHβ and a suite of rhodopsins. Isolated SVs respond to changing photoperiod in vitro, and, its surgical removal results in testicular growth. However, SVs are not evident in all teleosts, and this structure is absent from known photoperiodic species (O'Brien et al. 2012; Dardente et al. 2014). Also photoperiodic induction of Dio2 is not restricted to the SV, it is strongly induced in the optic tectum of the Atlantic salmon (Lorgen et al. 2015). The optic tectum also contains melatonin receptors and non-visual opsins, suggesting that photoperiodic control of thyroid hormone metabolism may be more decentralised and tissue-intrinsic in fish than higher vertebrates (Fig. 2.5). The drive to evolve a centralised system of seasonal physiological control may be related to the greater energetic demands of endothermy placed on organisms, requiring greater control and coordination.

Despite the strong focus on the *pars tuberalis* in this chapter, it is clear that the tanycytes lining the third ventricle of the hypothalamus require close consideration. There are maternal photoperiodic history effects programmed in the tanycytes of the 3rd ventricle that alter the offspring's sensitivity to photoperiodic signals, through changes in sensitivity to *pars tuberalis*-derived TSH in the tanycytes (Sáenz de Miera et al. 2017). Long-term control of energy balance is essential in seasonal mammals, and hypothalamic tanycytes are nutrient sensors and regulate the transport of hormones and metabolites into the hypothalamus (Lewis and Ebling 2017), and

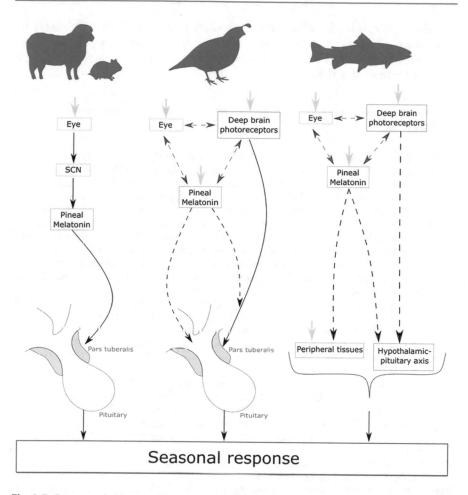

Fig. 2.5 In mammals (sheep and hamster exemplified here), light (yellow arrow) enters the eye and the photic input pathway from the retina to the SCN drives rhythmic melatonin production from the pineal gland and this melatonin signal is sculpted by photoperiod to provide an internal endocrine representation for external photoperiod. Melatonin is received by the *pars tuberalis*-specific thyrotroph, which has melatonin receptor 1, and drives seasonal outputs as described in the text and Fig. 2.2. In birds (exemplified by the Japanese quail), light is received by the eye and deep-brain photoreceptors (rhodopsin, melanopsin, VA-opsin, Opsin 5), currently OPN5 is the best characterised and contacts the paraventricular organ and the *pars tuberalis*, driving seasonal reproduction from the *pars tuberalis* using the same pathways as mammals. There is also a role for melatonin in the regulation of seasonal outputs. In fish, the neuroendocrine regulation of seasonal outputs is least well characterised and appears to have a decentralised system, with light reception by opsins in the pineal, deep-brain photoreceptors and directly in peripheral tissues. It is known that melatonin plays a role and that these outputs are coordinated through the hypothalamic pituitary axis but that the classic changes in thyroid hormone metabolism may be more decentralised and tissue-intrinsic in fish than higher vertebrates. Adapted from West and Wood (2018)

are also highly active in hibernators (Bratincsák et al. 2007). This highlights the importance of tanycytes as integrators of other environmental signals, and that a close consideration of *pars tuberalis*—tanycyte crosstalk in seasonal timekeeping in birds and mammals is required.

References

Akimoto M et al (2010) Hes1 regulates formations of the hypophyseal pars tuberalis and the hypothalamus. Cell Tissue Res 340(3):509–521. https://doi.org/10.1007/s00441-010-0951-2

Anderson GM, Barrell GK (1998) Pulsatile luteinizing hormone secretion in the ovariectomized, thyroidectomized red deer hind following treatment with dopaminergic and opioidergic agonists and antagonists. Biol Reprod 59(4):960–968. http://www.ncbi.nlm.nih.gov/pubmed/9746749

Anderson G et al (2003) Evidence that thyroid hormones act in the ventromedial preoptic area and the premammillary region of the brain to allow the termination of the breeding season in the ewe. Endocrinology 144(7):2892–2901. https://doi.org/10.1210/en.2003-0322

Bank JHH et al (2017) Gene expression analysis and microdialysis suggest hypothalamic triiodo-thyronine (T3) gates daily torpor in Djungarian hamsters (*Phodopus sungorus*). J Comp Physiol B 187(5–6):857–868. https://doi.org/10.1007/s00360-017-1086-5

Barrett P et al (2006) Photoperiodic regulation of cellular retinoic acid-binding protein 1, GPR50 and nestin in tanycytes of the third ventricle ependymal layer of the Siberian hamster. J Endocrinol 191(3):687–698. https://doi.org/10.1677/joe.1.06929

Barrett P et al (2007) Hypothalamic thyroid hormone catabolism acts as a gatekeeper for the seasonal control of body weight and reproduction. Endocrinology 148(8):3608–3617. https://doi.org/10.1210/en.2007-0316

Bartness TJ et al (1993) The timed infusion paradigm for melatonin delivery: what has it taught us about the melatonin signal, its reception, and the photoperiodic control of seasonal responses? J Pineal Res 15(4):161–190. http://www.ncbi.nlm.nih.gov/pubmed/8120796

Bechtold DA et al (2012) A role for the melatonin-related receptor GPR50 in leptin signaling, adaptive thermogenesis, and torpor. Curr Biol 22(1):70–77. https://doi.org/10.1016/j.cub.2011.11.043

Benoit J (1936) Role de la thyroide dans la gonado-stimulation par lumiere artificielle chez le canard domestique. C R Soc Biol 123:243–246

Beymer M et al (2016) The role of kisspeptin and RFRP in the circadian control of female reproduction. Mol Cell Endocrinol 438:89–99. https://doi.org/10.1016/j.mce.2016.06.026

Billings HJ et al (2002) Temporal requirements of thyroid hormones for seasonal changes in LH secretion. Endocrinology 143(7):2618–2625. https://doi.org/10.1210/endo.143.7.8924

Bittman EL, Dempsey RJ, Karsch FJ (1983) Pineal melatonin secretion drives the reproductive response to daylength in the ewe. Endocrinology 113(6):2276–2283. https://doi.org/10.1210/endo-113-6-2276

Bockmann J et al (1997) Thyrotropin expression in hypophyseal pars tuberalis-specific cells is 3,5,3'-triiodothyronine, thyrotropin-releasing hormone, and pit-1 independent. Endocrinology 138(3):1019–1028. https://doi.org/10.1210/endo.138.3.5007

Bratincsák A et al (2007) Spatial and temporal activation of brain regions in hibernation: c-fos expression during the hibernation bout in thirteen-lined ground squirrel. J Comp Neurol 505 (4):443–458. https://doi.org/10.1002/cne.21507

Brinklow BR, Loudon AS (1993) Evidence for a circannual rhythm of reproduction and prolactin secretion in a seasonally breeding macropodid marsupial, the Bennett's wallaby (Macropus rufogriseus rufogriseus). J Reprod Fertil 98(2):625–630. http://www.ncbi.nlm.nih.gov/pubmed/8410834

Bünning E (1936) Die endogene Tagesperiodik als Grundlage der photoperiodischen Reaktion. Ber Dtsch Bot Ges 54:590–608

Butler MP et al (2010) Seasonal regulation of reproduction: altered role of melatonin under naturalistic conditions in hamsters. Proc Biol Sci 277(1695):2867–2874. https://doi.org/10.1098/rspb.2010.0396

Carter DS, Goldman BD (1983) Antigonadal effects of timed melatonin infusion in pinealectomized male Djungarian hamsters (Phodopus sungorus sungorus): duration is the critical parameter. Endocrinology 113(4):1261–1267. https://doi.org/10.1210/endo-113-4-1261

Curlewis JD (1992) Seasonal prolactin secretion and its role in seasonal reproduction: a review. Reprod Fertil Dev 4(1):1–23. http://www.ncbi.nlm.nih.gov/pubmed/1585003

Dardente H (2012) Melatonin-dependent timing of seasonal reproduction by the pars tuberalis: pivotal roles for long daylengths and thyroid hormones. J Neuroendocrinol 24(2):249–266. https://doi.org/10.1111/j.1365-2826.2011.02250.x

Dardente H et al (2003) MT1 melatonin receptor mRNA expressing cells in the pars tuberalis of the European hamster: effect of photoperiod. J Neuroendocrinol 15(8):778–786. http://www.ncbi.nlm.nih.gov/pubmed/12834439

Dardente H et al (2010) A molecular switch for photoperiod responsiveness in mammals. Curr Biol 20(24):2193–2198. https://doi.org/10.1016/j.cub.2010.10.048

Dardente H, Hazlerigg DG, Ebling FJP (2014) Thyroid hormone and seasonal rhythmicity. Front Endocrinol 5:19. https://doi.org/10.3389/fendo.2014.00019

Dawson A (2015) Annual gonadal cycles in birds: modeling the effects of photoperiod on seasonal changes in GnRH-1 secretion. Front Neuroendocrinol 37:52–64. https://doi.org/10.1016/j.yfrne.2014.08.004

Dufourny L et al (2008) GPR50 is the mammalian ortholog of Mel1c: evidence of rapid evolution in mammals. BMC Evol Biol 8(1):105. https://doi.org/10.1186/1471-2148-8-105

Duncan MJ et al (1985) Testicular function and pelage color have different critical daylengths in the djungarian hamster, Phodopus sungorus sungorus. Endocrinology 116(1):424–430. https://doi.org/10.1210/endo-116-1-424

Dupré SM et al (2008) Identification of melatonin-regulated genes in the ovine pituitary pars tuberalis, a target site for seasonal hormone control. Endocrinology 149(11):5527–5539. https://doi.org/10.1210/en.2008-0834

Dupré SM et al (2010) Identification of Eya3 and TAC1 as long-day signals in the sheep pituitary. Curr Biol 20(9):829–835. https://doi.org/10.1016/j.cub.2010.02.066

Duston J, Bromage N (1991) Circannual rhythms of gonadal maturation in female rainbow trout (Oncorhynchus mykiss). J Biol Rhythm 6(1):49–53. https://doi.org/10.1177/074873049100600106

Falcón J et al (2010) Current knowledge on the melatonin system in teleost fish. Gen Comp Endocrinol 165(3):469–482. https://doi.org/10.1016/j.ygcen.2009.04.026

Follett BK, Nicholls TJ (1985) Influences of thyroidectomy and thyroxine replacement on photoperiodically controlled reproduction in quail. J Endocrinol 107(2):211–221. http://www.ncbi.nlm.nih.gov/pubmed/4067480

Frantzen M et al (2004) Effects of photoperiod on sex steroids and gonad maturation in Arctic charr. Aquaculture 240(1–4):561–574. https://doi.org/10.1016/j.aquaculture.2004.07.013

Freeman ME et al (2000) Prolactin: structure, function, and regulation of secretion. Physiol Rev 80 (4):1523–1631. https://doi.org/10.1152/physrev.2000.80.4.1523

Fustin JM et al (2009) Egr1 involvement in evening gene regulation by melatonin. FASEB J 23 (3):764–773. https://doi.org/10.1096/fj.08-121467

Goldman BD (2001) Mammalian photoperiodic system: formal properties and neuroendocrine mechanisms of photoperiodic time measurement. J Biol Rhythm 16(4): 283–301. http://www.ncbi.nlm.nih.gov/pubmed/11506375

Gross DS (1984) The mammalian hypophysial pars tuberalis: a comparative immunocytochemical study. Gen Comp Endocrinol 56(2):283–298. http://www.ncbi.nlm.nih.gov/pubmed/6510690. Accessed 27 Oct 2014

Gwinner E (1986) Circannual rhythms. Springer, Berlin

Hanon EA et al (2008) Ancestral TSH mechanism signals summer in a photoperiodic mammal. Curr Biol 18(15):1147–1152. https://doi.org/10.1016/j.cub.2008.06.076

Hanon EA et al (2010) Effect of photoperiod on the thyroid-stimulating hormone neuroendocrine system in the European hamster (Cricetus cricetus). J Neuroendocrinol 22(1):51–55. https://doi.org/10.1111/j.1365-2826.2009.01937.x

Hazlerigg D, Loudon A (2008) New insights into ancient seasonal life timers. Curr Biol 18(17): R795–R804. https://doi.org/10.1016/j.cub.2008.07.040

Hazlerigg D, Simonneaux V (2015) Seasonal reproduction in mammals. In: Plant T, Zeleznic A (eds) Knobil and Neill's physiology and reproduction, 4th edn. Academic Press, London, pp 1575–1660

Hazlerigg DG et al (1993) Prolonged exposure to melatonin leads to time-dependent sensitization of adenylate cyclase and down-regulates melatonin receptors in pars tuberalis cells from ovine pituitary. Endocrinology 132(1):285–292. https://doi.org/10.1210/endo.132.1.7678217

Hazlerigg D, Blix AS, Stokkan K-A (2017) Waiting for the sun: the circannual program of reindeer is delayed by the recurrence of rhythmical melatonin secretion after the arctic night. J Exp Biol 220(Pt 21):jeb.163741. https://doi.org/10.1242/jeb.163741

Heyland A, Hodin J, Reitzel AM (2005) Hormone signaling in evolution and development: a non-model system approach. BioEssays 27(1):64–75. https://doi.org/10.1002/bies.20136

Hoffman RA, Reiter RJ (1965) Pineal gland: influence on gonads of male hamsters. Science (New York, NY) 148(3677):1609–1611.http://www.ncbi.nlm.nih.gov/pubmed/14287606

Inoue K et al (1999) The structure and function of folliculo-stellate cells in the anterior pituitary gland. Arch Histol Cytol 62(3):205–218. http://www.ncbi.nlm.nih.gov/pubmed/10495875

Inoue M et al (2013) Detailed morphogenetic analysis of the embryonic chicken pars tuberalis as glycoprotein alpha subunit positive region. J Mol Hist 44(4):401–409. https://doi.org/10.1007/s10735-012-9479-y

Ivanova EA et al (2008) Altered metabolism in the melatonin-related receptor (GPR50) knockout mouse. Am J Physiol Endocrinol Metab 294(1). http://ajpendo.physiology.org/content/294/1/E176

Johnston JD et al (2006) Regulation of MT melatonin receptor expression in the foetal rat pituitary. J Neuroendocrinol 18(1):50–56. https://doi.org/10.1111/j.1365-2826.2005.01389.x

Kameda Y, Miura M, Maruyama S (2002) Effect of pinealectomy on the photoperiod-dependent changes of the specific secretory cells and à-subunit mRNA level in the chicken pars tuberalis. Cell Tissue Res 308(1):121–130. https://doi.org/10.1007/s00441-002-0537-8

Klosen P et al (2002) The mt1 melatonin receptor and RORbeta receptor are co-localized in specific TSH-immunoreactive cells in the pars tuberalis of the rat pituitary. J Histochem Cytochem 50 (12):1647–1657. http://www.ncbi.nlm.nih.gov/pubmed/12486087

Klosen P et al (2013) TSH restores a summer phenotype in photoinhibited mammals via the RF-amides RFRP3 and kisspeptin. FASEB J 27(7):2677–2686. https://doi.org/10.1096/fj.13-229559

Korf H-W (2018) Signaling pathways to and from the hypophysial pars tuberalis, an important center for the control of seasonal rhythms. Gen Comp Endocrinol 258:236–243. https://doi.org/10.1016/j.ygcen.2017.05.011

Król E et al (2012) Strong pituitary and hypothalamic responses to photoperiod but not to 6-methoxy-2-benzoxazolinone in female common voles (Microtus arvalis). Gen Comp Endocrinol 179(2):289–295. https://doi.org/10.1016/j.ygcen.2012.09.004

Lechan RM, Fekete C (2005) Role of thyroid hormone deiodination in the hypothalamus. Thyroid 15(8):883–897. https://doi.org/10.1089/thy.2005.15.883

Lewis JE, Ebling FJP (2017) tanycytes as regulators of seasonal cycles in neuroendocrine function. Front Neurol 8:79. https://doi.org/10.3389/fneur.2017.00079

Lincoln GA (2006) Melatonin entrainment of circannual rhythms. Chronobiol Int 23 (1–2):301–306. https://doi.org/10.1080/07420520500464452

Lincoln GA, Clarke IJ (1994) Photoperiodically-Induced cycles in the secretion of prolactin in hypothalamo-pituitary disconnected rams: evidence for translation of the melatonin signal in the pituitary gland. J Neuroendocrinol 6(3):251–260. https://doi.org/10.1111/j.1365-2826.1994. tb00580.x

Lincoln G et al (2002) Temporal expression of seven clock genes in the suprachiasmatic nucleus and the pars tuberalis of the sheep: evidence for an internal coincidence timer. Proc Natl Acad Sci U S A 99(21):13890–13895. https://doi.org/10.1073/pnas.212517599

Lincoln GA et al (2005) Photorefractoriness in mammals: dissociating a seasonal timer from the circadian-based photoperiod response. Endocrinology 146(9):3782–3790. https://doi.org/10. 1210/en.2005-0132

Lincoln GA et al (2006) Characterizing a mammalian circannual pacemaker. Science (New York, NY) 314(5807):1941–1944. https://doi.org/10.1126/science.1132009

Lorgen M et al (2015) Functional divergence of type 2 deiodinase paralogs in the Atlantic salmon. Curr Biol 25(7):936–941. https://doi.org/10.1016/j.cub.2015.01.074

Lu J et al (2012) The earliest known stem-tetrapod from the Lower Devonian of China. Nat Commun 3:1160–1167. https://doi.org/10.1038/ncomms2170

Maeda R et al (2015) Ontogeny of the saccus vasculosus, a seasonal sensor in fish. Endocrinology 156(11):4238–4243. https://doi.org/10.1210/en.2015-1415

Masumoto K et al (2010) Acute induction of eya3 by late-night light stimulation triggers TSHβ expression in photoperiodism. Curr Biol 20(24):2199–2206. https://doi.org/10.1016/j.cub.2010. 11.038

Maywood ES, Hastings MH (1995) Lesions of the iodomelatonin-binding sites of the mediobasal hypothalamus spare the lactotropic, but block the gonadotropic response of male Syrian hamsters to short photoperiod and to melatonin. Endocrinology 136(1):144–153. https://doi. org/10.1210/en.136.1.144

Meijer JH et al (1999) Functional absence of extraocular photoreception in hamster circadian rhythm entrainment. Brain Res 831(1–2):337–339. http://www.ncbi.nlm.nih.gov/pubmed/ 10412017

Migaud H, Davie A, Taylor JF (2010) Current knowledge on the photoneuroendocrine regulation of reproduction in temperate fish species. J Fish Biol 76(1):27–68. https://doi.org/10.1111/j.1095-8649.2009.02500.x

Morgan PJ, Williams LM (1996) The pars tuberalis of the pituitary: a gateway for neuroendocrine output. Rev Reprod 1(3):153–161. http://www.ncbi.nlm.nih.gov/pubmed/9414453

Morgan PJ et al (1994) Melatonin receptors: localization, molecular pharmacology and physiological significance. Neurochem Int 24(2):101–146. http://www.ncbi.nlm.nih.gov/pubmed/ 8161940. Accessed 19 Feb 2014

Morgan PJ et al (1996) The ovine pars tuberalis secretes a factor(s) that regulates gene expression in both lactotropic and nonlactotropic pituitary cells. Endocrinology 137(9):4018–4026. https:// doi.org/10.1210/endo.137.9.8756579

Murphy M et al (2012) Effects of manipulating hypothalamic triiodothyronine concentrations on seasonal body weight and torpor cycles in Siberian hamsters. Endocrinology 153(1):101–112. https://doi.org/10.1210/en.2011-1249

Nakane Y, Yoshimura T (2010) Deep brain photoreceptors and a seasonal signal transduction cascade in birds. Cell Tissue Res 342(3):341–344. https://doi.org/10.1007/s00441-010-1073-6

Nakane Y, Yoshimura T (2014) Universality and diversity in the signal transduction pathway that regulates seasonal reproduction in vertebrates. Front Neurosci 8:115. https://doi.org/10.3389/ fnins.2014.00115

Nakane Y et al (2010) A mammalian neural tissue opsin (Opsin 5) is a deep brain photoreceptor in birds. Proc Natl Acad Sci 107(34):15264–15268. https://doi.org/10.1073/pnas.1006393107

Nakane Y et al (2013) The saccus vasculosus of fish is a sensor of seasonal changes in day length. Nat Commun 4:2108. https://doi.org/10.1038/ncomms3108

Nakao N et al (2008) Thyrotrophin in the pars tuberalis triggers photoperiodic response. Nature 452 (7185):317–322. https://doi.org/10.1038/nature06738

Nelson RJ, Zucker I (1981) Photoperiodic control of reproduction in olfactory-bulbectomized rats. Neuroendocrinology 32(5):266–271. http://www.ncbi.nlm.nih.gov/pubmed/7242854

Nicholls TJ et al (1988) Possible homologies between photorefractoriness in sheep and birds: the effect of thyroidectomy on the length of the ewe's breeding season. Reprod Nutr Dev 28 (2B):375–385. http://www.ncbi.nlm.nih.gov/pubmed/3413338

O'Brien CS et al (2012) Conservation of the photoperiodic neuroendocrine axis among vertebrates: evidence from the teleost fish, *Gasterosteus aculeatus*. Gen Comp Endocrinol 178(1):19–27. https://doi.org/10.1016/j.ygcen.2012.03.010

Ono H et al (2008) Involvement of thyrotropin in photoperiodic signal transduction in mice. Proc Natl Acad Sci U S A 105(47):18238–18242. https://doi.org/10.1073/pnas.0808952105

Parkinson TJ, Follett BK (1994) Effect of thyroidectomy upon seasonality in rams. Reproduction 101(1):51–58. https://doi.org/10.1530/jrf.0.1010051

Pelletier J et al (1992) Localization of luteinizing hormone beta-mRNA by in situ hybridization in the sheep pars tuberalis. Cell Tissue Res 267(2):301–306.http://www.ncbi.nlm.nih.gov/pubmed/1600562

Pelletier J et al (1995) Changes in LHbeta-gene and FSHbeta-gene expression in the ram pars tuberalis according to season and castration. Cell Tissue Res 281(1):127–133. http://www.ncbi.nlm.nih.gov/pubmed/16358468

Pittendrigh CS, Minis DH (1964) The entrainment of circadian oscillations by light and their role as photoperiodic clocks. Am Nat 98:261–299

Reierth E, Van't Hof TJ, Stokkan K-A (1999) Seasonal and daily variations in plasma melatonin in the high-arctic svalbard ptarmigan (*Lagopus mutus hyperboreus*). J Biol Rhythm 14 (4):314–319. https://doi.org/10.1177/074873099129000731

Reiter RJ (1980) Photoperiod: its importance as an impeller of pineal and seasonal reproductive rhythms. Int J Biometeorol 24(1):57–63.http://www.ncbi.nlm.nih.gov/pubmed/7189183

Reppert SM (1997) Melatonin receptors: molecular biology of a new family of G protein-coupled receptors. J Biol Rhyth 12(6):528–31. http://www.ncbi.nlm.nih.gov/pubmed/9406026

Reppert SM et al (1996a) Cloning of a melatonin-related receptor from human pituitary. FEBS Lett 386(2–3):219–224. http://www.ncbi.nlm.nih.gov/pubmed/8647286

Reppert SM, Weaver DR, Godson C (1996b) Melatonin receptors step into the light: cloning and classification of subtypes. Trends Pharmacol Sci 17(3):100–102. https://doi.org/10.1016/0165-6147(96)10005-5

Revel FG et al (2006) Melatonin regulates type 2 deiodinase gene expression in the Syrian hamster. Endocrinology 147(10):4680–4687. https://doi.org/10.1210/en.2006-0606

Richter CP (1978) Evidence for existence of a yearly clock in surgically and self-blinded chipmunks. Proc Natl Acad Sci 75(7):3517–3521. https://doi.org/10.1073/pnas.75.7.3517

Rodríguez EM et al (2005) Hypothalamic tanycytes: a key component of brain-endocrine interaction. Int Rev Cytol 247:89–164. https://doi.org/10.1016/S0074-7696(05)47003-5

Ross AW et al (2011) Thyroid hormone signalling genes are regulated by photoperiod in the hypothalamus of F344 rats. In: Yamazaki S (ed) PLoS One 6(6):e21351. https://doi.org/10.1371/journal.pone.0021351

Sáenz de Miera C et al (2013) Circannual variation in thyroid hormone deiodinases in a short-day breeder. J Neuroendocrinol 25(4):412–421. https://doi.org/10.1111/jne.12013

Sáenz de Miera C et al (2014) A circannual clock drives expression of genes central for seasonal reproduction. Curr Biol 24(13):1500–1506. https://doi.org/10.1016/j.cub.2014.05.024

Sáenz de Miera C et al (2017) Maternal photoperiod programs hypothalamic thyroid status via the fetal pituitary gland. Proc Natl Acad Sci 114(31):8408–8413. https://doi.org/10.1073/pnas.1702943114

Simonneaux V et al (2013) Kisspeptins and RFRP-3 act in concert to synchronize rodent reproduction with seasons. Front Neurosci 7:22. https://doi.org/10.3389/fnins.2013.00022

Stirland JA et al (2001) Photoperiodic regulation of prolactin gene expression in the Syrian hamster by a pars tuberalis-derived factor. J Neuroendocrinol 13(2):147–157. http://www.ncbi.nlm.nih.gov/pubmed/11168840

Stoeckel E et al (1993) Early expression of the glycoprotein hormone alpha-subunit in the pars tuberalis of the rat pituitary gland during ontogenesis. Neuroendocrinology 58(6):616–624. https://doi.org/10.1159/000126600

Stokkan K-A, Tyler NJC, Reiter RJ (1994) The pineal gland signals autumn to reindeer (*Rangifer tarandus tarandus*) exposed to the continuous daylight of the Arctic summer. Can J Zool 72 (5):904–909. https://doi.org/10.1139/z94-123

Stokkan K-A et al (2007) Adaptations for life in the arctic: evidence that melatonin rhythms in reindeer are not driven by a circadian oscillator but remain acutely sensitive to environmental photoperiod. J Pineal Res 43(3):289–293. https://doi.org/10.1111/j.1600-079X.2007.00476.x

Strand JET et al (2008) Keeping track of time under ice and snow in a sub-arctic lake: plasma melatonin rhythms in Arctic charr overwintering under natural conditions. J Pineal Res 44 (3):227–233. https://doi.org/10.1111/j.1600-079X.2007.00511.x

Tsutsui K et al (2013) Review: regulatory mechanisms of gonadotropin-inhibitory hormone (GnIH) synthesis and release in photoperiodic animals. Front Neurosci 7:60. https://doi.org/10.3389/fnins.2013.00060

Ubuka T, Bentley GE, Tsutsui K (2013) Neuroendocrine regulation of gonadotropin secretion in seasonally breeding birds. Front Neurosci 7:38. https://doi.org/10.3389/fnins.2013.00038

Unfried C et al (2009) Impact of melatonin and molecular clockwork components on the expression of thyrotropin β-chain (Tshb) and the Tsh receptor in the mouse pars tuberalis. Endocrinology 150(10):4653–4662. https://doi.org/10.1210/en.2009-0609

Viguie C (1999) Thyroid hormones act primarily within the brain to promote the seasonal inhibition of luteinizing hormone secretion in the ewe. Endocrinology 140(3):1111–1117. https://doi.org/10.1210/en.140.3.1111

Watanabe M et al (2004) Photoperiodic regulation of type 2 deiodinase gene in djungarian hamster: possible homologies between avian and mammalian photoperiodic regulation of reproduction. Endocrinology 145(4):1546–1549. https://doi.org/10.1210/en.2003-1593

Watanabe T et al (2007) Hypothalamic expression of thyroid hormone-activating and -inactivating enzyme genes in relation to photorefractoriness in birds and mammals. Am J Phys Regul Integr Comp Phys 292(1):R568–R572. https://doi.org/10.1152/ajpregu.00521.2006

Webster JR, Moenter SM, Woodfill CJ et al (1991a) Role of the thyroid gland in seasonal reproduction. II. Thyroxine allows a season-specific suppression of gonadotropin secretion in sheep. Endocrinology 129(1):176–183. https://doi.org/10.1210/endo-129-1-176

Webster JR, Moenter SM, Barrell GK et al (1991b) Role of the thyroid gland in seasonal reproduction. III. Thyroidectomy blocks seasonal suppression of gonadotropin-releasing hormone secretion in sheep. Endocrinology 129(3):1635–1643. https://doi.org/10.1210/endo-129-3-1635

West AC, Wood SH (2018) Seasonal physiology: making the future a thing of the past. Curr Opin Physiol 5:1–8. https://doi.org/10.1016/j.cophys.2018.04.006

West A et al (2013) Npas4 is activated by melatonin, and drives the clock gene Cry1 in the ovine pars tuberalis. Mol Endocrinol 27(6):979–989. https://doi.org/10.1210/me.2012-1366

Woitkewitsch A (1940) Dependence of seasonal periodicity in gonadal changes on the thyroid gland. C R Dokl Acad Sci URSS 27:741–745

Wood S, Loudon A (2014) Clocks for all seasons: unwinding the roles and mechanisms of circadian and interval timers in the hypothalamus and pituitary. J Endocrinol 222(2):R39–R59. https://doi.org/10.1530/JOE-14-0141

Wood S, Loudon A (2017) The pars tuberalis: the site of the circannual clock in mammals. Gen Comp Endocrinol 258:222–235. https://doi.org/10.1016/j.ygcen.2017.06.029

Wood SH et al (2015) Binary switching of calender cells in the pituitary defines the phase of the circannual cycle in mammals. Curr Biol 25(20). https://doi.org/10.1016/j.cub.2015.09.014

Woodfill CJ et al (1994) Photoperiodic synchronization of a circannual reproductive rhythm in sheep: identification of season-specific time cues. Biol Reprod 50(4):965–76. http://www.ncbi.nlm.nih.gov/pubmed/8199277

Yasuo S, Korf H-W (2011) The hypophysial pars tuberalis transduces photoperiodic signals via multiple pathways and messenger molecules. Gen Comp Endocrinol 172(1):15–22. https://doi.org/10.1016/j.ygcen.2010.11.006

Yasuo S et al (2009) Melatonin transmits photoperiodic signals through the MT1 melatonin receptor. J Neurosci 29(9):2885–2889. https://doi.org/10.1523/JNEUROSCI.0145-09.2009

Yasuo S et al (2014) 2-Arachidonoyl glycerol sensitizes the pars distalis and enhances forskolin-stimulated prolactin secretion in Syrian hamsters. Chronobiol Int 31(3):337–342. https://doi.org/10.3109/07420528.2013.852104

Yoshimura T (2010) Neuroendocrine mechanism of seasonal reproduction in birds and mammals. Anim Sci J 81(4):403–410. https://doi.org/10.1111/j.1740-0929.2010.00777.x

Yoshimura T (2013) Thyroid hormone and seasonal regulation of reproduction. Front Neuroendocrinol 34(3):157–166. https://doi.org/10.1016/j.yfrne.2013.04.002

Yoshimura T et al (2003) Light-induced hormone conversion of T4 to T3 regulates photoperiodic response of gonads in birds. Nature 426(6963):178–181. https://doi.org/10.1038/nature02117

Zucker I (1985) Pineal gland influences period of circannual rhythms of ground squirrels. Am J Physiol 249(1 Pt 2):R111–R115. http://www.ncbi.nlm.nih.gov/pubmed/4014491

Recommended Further Reading

Dardente H, Wood S, Ebling FJ, Sáenz de Miera C (2019) An integrative view of mammalian seasonal neuroendocrinology. J Neuroendocrinol 31(5):e12729. https://doi.org/10.1111/jne.12729. A very recent detailed open access review of the *pars tuberalis* and associated mechanisms underlying seasonality in mammals.

David A. Freeman, Brett J. W. Teubner, Carlesia D. Smith, Brian J. Prendergast, (2007) Exogenous Tmimics long day lengths in Siberian hamsters. American Journal of Physiology-Regulatory, Integrative and Comparative Physiology 292 (6):R2368-R2372

Hazlerigg DG, Lincoln GA (2011) Hypothesis: cyclical histogenesis is the basis of circannual timing. J Biol Rhythms 26:471–485. https://doi.org/10.1177/0748730411420812. An influential review proposing the hypothesis that circannual rhythm generation depends on tissue-autonomous, reiterated cycles of cell division, functional differentiation, and cell death, using the *pars tuberalis* in mammals as a prime example.

Wood SH, Christian HC, Miedzinska K, Saer BR, Johnson M, Paton B, Yu L, McNeilly J, Davis JR, McNeilly AS, Burt DW, Loudon AS (2015) Binary switching of calendar cells in the pituitary defines the phase of the circannual cycle in mammals. Curr Biol 25: 2651–2662. https://doi.org/10.1016/j.cub.2015.09.014. A primary research paper providing substantial evidence that thyrotrophs in the sheep *pars tuberalis* transition between two states, resulting in a morphological plasticity that underpins circannual rhythmicity.

Tanycytes and Their Pivotal Role in Seasonal Physiological Adaptations

3

Perry Barrett and Peter J. Morgan

Abstract

Tanycytes are glial cells whose cell soma are embedded in the ependymal layer surrounding the ventral region of the third ventricle in the hypothalamus. They send projections into the surrounding hypothalamus, with processes terminating in the neuropil of the hypothalamus, or extended to contact portal blood vessels in the median eminence or the surrounding *pars tuberalis*. Photoperiodic regulation of gene expression occurs in tanycytes through local signals emanating in the *pars tuberalis*. Of considerable importance across vertebrate taxa is photoperiodic regulation of type II (*Dio2*) and type III (*Dio3*) deiodinase enzyme gene expression in tanycytes as these regulate local thyroid hormone availability. This chapter explores the evidence for photoperiodic regulation of thyroid hormone and retinoic acid signalling by tanycytes, and considers this in relation to their other key functions, including their potential as a stem cell niche in the adult brain, their role as part of the blood brain barrier in transporting nutrients and hormones into the brain, and their role in regulating neuroendocrine secretion in the median eminence by virtue of their anatomical proximity to neuronal terminals.

Keywords

Hypothalamus · Seasonality · Neurogenesis · Melatonin · Thyroid hormone

P. Barrett (✉) · P. J. Morgan
Rowett Institute, Foresterhill Campus, University of Aberdeen, Aberdeen, Scotland
e-mail: p.barrett@abdn.ac.uk; p.morgan@abdn.ac.uk

© The Editor(s) (if applicable) and The Author(s), under exclusive license to Springer Nature Switzerland AG 2020
F. J. P. Ebling, H. D. Piggins (eds.), *Neuroendocrine Clocks and Calendars*, Masterclass in Neuroendocrinology 10, https://doi.org/10.1007/978-3-030-55643-3_3

3.1   Introduction

The study of tanycyte biology originated in the early 1950s with the term tanycyte coined in 1954 (Horstmann 1954) to describe cells in a layer separating the third ventricle from neuropil of the hypothalamus with an extended distal process contacting portal blood vessels in the median eminence (Fig. 3.1). Up until the 1980s, tanycytes were a large focus of neuroendocrine research investigating the interaction between the brain and pituitary. However, with the advent of tools and techniques, which facilitated detailed analysis of the cellular and molecular interactions in specific neurons of the hypothalamus, research on these cells diminished. Nevertheless, in the absence of the many technical advances, which are taken for granted today, the early work uncovered substantial information about tanycyte cytology and ultrastructure, including responses to variations in environmental conditions. Even during the early years of tanycyte research, studies revealed that structural changes occur in response to the season of the year, hinting at their likely involvement in hypothalamic mechanisms related to seasonal physiology (Hagedoorn 1965; Wittkowski and Muller 1976; Brawer and Gustafson 1979).

Much of our knowledge about tanycytes to date has been derived from studies using non-seasonal rodents, in particular studies utilising mice, where the advantages of transgenic technologies have been applied to further our understanding of tanycyte functions. Tanycytes are a component of the ependyma (a single layer of cells) lining the third ventricle, forming a barrier between the cerebrospinal fluid (CSF) of the ventricle and the neuropil of the hypothalamus. Morphologically, tanycytes are similar among species and share common characteristics such as expression of thyroid hormone deiodinase proteins and intermediate filament proteins. Therefore, it is likely that the role and function of tanycytes is similar among species. However, there may be adaptations for specific functions, for example in seasonal mammals, physiological adaptations may be dependent on co-ordinated photoperiodic regulation in tanycytes of type II (*Dio2*) and type III (*Dio3*) deiodinase enzyme gene expression (Sect. 3.5).

3.1.1   Structure of Tanycytes

The developmental origins of tanycytes are radial glial cells, formed as part of the neuroepithelium in the early stages of brain development. Even after differentiation, tanycytes retain some markers of their origin, including expression of the intermediate filament protein nestin (Hartfuss et al. 2001). Tanycytes comprise the floor of the infundibular recess and extend dorsally for about one-third of the ventricular wall where they give way to ependymocytes (a.k.a. ependymal cells) (Fig. 3.1b). Ependymocytes are readily distinguishable from tanycytes, being cube-like cells with a tuft of cilia projecting into the ventricle and lacking a projection into the adjacent parenchyma (Rodriguez et al. 2005). The tanycyte cell body resides in the ventricular wall with an extended basal process arching into the hypothalamic parenchyma (Fig. 3.1c), terminating at locations ranging from portal blood vessels

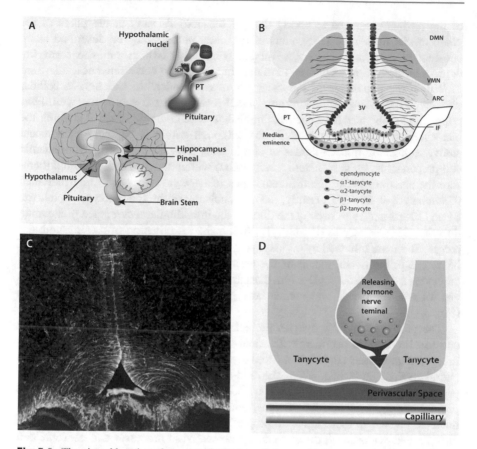

Fig. 3.1 The pivotal location of tanycytes in the hypothalamus. (**a**) diagrammatic view of a sagittal section through the human brain. The projected region from this section enlarges the area containing the pituitary gland at the base of the hypothalamus giving relative location of hypothalamic structures of the arcuate nucleus (ARC), dorsomedial nucleus (DMN), ventromedial nucleus (VMN), paraventricular nucleus (PVN), supraoptic nucleus (SON), suprachiasmatic nucleus (SCN) together with the pituitary gland and *pars tuberalis* (PT). (**b**) diagrammatic view of a coronal section across the hypothalamus, revealing hypothalamic nuclei, the third ventricle (3V), infundibular recess (IF), median eminence and *pars tuberalis* (PT) surrounding the median eminence. (**c**) A coronal section through the hypothalamus of a rat brain immunostained with antibodies to the intermediate filament proteins vimentin (red) and glial fibrillary acidic protein [GFAP] (green). Both proteins are co-expressed in the majority of tanycytes giving rise to yellow/orange colour in the merged image. The extended processes radiating outwards from tanycyte cell bodies can be seen mostly in tanycytes comprising α1 and β2 tanycytes. (**d**) Diagrammatic view of tanycyte end-feet surrounding the terminal of a nerve conveying a hypophysiotrophic hormone targeting the pituitary gland. The tanycyte end-feet are shown surrounding the nerve terminal blocking access of a releasing hormone to the perivascular space. Upon retraction of the end-feet, access is permitted and the hormone can enter the portal blood system for transport to the pituitary gland. Panel (**c**) is reproduced from Bolborea et al. (2015)

of the median eminence to poorly defined locations dorsally in the plane of the ventromedial nucleus. The terminus of the basal process may be described as an end-foot surrounding neuronal terminals (Fig. 3.1d), which can show varying degrees of interaction with these terminals in response to endocrine cues.

Within the population of tanycytes, there is considerable variation in cellular phenotype depending on their ventro-dorsal location in the ventricular wall. Four populations (subtypes) have been distinguished based on morphological features and histochemistry (Rodriguez et al. 2005), although within these subtypes a recent study, sequencing transcriptomes of single cells from a mixture of hypothalamic cell preparations, suggests heterogeneity exists within tanycyte subtypes, and therefore the classification of the different types of tanycyte may need to be redefined (Campbell et al. 2017). Currently, the nomenclature of the four subtypes is α1, α2, β1 and β2. β2 tanycytes occupy the floor of the infundibular recess, then proceeding dorsally, β2 give way to β1 tanycytes lining the invagination of the infundibular recess. These are followed by α2 tanycytes that extend dorsally from the infundibular recess to the dorsal extent of the arcuate nucleus. The most dorsally located tanycytes are the α1 tanycytes, which occupy the ventricular wall in the plane of the ventromedial nucleus, and which are gradually replaced by ependymocytes (Fig. 3.1).

The processes of β2 tanycytes project into the median eminence where their end-feet lie between peptidergic neuronal termini and endothelial cells comprising the portal capillaries (Fig. 3.1b). Similar processes of β1 tanycytes project to the lateral median eminence where the end-feet can also surround nerve terminal projections to the portal capillaries (Fig. 3.1d). The basal processes of α1 tanycytes project into the ventromedial nucleus, while those of α2 project into the arcuate nucleus, but where these tanycyte projections terminate is largely unknown with only limited evidence for direct contact between basal processes and neuronal cell bodies (β1/2 tanycyte interacting with AgRP/NPY neuron—Coppola et al. 2007). However, electron microscopy shows the interaction of tanycyte end-feet with hypophysiotrophic nerve terminals (Clasadonte and Prevot 2017) with more ventrally localised tanycytes making contact with fenestrated (having pores) parenchymal microcapillaries (Mullier et al. 2010).

3.1.2 Tanycytes as a Barrier Between the Periphery and Hypothalamus

The brain is isolated from the array of hormones circulating in the peripheral blood supply by the blood brain barrier (BBB), but at privileged regions, known as circumventricular organs located next to ventricular cavities, hormones from the periphery are able to gain regulated access to the brain through a highly permeable fenestrated microvasculature. The median eminence, comprising axon terminals of releasing hormone neurons and axons of magnocellular neurons, end-feet of tanycytes and microvessels, constitutes such a circumventricular organ. The barrier to diffusion posed by tanycytes to circulating hormones and metabolites into the hypothalamus is provided by a honeycomb formation of proteins known as tight junction proteins, specifically claudin 1, occludin and zonula occludens-1, encircling β1 and β2 tanycytes (Langlet et al. 2013). This is evident by restriction of the azo dye, Evans blue, when injected into the hypothalamus from reaching the periphery. More dorsally in the region of the α1 and α2 tanycytes, there is a more diffuse pattern of tight junction proteins where Evans blue dye administered in the ventricular system gains access to the arcuate nucleus. This indicates in the vicinity of these tanycytes there is no barrier function, so hormones present in CSF of the ventricular space will gain access to neurons within the arcuate nucleus (Mullier et al. 2010).

In response to food restriction, there is enhanced organisation of tight junction proteins in tanycytes in the vicinity of the arcuate nucleus and median eminence, which reverts to a less organised state when mice are refed. This reversible function of the BBB is also mimicked by glucose deprivation and repletion, indicating the important role glucose plays in barrier organisation (Langlet et al. 2013). The altered organisational plasticity is dependent upon increased VEGF-A synthesis by tanycytes acting on VEGFR2 receptors (Langlet et al. 2013). Inhibition of BBB plasticity through receptor inactivation significantly decreases food intake, which demonstrates the importance of tanycytes in food intake control and energy balance regulation (Langlet et al. 2013).

The neural parenchyma of the hypothalamus houses several key neuronal groups involved in appetite and energy balance regulation, such as neuropeptide Y (NPY) and agouti-related peptide (AgRP) co-expressing neurons, and neurons co-expressing pro-opiomelanocrtin (POMC) and cocaine and amphetamine-regulated transcript (CART) neuropeptides. Both these groups of cells are located in close proximity to the ventricular wall. Nevertheless, with a direct role in food intake control, tanycytes should be considered as an integral part of the overall hypothalamic consortium contributing to nutrient sensing and appetite regulation. Further evidence for the involvement of tanycytes in appetite regulation is demonstrated by responses to fasting, which induces *Dio2* expression encoding the enzyme type 2 deiodinase (DIO2) responsible for the conversion of thyroxine (T4) to thyroid hormone (T3, see Sect. 3.5). This leads to increased T3 synthesis in tanycytes that communicate with NPY/AgRP neurons. The fasting-induced increase in T3 drives mitochondrial proliferation in NPY/AgRP neurons leading to rebound feeding (Coppola et al. 2007), and provides one example of the importance of tanycytes to a neuron-mediated homeostatic function.

Recent studies have shown that tanycytes express the molecular machinery to enable nutrient sensing, and such a property is consistent with an involvement in homeostatic regulation of energy balance. The molecular machinery to sense nutrients includes the umami taste receptor (heterodimeric complex of taste receptors Tas1r1 and Tas1r3) and the metabotropic glutamate receptor mGlu4, which confer the ability to sense and respond to a variety of amino acids (Lazutkaite et al. 2017). Tanycytes also constitute a part of the central mechanism of glucose sensing (Benford et al. 2017), responding to glucose through a mechanism involving an intracellular rise in $[Ca^{2+}]$. This is followed by a release of ATP, which subsequently acts on adjacent tanycytes via P2Y1 receptors to increase intracellular Ca^{2+}, creating a large wave of Ca^{2+} (Frayling et al. 2011). Tanycytes also express GLUT1 and GLUT2 glucose transporters and the sweet taste receptor, which is a heterodimeric complex of the taste receptor subunits Tas1r2 and Tas1r3, so it seems likely that glucose sensing and organisational transition of the BBB by glucose occur via these glucose receptive proteins (Langlet et al. 2013). This raises an interesting question in the context of seasonal mammals: could nutrient sensing by tanycytes be part of a mechanism to adjust food intake in relation to seasonal food availability?

Although acting as a barrier, tanycytes also act as a conduit for the transport (transcytosis) of bioactive molecules from the circulation into the ventricular space and neuronal parenchyma. Absorption of bioactive molecules takes place through a clathrin- or caveolin-dependent endocytosis mechanism. The former has been shown to be involved in the entry of leptin from the periphery into the hypothalamus, involving a mechanism that requires the presence of the leptin receptor on tanycytes for uptake and activation of an extracellular regulated kinase for leptin release from tanycytes (Balland et al. 2014). This could be an interesting line of inquiry in the context of seasonal animals, and specifically could tanycytes be involved in a photoperiod-dependent sensitivity to leptin as evident in sheep and Siberian hamsters, to allow accumulation of fat at the appropriate time (Rousseau et al. 2002; Adam et al. 2006; Tups et al. 2012)?

3.2   Tanycytes as a Neural Stem Cell Niche

There is a growing body of evidence that tanycytes have the potential to be neurogenic progenitor cells (Yoo and Blackshaw 2018), a property that seems to have been retained from their origin as radial glial cells, of which both give rise to neurons during the course of development and serve as paths for migrating neurons. Indicative of neuroprogenitor potential is the expression of neural stem cell markers, including *Nestin*, *Rax*, *Sox2*, *Notch* and components of the *Wnt*-signalling pathway (Rodriguez et al. 2005; Miranda-Angulo et al. 2014; Helfer and Tups 2016). The principal technique for the identification of tanycytes as stem cells has been the incorporation of the nucleotide BrdU into DNA of dividing cells, with subsequent detection of the incorporated label using antibodies raised to BrdU, but more recently transgenic mouse technology has come to the aid of the tanycyte research field, enabling lineage tracing expressing a marker protein (such as LacZ or green fluorescent protein) that specifically labels tanycytes (Fig. 3.2).

The use of transgenic mice to label tanycyte cells has identified two apparently distinct populations with stem cell activity. The promoter of the glutamate transporter, *Glast2*, was used to label α2 tanycytes, which were found to yield neurospheres in vitro, particularly in the presence of FGF2 (Robins et al. 2013). This approach also identified self-proliferation of tanycyte cell number in the α2 layer and migration dorsally to become an α1 subtype, or migrating ventrally to contribute to the β1 population. Chase experiments also showed tanycytes migrating into the neural parenchyma that then differentiate into either astrocytes or neurons (Robins et al. 2013). The lineage of a second niche can be traced with a

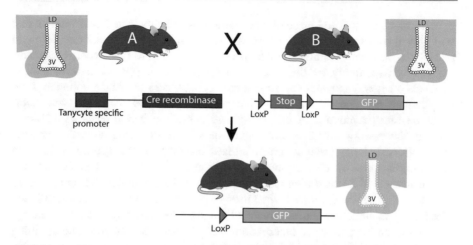

Fig. 3.2 Schematic outline of the generation of mice with tanycyte specific expression of green fluorescent protein (GFP). One transgenic mouse 'A' expresses a CRE recombinase from a promoter localised to the cell type of interest (tanycytes). A second transgenic mouse 'B' harbours GFP downstream of the universally expressed promoter, ROSA26, but expression of the protein is blocked by a stop codon in the sequence upstream of the GFP-coding region. The stop codon is flanked by two lox P sites. To remove the stop codon, the transgenic mice are crossed giving rise to offspring, which will express CRE recombinase in tanycytes harbouring GFP in the ROSA26 locus. This will result in excision of the stop coding preceding GFP-coding sequence and permit production of a fluorescent protein specifically in tanycytes. *3V* third ventricle

marker protein driven by the promoter for FGF10 or nestin (Hann et al. 2013; Chaker et al. 2016), where expression is largely confined to β1 and β2 tanycytes. Tanycytes from this population (mostly β2) give rise to new neurons or less frequently astrocytes, then migrate to regions of the hypothalamus important for energy balance. This includes the arcuate nucleus, ventromedial nucleus, dorsomedial nucleus and the lateral hypothalamus. In the arcuate nucleus, neurons derived from tanycytes have been identified with expression of orexigenic NPY or anorexigenic POMC-derived neuropeptides, both being important to energy balance homeostasis. The same population of tanycytes can also contribute to neuronal expansion within the median eminence, and interestingly neural progenitor activity of tanycytes in this region can be affected by a high-fat diet, promoting a fourfold increase in neurogenesis (Lee et al. 2012). Neuroprogenitor activity of tanycytes may also be of importance in the context of the seasonal animal and is discussed in Sect. 3.8.

3.3 Animal Models for Studying Seasonal Changes in Tanycyte Function

Mammals living in temperate zones experience a large variation in environmental conditions over the course of a year, notably day length, temperature and availability of food supply. Accordingly, many mammals living in these temperate zones have evolved physiological and metabolic adaptations to the anticipated environment that will prevail over the course of the year. In doing so, mammals have prioritised and partitioned energy expenditure to vital processes, serving to tailor energy expenditure to food availability and their survival. Reproduction imposes one of the highest demands on energy expenditure, so is therefore a process for which abundant food supplies are necessary for reproductive success. Seasonal mammals with short gestation times reproduce in the spring and summer when food is available to support the energy demands for rapid foetal and offspring growth, whereas mammals with long gestation times initiate breeding in the autumn with birth occurring in spring when food availability is increasing. Seasonal mammals may also increase food intake during the summer months to accumulate fat for an energy source during the winter months when food may be scarce, this being exemplified in hibernating mammals when accumulated fat may be the only source of energy during the entire period of hibernation. The central mechanisms underpinning physiological and behavioural adaptations in seasonal mammals are not well understood, but it has become increasingly clear that tanycytes play a pivotal role.

Much of our limited understanding of the molecular mechanisms regulating seasonal physiology has been derived mostly from four animal models—the sheep, Siberian hamster, Fischer F344 rat and the Japanese quail (Fig. 3.3), although other models have made a contribution such as the Syrian hamster, European hamster, ground squirrel, vole and salmon. Each of the most common models used in research investigating the molecular mechanism underpinning physiological adaptations have been chosen for different reasons. The rapidity of response of the reproductive axis to photoperiodic change in the Japanese quail established this bird as an excellent avian model of a long-day breeder. The sheep has proved useful because of its size, providing ample tissue and blood for analysis, and represents an example of a short-day breeding mammal with a gestation period of approximately 150 days. Among breeds of sheep responding to seasonal variation in photoperiod, many of the cellular and molecular investigations have been performed using the Soay sheep, as this semi-domesticated breed shows robust physiological adaptations to summer and winter photoperiod, including a change in food intake, body weight, adiposity and reproductive status.

The Siberian hamster is an example of a long-day breeder with a short gestation period of 19–21 days, which has also been extensively used as a model of seasonality. The Siberian hamster shows involution of the reproductive axis, a reduction of food intake and loss of body weight when switched from long to short photoperiod. While both the sheep and hamster are both good models of photoperiodic regulation of energy balance and reproduction, the Siberian hamster has the advantage of a shorter gestation time and lower animal husbandry costs.

The Fisher 344 rat is a recent addition to the family of photoresponsive mammals. While laboratory strains of rats are not generally considered as seasonal, F344 rats have retained responsiveness to photoperiod, so that short-day exposure (8 h light:16 h dark) causes a small but significant reduction in somatic growth, food intake and a transient regression of testes in males (Heideman and Sylvester 1997; Ross et al. 2009). The discovery of seasonal photoperiod responsiveness in the F344

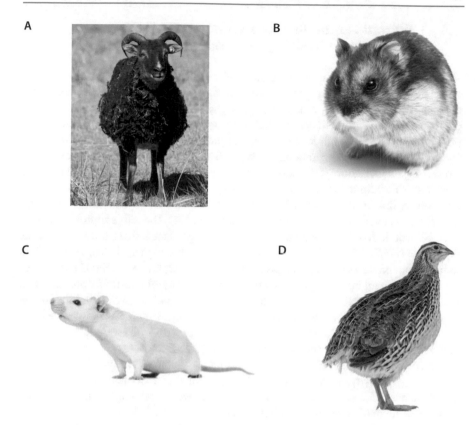

Fig. 3.3 Research models for investigating the molecular mechanisms underpinning seasonal physiological adaptations. (**a**) Soay sheep, (**b**) Siberian hamster, (**c**) Fisher F344 rat, (**d**) Japanese quail

rat has been advantageous to investigation of the molecular mechanisms in the brain underpinning physiological adaptations, as this model has benefited from the availability of genome data for microarray fabrication, enabling high-throughput transcriptome analysis of hypothalamic tissue in different photoperiodic states (Ross et al. 2011).

In a natural environment, seasonal animals alter their physiological status in response to a changing day length. The day length at which physiological adaptations are initiated varies according to species and latitude of origin (Goldman et al. 2004). Nevertheless, in laboratory conditions, this can be mimicked by placing animals in artificially generated photoperiods representing either long day or short days. Consequently, many studies have been performed using a square-wave paradigm (see Sect. 3.8) with artificial light to mimic long-day exposure (generally >14-h light in a 24-h period) and short-day exposure (generally <10-h light in a 24-h period).

3.4   Thyroid Hormone as the Common Denominator to Seasonal Physiological Responses

Work to understand the mechanistic basis of seasonal reproduction in the Japanese quail provided the first major advance in the quest to unravel the molecular mechanisms underpinning seasonal physiology. A comparative analysis of genes expressed in the hypothalamus between quails housed in long and short photoperiods showed high levels of gene expression for type II deiodinase (*Dio2*) and low levels of gene expression for type III deiodinase (*Dio3*) under long days. Conversely, under short photoperiod, gene expression of *Dio2* was low and *Dio3* was high (Yoshimura et al. 2003; Yasuo et al. 2005). The significance of this observation lies in the functional activity of DIO2 and DIO3 enzymes to regulate hypothalamic availability of thyroid hormone (Fig. 3.4). Bioactive thyroid hormone (L-3,5,3′-triiodothyronine—abbreviated as T3) is produced from the prohormone, thyroxine (L-3,5,3′,5′-tetraiodothyronine—abbreviated as T4) by removal of an iodine group on the outer of two benzene rings by DIO2; however, DIO3 catabolises T3 and T4 with an inner ring deiodination to produce thyroid hormone products that are biologically inactive, L-3,3′-diiodothyronine (T2) and L-3,3′5′ triiodothyronine (reverseT3 or rT3), respectively. In the quail, switching reproductively inactive birds held on short days to long days stimulates a rapid and measurable increase in luteinising hormone (LH) secretion, which is sufficient to drive reproductive recrudescence. Several lines of evidence support the notion of a pivotal role for T3 produced by tanycytes in the seasonal response; this includes measurement of hypothalamic T3 and T4 concentrations, which were both higher in long days; infusion of iopanoic acid, an inhibitor of DIO2, into the third ventricle of long-day housed quails induced testicular regression, and T3 infusion into the hypothalamus in short-day housed birds induced testicular growth (Yoshimura et al. 2003). In addition to the synthesis of T3 as a pivotal hormone, a physical role of the tanycytes in this process was also shown by delivery of exogenous T3 into the hypothalamus in short-day housed quails. This treatment stimulated testicular growth and caused morphological changes of tanycyte end-feet to allow GnRH nerve terminals to contact the portal capillaries supplying blood to the neighbouring pituitary gland, which are normally surrounded by tanycyte end-feet in the short-day condition (Yamamura et al. 2006). This suggests that T3 acts within tanycytes to facilitate a physiological response and the enzymes responsible for the synthesis (DIO2) and catabolism of T3 (DIO3) are found in tanycytes where they are regulated by photoperiod, giving tanycytes a critical role in the seasonal physiological response.

Subsequent studies in other photoperiodically sensitive species have shown the central importance of thyroid hormone to the co-ordination of seasonal physiological adaptations irrespective of the time of year the animal may breed. In sheep, a short-day breeder, thyroidectomy with T3 replacement via T3-releasing implants has shown the requirement for thyroid hormone to terminate the breeding season (Anderson et al. 2003). Like quail, the location of the deiodinase enzymes responsible for the conversion of T4 to T3 (DIO2) and the catabolism of T3 or T4 (DIO3) are located in tanycytes surrounding the 3rd ventricle (Sanez de Miera et al. 2013).

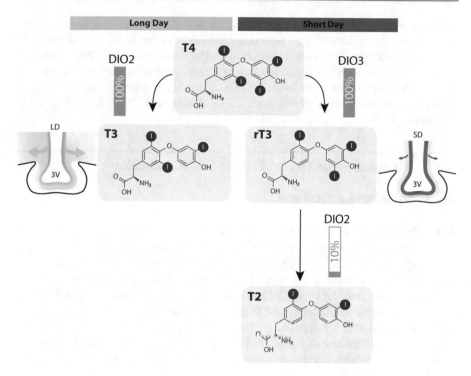

Fig. 3.4 Metabolism of T4 in long- and short-day tanycytes. The fate of thyroid hormone (thyroxine: T4) transported into tanycytes depends upon the presence of the subtype of deiodinase (DIO) present. In long days (LD) only DIO2 is present, so T4 will be converted to T3 and made available to the tanycyte and surrounding hypothalamic neurons. In short days (SD), the principal DIO present is DIO3. This will convert T4 to reverse T3 (rT3). A small amount of DIO2 may still be present in tanycytes of short-day hamsters and could convert rT3 to T2. Both these compounds could be potentially exported into the surrounding hypothalamus, but there is no evidence to date that rT3 or T2 is involved in seasonal physiological adaptations. Bars with percentage represent values of mRNA expression in each photoperiod up to a full expression value of 100%. *3V* third ventricle

Further evidence for the universality of thyroid hormone in the seasonal response was provided by studies using microimplants to deliver T3 into the hypothalamus of the male Siberian hamster. When long-day male hamsters were implanted with microimplants releasing T3 into the hypothalamus and then switched to short days, the expected decrease in food intake, decline in body weight and testicular regression were blocked (Barrett et al. 2007). Conversely, in male hamsters adapted to short days with reduced body weight and adiposity and regressed testes, T3 implants stimulated a rapid increase in food intake, body weight and testicular growth (Murphy et al. 2012). These data imply that in hamsters, high levels of hypothalamic T3 are required for the long-day response and low levels of T3 facilitate the short-day response. Consistent with this, in situ hybridisation experiments have shown high levels of *Dio2* and an absence of *Dio3* gene expression in tanycytes in long days, yet low levels of *Dio2* and high levels of *Dio3* gene expression in short days generating high and low levels of hypothalamic T3 under long and short days, respectively (Fig. 3.4) (Barrett et al. 2007; Watanabe et al. 2007). The involvement of deiodinases and thyroid hormone in seasonal adaptations is also evident in other seasonal animals, including Syrian hamster, European hamster, vole and Salmon (Revel et al. 2006; Hanon et al. 2009; Krol et al. 2012; Nakane et al. 2013).

3.5   Regulation of Thyroid Hormone Availability

3.5.1   Deiodinase Enzymes

The consensus view of evidence from several models of seasonality is that T3 availability to the hypothalamus has a pivotal role in seasonal physiology. Therefore, the mechanism by which deiodinase enzymes are regulated is clearly important. In both birds and mammals, the thyroid-stimulating hormone (TSH) synthesis and secretion by the *pars tuberalis* (PT) is central to this regulation, only differing in these species in the regulatory input to the *pars tuberalis*. In birds, seasonal photoperiod is transmitted by deep-brain photoreceptors present in the paraventricular organ, whereas in mammals, melatonin provides a hormonal cue via the periphery to regulate TSH synthesis in the *pars tuberalis* to reflect seasonal photoperiod (Nakane and Yoshimura 2014).

Melatonin is synthesised by the pineal gland during the hours of darkness and is therefore elevated in the circulation for longer during short days. Pinealectomy (removal of the pineal gland) and timed melatonin infusion paradigms clearly demonstrate that melatonin is required for the generation of short-day physiology (Arendt et al. 1988; Bartness and Goldman 1989). However, melatonin does not regulate *Dio2* gene expression directly, as melatonin receptors are not found on tanycytes. Instead melatonin receptors are present on cells of the neighbouring *pars tuberalis* of the pituitary stalk (Morgan et al. 1994). Here, melatonin through a sequence of molecular events regulates synthesis and secretion of TSH, which, in turn, stimulates tanycytes to increase *Dio2* expression to alter the balance of deiodinase enzymes in favour of T3 synthesis. The mechanism of melatonin action governing TSH synthesis involves utilising components of the circadian clock to regulate a transcriptional coactivator that is required for the transcription of the *Tshβ* subunit, called EYA3 (*eyes absent 3*). In brief, PER1, a component of the clock and a transcriptional repressor is induced at the beginning of the light phase. However, PER1 requires the clock protein CRY1 to form a transcriptional repressor (Reppert and Weaver 2001). Melatonin induces the expression of CRY1 at the onset of the dark phase, but PER1 is induced in the early light phase and degrades slowly. In long days CRY1 transcription occurs after PER1 has been degraded and therefore does not form a repressor with CRY1, but in short days transcriptional activation of CRY1 by melatonin occurs earlier relative to the beginning of the light phase before PER1 has been degraded. Thus, PER1 and CRY1 proteins are present at the same time and form a transcriptional repressor for *Eya3*. Therefore, in long days, EYA3 transcription factor is able to participate in the activation of *Tshβ* subunit gene expression resulting in elevated TSH synthesis and secretion from the *pars tuberalis* to stimulate *Dio2* transcription in tanycytes (Wood and Loudon 2018).

During long days newly synthesised TSH will require access to the ventricular tanycytes to stimulate *Dio2* expression—so how is this achieved? In situ hybridisation studies indicate TSH receptors may be largely localised to α1, α2 and β1 tanycytes (Hanon et al. 2008; Herwig et al. 2013). Tracing and high-resolution electron microscopy studies of the basal hypothalamus in the rat have uncovered two possible routes. The first route is via CSF and could be a route to facilitate access to all three tanycyte subtypes expressing TSH receptors. Electron microscopy shows the ventricular system in the region of the arcuate nucleus is open to the *pars tuberalis* and shares CSF of the ventricular system. Therefore, secreted TSH may gain access via this route by diffusion. The second route may be even more direct as β1 tanycytes appear to establish contact with the secretory cell types of the *pars tuberalis* (Guerra et al. 2010). Therefore, during long days, when βTSH synthesis and secretion ensues in the *pars tuberalis*, βTSH has access to TSH receptors expressed in tanycytes either through direct communication or via the CSF. Once engaged with receptor, βTSH activates a stimulatory G-protein-signalling transduction pathway (Gs-coupled pathway) leading to the generation of cAMP and a G-protein-coupled pathway leading to the activation of MAPK (Bolborea et al. 2015). *Dio2* mRNA expression increases with activation of a cAMP signal transduction pathway (Hanon et al. 2008), making this signal transduction pathway the likely mediator of stimulated *Dio2* gene expression subsequently leading to increased hypothalamic T3 concentrations. It is also worth bearing in mind that there may be other *pars tuberalis*-derived hormones, which may affect tanycyte function. One such hormone is Neuromedin U (NMU), which is under strong photoperiodic regulation in the *pars tuberalis*. NMU is able to stimulate expression of *Dio2* and genes of the *Wnt*-signalling pathway in ventricular tanycytes of the F344 rat and therefore may have a role to play in seasonal physiology (Helfer et al. 2013).

Although high levels of T3 produced by elevated *Dio2* gene expression drive long-day physiology, the converse is not necessarily sufficient to initiate short-day physiology; this is exemplified in the Siberian hamster and discussed in Sect. 3.8. Therefore, catabolism of T4 and T3 to biologically inactive rT3 or T2, respectively, by DIO3 may be equally important for the induction of short-day physiology. However, the mechanism of regulation of *Dio3* gene expression is not yet clear. In the F344 rat, it has been shown that TSH administered by intracerebral ventricular injection (ICV) suppresses *Dio3* gene expression (Helfer et al. 2013), suggesting that TSH plays an important role as a negative regulator of seasonal expression of *Dio3*, but in other seasonal mammals down-regulation of *Dio3* occurs in the absence of TSH (Bockers et al. 1997; Barrett et al. 2007; Watanabe et al. 2007).

The mechanism to promote *Dio3* gene is equally enigmatic. One study in Siberian hamsters indicates that photoperiod-mediated epigenetic regulation in the form of DNA methylation may be involved in regulating *Dio3* gene expression. DNA methylation of cytosine residues in CpG dinucleotides present in the promoter region of a gene is an established mechanism limiting access of the promoter to transcription factors. Thus, enhanced rates of gene transcription take place with reduced methylation of CpG dinucleotides in the promoter region, and conversely transcription is suppressed when there is a high degree of CpG methylation in the promoter. In the genome of a long-day housed Siberian hamster, there are 17 methylated CpG dinucleotide sites within the first 250-bp proximal promoter of the *Dio3*-coding region, of which 9 show reduced methylation in hypothalamic DNA preparations in short days (Stevenson and Prendergast 2014). This is consistent with a short-day reduction in DNA methyltransferases (DNMT) 1 and 3b, enzymes involved in creating and maintaining genomic methylation marks.

After extended periods in short days, seasonal mammals will revert to the physiology of the long day state, a phenomenon known as the photorefractory response. It is likely that this phenomenon is a manifestation of an underlying circannual rhythm, which facilitates the establishment of long-day physiology in anticipation of a favourable climate as time progresses towards spring. The photorefractory state poses some interesting questions regarding the regulation of deiodinase enzymes and T3 availability. In both the Siberian hamster and sheep, *Dio2* mRNA shows a small increase in the short-day refractory state (Herwig et al. 2014; Sanez de Miera et al. 2013). However, in both species, the short-day absence of TSH in the *pars tuberalis* continues (Bockers et al. 1997; Sanez de Miera et al. 2013), suggesting that the small rise in *Dio2* expression is independent of TSH secretion from the *pars tuberalis*.

Whether a small rise in T3 is involved in promoting long-day physiology in short-day photorefractory animals remains to be established, but consistent with this idea is the temporal kinetics of the mRNA expression for the catabolic deiodinase DIO3. In the Siberian hamster, *Dio3* mRNA shows a peak of expression approximately 8 weeks after transfer from long to short days and then declines to undetectable levels by around 14 weeks, a few weeks prior to hamsters initiating a reversion to long-day physiology (Barrett et al. 2007; Watanabe et al. 2007; Milesi et al. 2017). This could be considered to be first event in the initiation of photorefractoriness, leading to the hypothesis that tanycytes possess an endogenous circannual clock and that the function of the PT is to record changes in day length through durational melatonin action as well as synchronise this circannual clock. Epigenetic regulation of the *Dio3* promoter may have a role in this response as the DNA methylation status of CpG dinucleotides in the photorefractory state reflects the methylation status of the promoter in long-day hamsters when *Dio3* is absent (Stevenson and Prendergast 2014). This supports a role for a dynamic regulation of *Dio3* promoter methylation as a component of the regulatory mechanism of *Dio3* expression.

3.5.2 Thyroid Hormone Transporters

In addition to the balance of anabolic and catabolic deiodinase enzymes, T3 availability also depends on thyroid hormone transporters to import T4 from the bloodstream into tanycytes for T3 synthesis. A number of proteins have been identified with the capacity to transport thyroid hormones across the plasma membrane; however, many of these transporters also transport other small molecules. These transport proteins fall into two groups. One group is the monocarboxylate transport proteins (MCTs), of which MCT8 and MCT10 have the capacity to transport thyroid hormones. MCT8 is highly specific for thyroid hormones and does not transport other monocarboxylate molecules. Furthermore MCT8 is expressed in tanycytes, whereas MCT10, which is also involved in cellular export of amino acids, has no distinct expression in tanycytes (Muller and Heuer 2014). The other group of proteins with the ability to transport thyroid hormone are a large family of organic anion transporting polypeptides (OATPs). Among these is OATP1c1, whose expression is found only in tanycytes and blood vessels constituting the blood brain barrier (Roberts et al. 2008).

In the context of seasonal physiology, MCT8 and OATP1c1 have provided the focus for a transport mechanism for regulating T3 availability to the hypothalamus. In the quail, although *OAPT1c1* is expressed in ventricular tanycytes, it is not photoperiodically regulated and therefore not likely to constitute a part of a seasonal mechanism (Nakao et al. 2006). However, short days decrease *OATP1c1* in ventricular tanycytes of the F344 rat and sheep and therefore may constitute a component of the mechanism in these species (Ross et al. 2011; Lomet et al. 2018). Regulation of *Mct8* mRNA on the other hand contrasts with *OATP1c1* mRNA expression. In sheep, *Mct8* mRNA shows a transient decrease in response to decreasing day length (Lomet et al. 2018) while in both Siberian hamsters and the F344 rat, short days increase *Mct8* mRNA (Herwig et al. 2009; Ross et al. 2011). This may seem counterintuitive particularly in the F344 rat where *OATP1c1* mRNA is decreased, potentially abrogating the impact of the decrease in OATP1c1. However, it should be noted that in the F344 rat, *Mct8* expression shows the same spatial and temporal regulation as *Dio3* expression (localising mostly to α1/2 subtypes), whereas *OATP1c1* mRNA is down-regulated in all tanycyte groups (Ross et al. 2011). While we do not know the precise function of MCT8 in the context of thyroid hormone transport, one hypothesis for increased *Mct8* mRNA is that MCT8 increases T4 transport in DIO3 expressing tanycytes where it is subsequently converted to rT3 (Fig. 3.5). Because rT3 is inhibitory to DIO2 enzyme activity, this would serve to further decrease or eliminate T3 synthesis, enhancing the promotion of short-day physiology.

3.6   Regulated Non-thyroid Hormone Signalling Genes Present in Tanycytes

In addition to components of the thyroid hormone signalling system, there are a number of other genes expressed in tanycytes that are altered by day-length exposure and function in nutrient sensing and signalling cascades. Some of these genes have been identified by a candidate gene approach, while two studies have undertaken analysis of the hypothalamic transcriptome to identify photoperiodically regulated genes that may underpin seasonal physiology (Ross et al. 2011; Lomet et al. 2018).

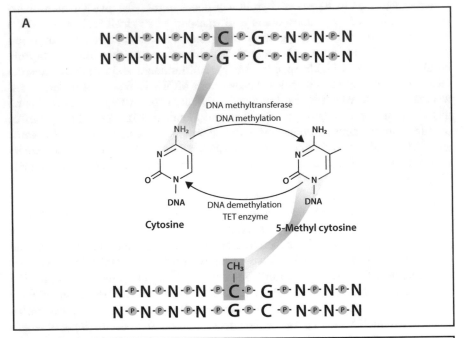

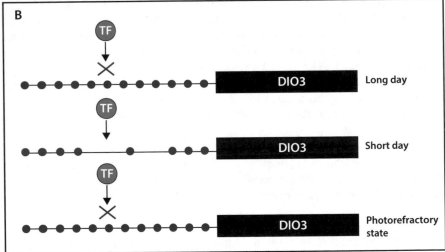

Fig. 3.5 Epigenetic regulation by cytosine methylation. (**a**) DNA methyltransferases may methylate cytosine nucleotides when present as a CpG dinucleotide in a DNA sequence. Reversal can be performed by 10–11 translocation methylcytosine dioxygenase (TET) enzymes. DNA methylation results in suppression of transcription by blocking transcription factor binding to promoters. (**b**) Methylation status of a 250-bp sequence upstream of the gene for deiodinase 3 (*Dio3*) in long days and short days. In long days, CpG dinucleotides are fully methylated in the upstream regulatory sequence of the *Dio3*-coding sequence. However, in short days, a number of CpG dinucleotides are demethylated enabling access of transcription factors (TF) to the promoter region to initiate mRNA transcription. In photorefractory hamsters, the upstream regulatory region of the *Dio3* gene largely

These studies have identified a large number of gene expression changes in RNA extracted from heterogeneous tissue composed of the hypothalamus together with the *pars tuberalis* (Ross et al. 2011; Lomet et al. 2018). A significant number of these photoperiodically regulated genes have been previously identified to originate from the *pars tuberalis*, including as discussed earlier, genes involved in the pathway regulating *Tshβ* expression. Of the remaining genes, of which there are many, in situ hybridisation will be needed to determine the origin of expression, particularly if they are exclusively located in tanycytes, and their potential role in seasonal physiology.

3.6.1 Metabolic Sensing

Nutrient sensing, such as glucose and amino acid sensing, is an emerging important function of tanycytes (Frayling et al. 2011; Lazutkaite et al. 2017), but there are no studies to date that have addressed whether there are any adaptations of nutrient-sensing mechanisms in relation to seasonal photoperiod. Evidently, photoperiod-regulated expression of deiodinase enzymes is responsive to food restriction in the Siberian hamster, with partial reversal of a decrease in *Dio2* gene expression and a partial reversal of the increase in *Dio3* gene expression in short-day exposed Siberian hamsters (Herwig et al. 2009). This would be consistent with the need to drive an increase in hypothalamic T3 in response to fasting and thence reduce the catabolic arm of the regulatory mechanism (Coppola et al. 2007).

Genes for enzymes involved in glycogen mobilisation (glycogen phosphorylase and phosphofructose kinase C) have been shown to be upregulated in tanycytes of the Siberian hamster in short days, suggesting tanycytes are utilising stored glycogen. But this event may be unrelated to nutrient sensing of glucose, as glucose levels do not change in long- or short-day housed hamsters (Murphy et al. 2013). In conjunction with a short-day stimulated reduction in the lactate transporter MCT2, glutamate transporter GLAST and glutamine synthetase in tanycytes, enhanced glycogen mobilisation is more likely to be involved with facilitating lactate and neurotransmitter supply to surrounding neurons (Nilaweera et al. 2011).

One of the more intriguing genes that is regulated by photoperiod in tanycytes is the gene for the orphan G-protein-coupled receptor, GPR50. Evidence from knock-out studies in mice supports a role for GPR50 in metabolic sensing. *Gpr50* knockout mice are resistant to weight gain on a high-energy diet, and have a lower night-time body temperature when fasted. This can develop into physiological torpor, a mechanism to reduce energy expenditure, characterised by hypometabolism and markedly reduced body temperature (Bechtold et al. 2012). Daily torpor is also a characteristic of the Siberian hamster, which enters the torpor state approximately 12 weeks after

Fig. 3.5 (continued) reflects the methylation status of the promoter in long-day housed hamsters. This demethylation and remethylation may constitute a part of the mechanism to regulate expression of *Dio3* mRNA switching from long to short days or with natural day length approaching the winter solstice (Petri et al. 2016). In artificial short days, *Gpr50* mRNA shows a reduction in expression in all tanycyte groups consistent with the propensity to engage torpor in *Gpr50* null mice (Barrett et al. 2006).

3.6.2 Hypophysiotrophic Hormone Gatekeeping

Short-day photoperiods initiate a down-regulation of mRNA for the intermediate filament proteins nestin and vimentin in tanycytes of several seasonal animals, which is manifest as changes to organisation of these proteins (Kameda et al. 2003; Yamamura et al. 2006; Barrett et al. 2006; Helfer et al. 2016; Butruille et al. 2018). All these changes are indicative of morphological changes in tanycyte end-feet and their relationship to the hypophysiotrophic axon terminals. In several species (quail, Siberian hamster, bat), clear differences have been visualised in end-feet ensheathment of hypophysiotrophic axon terminals between long and short days or after T3 infusions into the third ventricle (Kameda et al. 2003; Yamamura et al. 2006; Brawer and Gustafson 1979). Based on observations of ensheathment or retraction of tanycyte end-feet from axon terminals over the course of an oestrous cycle in rats (Prevot et al. 1999), the current view of the functional significance of ensheathment and retraction from hypophysiotrophic axon terminals is to either occlude or facilitate access to the terminals that project to the basal lamina adjacent to the portal blood vessels, respectively. This controls access of hypophysiotrophic hormones such as GnRH to the pituitary gland. However, the relationship between axonal ensheathment and hormonal profiles needs to be established in seasonal animals. The situation in the quail appears straightforward; in long days, there is minimal ensheathment of axon terminals with many abutting the basal lamina. Long-day morphology can be mimicked in short-day housed quails where nerve terminals are mostly ensheathed, by infusion of an optimal amount of T3 into the third ventricle, which causes retraction of end-feet (Yamamura et al. 2006). In the Siberian hamster, however, the situation is less clear, as hamsters held in continuous light for 1-month or a 16 h:8 h light:dark cycle for 2 months had ensheathment of axonal processes, with the contrary situation in the opposite light regime (Kameda et al. 2003). This would imply an inhibition of hypophysiotrophic hormone release in long days, but release in short days. However, timing relative to the initial exposure to long days may be an important factor as initiation of photorefractory mechanisms in preparedness for the anticipated season ahead may already be underway, and such preparation could include ensheathment of axon processes. Further work on the role of the relationship of tanycyte end-feet with axonal processes is required.

3.6.3 Retinoic Acid Signalling

Components of the retinoic acid (RA) signalling system were among the first hypothalamic genes to be identified in the Siberian hamster under the control of photoperiod (Ross et al. 2004). This includes the gene for cellular retinol–binding protein 1 (*Crbp1*), a component of the retinol transport mechanism localised to the ventricular layer. mRNA for other components of retinol transport, or enzymes for the conversion of retinol to retinoic acid transport and degradation have been subsequently localised to tanycytes, including *Stra6*, a receptor for retinol uptake, transthyretin (*Ttr*, a retinol-binding protein), *Raldh1* (RA synthesis), *Crapb1* (transport) and *Cyp26 B1* (degradation), all of which are elevated in long days (Helfer et al. 2012; Shearer et al. 2010, 2012).

The functional significance of retinoic acid production in tanycytes is yet to be established, but in the photoperiodic F344 rat where the effect of retinoic acid has been investigated in most detail, evidence would suggest retinoic acid may regulate chemerin (*Rarres2*), a cytokine and a target of retinoic acid signalling. Chemerin is expressed in tanycytes of F344 rats with higher expression in long compared to short days. In short-day exposed F344 rats, chemerin administered intracerebroventricularly for 28 days increases *vimentin* mRNA and protein levels, and produces a transient increase in food intake, all consistent with the transition to, and establishment of, the long-day state (Helfer et al. 2016). Retinoic acid may also have a role in regulating neurogenesis (see Sect. 3.7).

3.7 Tanycytes: A Seasonal Neural Stem Cell Niche

There is now good evidence that tanycytes are a stem cell niche, and an important question is whether this is of relevance to the control of physiology and behaviour in seasonal animals. In mice, neural stem cell (NSC) activity of β2 tanycytes is enhanced by a high-fat diet (Lee et al. 2012), setting a precedent for NSC responsiveness to an environmental factor. Annual change in photoperiod is a universal environmental factor and therefore it is not surprising that seasonal photoperiod may influence NSC activity.

There are several lines of evidence to support the potential for differential NSC activity in relation to photoperiod. It has been known for some time that in the Syrian hamster, short-day exposure increases the incorporation of the uridine analogue BrdU into newly synthesised DNA of actively dividing cells in several regions of the brain, including the hypothalamus (Huang et al. 1998; the location not defined in this early study). In the F344 rat, immunohistochemical detection of the proliferation marker Ki67 shows significantly more Ki67-labelled cells located in the ependymal layer in a short-day photoperiod (Shearer et al. 2012). In the Siberian hamster *vimentin* and *nestin*, markers associated with neural stem cells, decrease with short-day exposure (Kameda et al. 2003; Barrett et al. 2006). Moreover, in sheep, several markers of NSC cells can be detected in tanycytes, including *vimentin*, *nestin*, *Dcx* (doublecortin) and *Sox2*. The expression of these markers and BrdU incorporation in tanycytes have been shown to change across the year, with the highest stem cell activity in the months of autumn and winter (Migaud et al. 2011; Batailler et al. 2016; Butruille et al. 2018)—see Chap. 4. Furthermore, expression of PSA-NCAM, a protein found in migratory neuroblasts, is highest in the arcuate nucleus in autumn, which may be indicative of active migration (Butruille et al. 2018). Of course once derived, new neurons must migrate to specific brain regions and differentiate to neuronal cells to facilitate physiological adaptations. This poses important questions, such as: what permits or stimulates NSC activity, how many neurons are generated and to which regions of the hypothalamus do they migrate? Retinoic acid produced by tanycytes may be involved as it is known to inhibit NSC activity and induce differentiation. Consistent with this is the up-regulation of retinoic acid signalling components in tanycytes in long days and the observation that retinoic acid inhibits EGF stimulated NSC activation in the ependymal layer of F344 rats (Shearer et al. 2012).

Notably, seasonal variation in neurogenesis may be more extensive than the tanycyte stem cell niche; the brain of male meadow voles varies in weight and DNA content according to photoperiod (Dark et al. 1990), so it is unlikely that one source of proliferation accounts for a measurable difference in these parameters; seasonal variation in neurogenesis has been shown in the hippocampus of birds (Sherry and Hoshooley 2010), and in the Syrian hamster where photoperiod-dependent neurogenesis occurs in several areas of the brain, including the sub-ependymal layer of the lateral ventricles, cingulate/retrosplenial cortex and dentate gyrus of the hippocampus with NSC activity detected within 10 days of transfer from long to short days (Huang et al. 1998). This raises important questions including—how is neural stem cell activity regulated at such diverse regions of the brain? Is it the same mechanism of activation and how is a change in photoperiod length communicated to these spatially unrelated regions of the brain?

3.8 Regulation of Tanycyte Functions in a Natural Environment

To date the vast majority of experimental data has been derived from animals housed in laboratory settings and kept in artificial, fixed-length photoperiods, representing long and short days, with seasonal adaptations brought about by switching animals between these two photoperiods for an appropriate duration (square wave paradigm, Fig. 3.6a). These experiments often have a defined duration that is determined by a measurable physiological adaptation, e.g. body weight or testis mass. This experimental convenience has the advantage that studies can be performed at any time of the year and allows experiments to be conducted within animal facilities where temperature is held constant. This means that temperature as a potential variable can be ruled out as contributing to the physiological adaptations. Thus, data gathered from experiments performed using the square-wave paradigm have been used to infer and derive hypotheses as to the role of a specific genes in the context of seasonal and physiological adaptations. However, an abrupt transition between

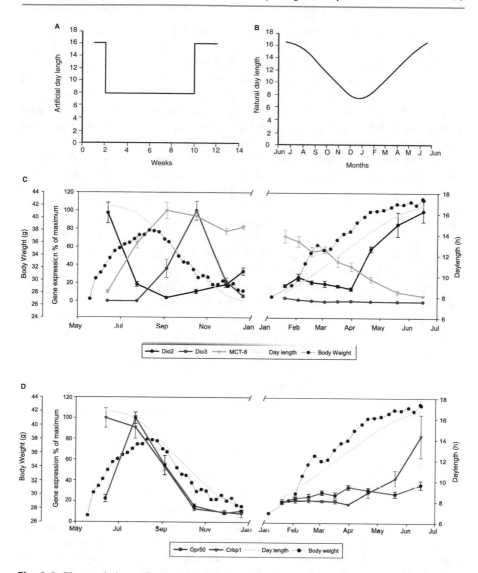

Fig. 3.6 Photoperiod paradigms and gene expression in tanycytes across a seasonal cycle. The duration of the light exposure received (y-axis) using: (**a**) 'square wave' paradigm where animals are exposed to artificial fixed photoperiods for defined lengths of time, (**b**) the decremental/incremental changes in day length over the course of a year in natural photoperiod, animals experience a small change every day in a natural environment. (**c**) Temporal expression profile for thyroid hormone–signalling components deiodinase 2 (*Dio2*), deiodinase 3 (*Dio3*) and monocarboxylate transporter 8 (*Mct8*) mRNAs over the course of one annual cycle in natural day length. (**d**) Temporal expression profile of *Gpr50* and cellular retinol-binding protein (*Crbp1*) mRNA expression in tanycytes over the course of one annual cycle of natural day length. Panels (**c**) and (**d**) are modified from Petri et al. 2016, *Scientific reports* 6:29689

fixed-length photoperiods to mimic long and short days is not representative of the natural environment where photoperiod changes occur in increments or decrements of seconds to minutes on a daily basis (Fig. 3.6b). Photoperiodic history is also a key element of the physiological response to a change in photoperiod length; i.e. the animal detects whether a day with 10-h light and 14-h darkness occurs when day length is increasing in spring or decreasing in autumn. So how do transcriptional changes in tanycytes reflect incremental changes in photoperiod and does this alter our thinking on the roles of specific genes, for example the deiodinases?

Only a limited number of experiments have investigated transcriptional events in tanycytes in natural photoperiod, but only one study in Siberian hamsters has comprehensively sampled at frequent time points throughout the course of the year (Petri et al. 2016). This study has provided some surprising new information about the temporal expression patterns of a limited number of tanycyte-expressed genes, including components of the thyroid hormone–signalling system (*Dio2*, *Dio3* and *Mct8*), retinoic acid system (*Crbp1*), intermediate filament proteins (*nestin* and *vimentin*) and the orphan receptor *Gpr50* (Fig. 3.6c, d).

In these experiments, hamsters were born from late February and raised in natural photoperiod and climate in outdoor facilities in the Northern hemisphere (52° N latitude). Male hamsters were assessed for gene expression in the hypothalamus from approximately 3 months old (late May onwards), over time points extending to mid-June of the following year. In situ hybridisation was used to analyse gene expression in tanycytes and neurons. The temporal gene expression pattern revealed would not have been discovered using the square-wave paradigm normally used in standard laboratory conditions. Importantly, the data raise fundamental questions about the role and function the genes analysed and challenge previous assumptions about their role in the photoperiodic response.

Given the current consensus that thyroid hormone signalling is the determinant of seasonal physiology, a key question was how do thyroid hormone–signalling components respond in natural photoperiod? In natural photoperiod, *Dio2* mRNA showed a high level of expression in late May, the first time point assessed, yet by mid-July it had decreased to less than 20% of the measured maximal expression (Petri et al. 2016). In a second experiment, the decline in *Dio2* occurred before the summer solstice (Petri et al. 2016), suggesting that *Dio2* gene expression shows a long-day photorefractory response, as in sheep. However, body weight and testis weight still continued to increase as *Dio2* mRNA approached minimal expression (~4% of maximum, Fig. 3.6b). Between mid-July and the beginning of April of the following year (i.e. after the vernal equinox, when day length has exceeded 12 h), *Dio2* mRNA levels remained at near-minimal expression values. However, from early February, body weight increased and reproductive recrudescence was re-established. Hence, does this mean thyroid hormone is not responsible for driving long-day physiology? *Dio2* mRNA level did not show a significant increase in expression until mid-April onwards or approximately 6 weeks after the vernal equinox. This time point may be significant as day length at mid-April exceeds the value at which exogenous melatonin or transfer to back to short days is able to re-initiate winter physiology (Butler et al. 2010). This might suggest that although

T3 can drive long-day physiology when administered exogenously, endogenously it acts to reset a mechanism to allow the hamster to respond to short days once more (i.e. melatonin).

In natural photoperiod, *Dio3* mRNA expression increased late August to early September. This coincides with the onset of body weight loss and testicular regression. At peak expression of *Dio3* mRNA, body weight and testis weights decreased to close to their minimal values. This suggests body weight and other short-day physiological adaptations may not occur until *Dio3* gene expression has been initiated. One explanation may be that even though *Dio2* mRNA is at a very low level, there is sufficient T3 present to maintain long-day characteristics until *Dio3* is expressed. Similar to experiments using the square-wave paradigm, *Dio3* gene expression becomes photorefractory (Barrett et al. 2007), i.e. expression decreases over a period of approximately 8 weeks becoming absent during the month of December despite the further decrease in day length approaching the winter solstice. One hypothesis for the initiation of the reversal of the short-day physiological state in late January or early February while day length is still much less than 12 h, would be that this is when *Dio3* expression has been completely silenced. The measurable, yet low level of *Dio2* mRNA, may then be sufficient to produce enough DIO2 enzyme to drive the development of long-day physiology in early spring—a hypothesis to be tested!

In natural photoperiod *Mct8* mRNA was almost absent in May, which contrasts to a measurable level of expression in long-day hamsters using the square-wave paradigm. Thereafter, *Mct8* mRNA quickly increased to achieve a peak value by early September. Subsequently, *Mct8* mRNA gradually declined reaching significance in late January, shortly before the start of a body weight increase and continued to decline, reaching absence in late May to early June the following year. This raises the question whether there is a direct link between the decline of *Mct8* mRNA and the advent of spring physiology. Could the increase in *Mct8* mRNA in early September followed by the gradual decline be the key event in seasonal physiological adaptations? These natural photoperiod experiments have revealed a temporal relationship between thyroid hormone–signalling components and seasonal physiology, which have not been observed using a square-wave paradigm. The regulation of *Dio2* expression in natural photoperiod contrasts (but does not contradict) with the expression data using the square-wave paradigm. In the latter paradigm, *Dio2* expression may not show any difference in expression between long- and short-day exposure (Barrett et al. 2007), but when hamsters are switched from short to long photoperiod, *Dio2* expression is substantially increased (Herwig et al. 2013). One explanation for this difference may lie in the length of time the hamsters have been housed in long days prior to use in experiment. If as suggested *Dio2* expression declines as a result of a long-day refractory response, which may happen at a relatively early age in a static long photoperiod (Herwig et al. 2012), at 3 months of age, when hamsters are generally used in experiments, *Dio2* may already be at or near a minimal level of expression and thus show little or no further reduction when transferred to short days. Similarly, the low level of expression of *Mct8* in May after birth and subsequent rise in expression, contrasts with a more established expression level in 3-month-old hamsters in long days and a relative small increase in *Mct8* expression, which can be observed on switch to short days (Herwig et al. 2013).

The retinol transport protein, *Crbp1,* was maximally expressed in late-May (similar to long-day fixed-length photoperiod), then showed a gradual decline from late August to near absence by late October (similar to hamsters housed in long day switched to short day). Thereafter, *Crbp1* expression remains at near absence until late-May of the following year when expression gradually increases. However, this temporal response of *Crbp1* is surprising as there are high levels of expression in long days (Ross et al. 2004). Thus, it is of interest to note that this gene only regained 50% of maximal expression after 6 weeks following a return to long-day from a short-day exposure using the square-wave paradigm (Ross et al. 2005). These data might infer the retinoic acid system does not play a significant role in driving long-day seasonal physiology in the hamster. However, a limited response of the retinoic acid system in the spring of the second year may reflect that the hamster is a short-lived species, generally not surviving more than 2 years in captivity and hence an ageing hamster having survived one winter, does not have the need to implement the activity of the retinoic acid system for a second year.

mRNA for the orphan G-protein coupled receptor, GPR50, showed a highly discrete interval of expression, rising from near absence in June of young adult hamsters to peak in early September before returning to absence by mid-October and remaining at near absent up to June of the following year. This contrasts with hamsters deployed in the square-wave paradigm, where *Gpr50* might be considered as a long-day expressed gene, but from the experiment in natural photoperiod, *Gpr50* expression is initiated in decreasing day lengths and becomes photorefractory, similar to *Dio3* mRNA expression. From gene knockout studies in mice, the absence of *Gpr50* is implicated in food-restricted-induced torpor (Bechtold et al. 2012). The timing of the peak of *Gpr50* expression in natural photoperiod in the hamster is interesting as this occurs approximately 12 weeks before the onset of torpor in mid-December, approximately the same interval of time for the induction of torpor in hamsters using the square-wave paradigm when transferred from long days to short days. Do these data point to a transient rise and then decline in GPR50 as the initiator of a process leading to torpor? This becomes a very intriguing question in light of recent evidence, which indicates a ligand-independent cleavage of the carboxy-terminal tail between amino acids 408 and 409 by a calcium-dependent calpain protease, generates a protein fragment, which translocates to the nucleus and can activate transcription (Ahamad et al. 2020).

3.9 Perspectives

Tanycytes were overlooked in a surge of research that has focussed on the role of neurons of the hypothalamus. However, a few key findings have transformed the status of these cells to parity with neurons. They are a vital component of the hypothalamic architecture, forming a BBB-regulating transport for permissive molecules, while excluding others and functioning as nutrient sensors to communicate information about metabolic status. They also play an important role in regulating neuropeptide access to the pituitary. In seasonal animals, thyroid hormone synthesis or degradation by tanycytes may be a pivotal element in the timing of physiology to take advantage of favourable environmental conditions in spring and summer and protect against adverse conditions from the onset of autumn into winter. Although in situ hybridisation studies have revealed many gene expression changes, much of our interpretation of the role of these genes in the mechanism underpinning the physiological responses has come from experiments using fixed-length photoperiod representing long and short days in a square-wave paradigm. However, a natural photoperiod experiment reveals the temporal relationship of a restricted set of tanycyte genes. The temporal expression in natural photoperiod is not aligned to predictions from experiments using square-wave paradigms, indicating that photoperiodic history and timing are likely to be important factors in the function of photoperiod-regulated genes. More studies conducted in natural photoperiod conditions are clearly required, in order to gain insight into the relationship between hypothalamic gene expression and physiology. This is also an important consideration for gene manipulation studies, where viral technologies or CRISPR are to be undertaken. In summary, tanycytes are a highly dynamic cell type producing a physiological pivotal hormone regulated by photoperiod and constitute a key element of seasonal physiology.

Acknowledgments We would like to thank Pat Bain at the Rowett Institute for the constructing the figures for this chapter. This work was supported by the Scottish Government Rural and Environment Science and Analytical Services Division to the Rowett Institute.

References

Adam CL, Findlay PA, Miller DW (2006) Blood-brain leptin transport and appetite and reproductive neuroendocrine responses to intracerebroventricular leptin injection in sheep: influence of photoperiod. Endocrinology 147:4589–4598

Ahamad R, Lahuna O, Sidibe A, Daulat A, Zhang Q, Luka M, Guillaume J-L, Gallet S, Guillonneau F, Hamroune J, Polo S, Prévot V, Delagrange P, Dam J, Jockers R (2020) GPR50-Ctail cleavage and nuclear translocation: a new signal transduction mode for G protein-coupled receptors. Cell Mol Life Sci. https://doi.org/10.1007/s00018-019-03440-7

Anderson GM, Hardy SL, Valent M, Billings HJ, Connors JM, Goodman RL (2003) Evidence that thyroid hormones act in the ventromedial preoptic area and the premammillary region of the brain to allow the termination of the breeding season in the ewe. Endocrinology 145:5252–5258

Arendt J, Symons AM, English J, Poulton AL, Tobler I (1988) How does melatonin control seasonal reproductive cycles. Reprod Nutr Dev 28:387–397

Balland E, Dam J, Langlet F, Caron E, Steculorum S, Messina A, Rasika S, Falluel-Morel A, Anouar Y, Dehouck B, Trinquet E, Jockers R, Bouret SG, Prevot V (2014) Hypothalamic tanycytes are an ERK-Gated conduit for leptin into the brain. Cell Metab 19:293–301

Barrett P, Ivanova E, Graham ES, Ross AW, Wilson D, Ple H, Mercer JG, Ebling FJP, Schuhler S, Dupre SM, Loudon A, Morgan PJ (2006) Photoperiodic regulation of cellular retinoic acid binding protein 1, GPR50 and nestin in tanycytes of the third ventricle ependymal layer of the Siberian hamster. J Endocrinol 191:687–698

Barrett P, Ebling FJP, Schuhler S, Wilson D, Ross AW, Warner A, Jethwa P, Boelen A, Visser TJ, Ozanne DM, Archer ZA, Mercer JG, Morgan PJ (2007) Hypothalamic thyroid hormone catabolism acts as a gatekeeper for the seasonal control of body weight and reproduction. Endocrinology 148:3608–3617

Bartness TJ, Goldman BD (1989) Mammalian pineal melatonin: a clock for all seasons. Experientia 45:939–945

Batailler M, Derouet L, Butruille L, Migaud M (2016) Sensitivity to the photoperiod and migratory features of neuroblasts in the adult sheep hypothalamus. Brain Struct Funct 221:3301–3314

Bechtold DA, Sidibe A, Saer BRC, Li J, Hand LE, Ivanova EA, Darras VM, Dam J, Jockers R, Luckman SM, Loudon ASI (2012) A role for the melatonin-related receptor GPR50 in leptin signalling, adaptive thermogenesis and torpor. Curr Biol 22:70–77

Benford H, Boborea M, Pollatzek E, Lossow K, Hermans-Borgmeyer I, Liu B, Meyherf W, Kasparov S, Dale N (2017) A sweet taste receptor-dependent mechanism of glucosensing in hypothalamic tanycytes. Glia 65:773–789

Bockers TM, Bockman J, Salem A, Nikowitz P, Lerchl A, Huppertz M, Wittkowski W, Kreutz MR (1997) Initial expression of the common α-chain in hypophyseal pars tuberalis-specific cells in spontaneous recrudescent hamsters. Endocrinology 138:4101–4108

Bolborea M, Helfer G, Ebling FJP, Barrett P (2015) Dual signal transduction pathways activated by TSH receptors in rat primary tanycyte cultures. J Mol Endocrinol 54:241–250

Brawer JR, Gustafson AW (1979) Changes in the fine structure of tanycytes during the annual reproductive cycle of the male little brown bat Myotis lucifugus lucifugus. Am J Anat 154:497–507

Butler MP, Turner KW, Park JH, Schoomer EE, Zucker I, Gorman MR (2010) Seasonal regulation of reproduction: altered role of melatonin under naturalistic conditions in hamsters. Proc R Soc Lond B 277:2867–2874

Butruille L, Bataliller M, Mazur D, Prevot V, Miguad M (2018) Seasonal reorganization of hypothalamic neurogenic niche in adult sheep. Brain Struct Funct 223:91–109

Campbell JN, Maccosko EZ, Fenselau H, Pers TH, Lyubetskaya A, Tenen D, Goldman M, Verstegen AMJ, Resch JM, McCarroll SA, Rosen ED, Lowell BB, Tsai LT (2017) A molecular census of arcuate hypothalamus and median eminence cell types. Nat Neurosci 20:484–496

Chaker Z, George C, Petrovska M, Caron J-P, Lacube P, Caille I, Holzenberger M (2016) Hypothalamic neurogenesis persists in the aging brain and is controlled by energy-sensing IGF-1 pathway. Neurobiol Aging 41:64–72

Clasadonte J, Prevot V (2017) The special relationship: glia-neuron interactions in the neuroendocrine hypothalamus. Nat Rev Endocrinol 14:25–44

Coppola A, Liu Z-W, Andrews ZB, Paradis E, Roy M-C, Friedman JM, Ricquier D, Richard D, Horvath TL, Gao X-B, Sabrina D (2007) A central thermogenic-like mechanism in feeding regulation: an interplay between the arcuate nucleus, T3 and UCP2. Cell Metab 5:21–33

Dark J, Spears N, Whaling CS, Wade GN, Meyer JS, Zucker I (1990) Long day lengths promote brain growth in meadow voles. Dev Brain Res 53:264–269

Frayling C, Britton R, Dale D (2011) ATP-mediated glucosensing by hypothalamic tanycytes. J Physiol 589:2275–2286

Goldman BD, Gwinner E, Karsch FJ, Saunders D, Zucker I, Ball GF (2004) Circannual rhythms and photoperiodism. In: Dunlap JC, Loros JJ, DeCoursey PJ (eds) Chronobiology—biological timekeeping. Sinauer Associates, Sunderland, MA, pp 107–142

Guerra M, Blazquez JL, Peruzzo B, Pelaez B, Radriguez S, Toranzo D, Pastor F, Rodriguez EM (2010) Cell organization of the rat pars tuberalis. Evidence for open communication between pars tuberalis, cerebrospinal fluid and tanycytes. Cell Tissue Res 339:359–381

Hagedoorn J (1965) Seasonal changes in the ependymal of the third ventricle of the skunk, Mephitis mephitis nigra. Anat Rec 151:453. (Abstract)

Hann N, Goodman T, Najdl-Samiei A, Stratford CM, Rice R, El Agha E, Bellusci S, Hajihosseini MK (2013) Fgf10-expressing tanycytes add new neurons to the appetite/energy-balance regulating centers of the postnatal and adult hypothalamus. J Neurosci 33:6170–6180

Hanon EA, Lincln GA, Fustin J-M, Dardente H, Masson-Pevet M, Morgan PJ, Hazlerigg DG (2008) Ancestral TSH mechanism signals summer in a photoperiodic mammal. Curr Biol 18:1147–1152

Hanon EA, Routledge H, Dardente M, Masson-Pevet M, Morgan PJ, Hazlerigg DG (2009) Effect of photoperiod on the thyroid stimulating hormone neuroendocrine system in the European hamster (Cricetus cricetus). J Neuroendocrinol 22:51–55

Hartfuss E, Galli R, Heins N, Gotz M (2001) Characterization of CNS precursor subtypes and radial glia. Dev Biol 229:15–30

Heideman PD, Sylvester CJ (1997) Reproductive photoresponsiveness in unmanipulated male Fischer F344 laboratory rats. Biol Reprod 57:134–138

Helfer G, Tups A (2016) Hypothalamic Wnt signalling and its role in energy balance regulation. J Neuroendocrinol 28:12368

Helfer G, Ross AW, Russell L, Thomson LM, Shearer KD, Goodman TH, McCaffery PJ, Morgan PJ (2012) Photoperiod regulates Vitamin A and Wnt/β-catenin signalling in F344 rats. Endocrinology 153:815–824

Helfer G, Ross AW, Morgan PJ (2013) Neuromedin U partly mimics thyroid-stimulating hormone and triggers Wnt/β-Catenin signalling in the photoperiodic response of F344 rats. J Neuroendocrinol 25:1264–1272

Helfer G, Ross AW, Thomson LM, Mayer CD, Stoney PN, McCaffery PJ, Morgan PJ (2016) A neuroendocrine role for chemerin in hypothalamic remodelling and photoperiodic control of energy balance. Sci Rep 6:e26830

Herwig A, Wilson D, Logie TJ, Boelen A, Morgan PJ, Mercer JG, Barrett P (2009) Photoperiod and acute energy deficits interact on components of the thyroid hormone system in hypothalamic tanycytes of the Siberian hamster. Am J Physiol Regul Integr Comp Physiol 296:R1307–R1315

Herwig A, Petri I, Barrett P (2012) Hypothalamic gene expression rapidly changes in response to photoperiod in juvenile Siberian hamsters (Phodopus sungorus). J Neuroendocrinol 24:991–998

Herwig A, de Vries EM, Bolborea M, Wilson D, Mercer JG, Ebling FJP, Morgan PJ, Barrett P (2013) Hypothalamic ventricular ependymal thyroid hormone deiodinases are an important element of circannual timing in the Siberian hamster (Phodopus sungorus). PLoS One 8:e62003

Horstmann E (1954) Die Faserglia des Salachiergehirns. Z Zellforsch 39:588–617

Herwig A, Campbell G, Mayer CD, Boelen A, Anderson R, Ross AW, Mercer JG, Barrett P (2014) A thyroid hormone challenge in hypothyroid rats identifies T3 regulated genes in the hypothalamus and in models with altered energy balance and glucose homeostasis. Thyroid 24:1575–1593

Huang L, DeVries GJ, Bittman EL (1998) Photoperiod regulates neuronal bromodeoxyuridine labelling in the brain of a seasonally breeding mammal. J Neurobiol 36:410–420

Kameda Y, Arai Y, Nishimaki T (2003) Ultrastructural localization of vimentin immunoreactivity and gene expression in tanycytes and their alterations in hamsters kept under different photoperiods. Cell Tissue Res 314:251–262

Krol E, Douglas A, Dardente H, Birnie MJ, Van der Vinne V, Eijer WG, Gerkema MP, Hazlerigg DG, Hut RA (2012) Strong pituitary and hypothalamic responses to photoperiod but not 6-methoxy-2-benzoxalinone in female common voles (Microtus arvalis). Gen Comp Endocrinol 179:289–295

Langlet F, Levin BE, Luquet S, Mazzone M, Messina A, Dunn-Myenell AA, Balland E, Lacome A, Mazur D, Carmeliet P, Bouret SG, Prevot V, Dehouck B (2013) Tanycytic VEGF-A boosts blood-hypothalamus barrier plasticity and access of metabolic signal to the arcuate nucleus in response to fasting. Cell Metab 17:607–617

Lazutkaite G, Solda A, Lossow K, Meyherhof W, Dale N (2017) Amino acid sensing in hypothalamic tanycytes via umami taste receptors. Mol Metab 6:1480–1492

Lee DA, Bedont JL, Pak T, Wang H, Song J, Miranda-Angulo A, Takiar V, Charubhumi V, Balordi F, Takebayashi H, Aja S, Ford E, Fishell G, Blackshaw S (2012) Tanycytes of the hypothalamic median eminence form a diet-responsive neurogenic niche. Nat Neurosci 15:700–702

Lomet D, Cognie J, Chesneau D, Dubois E, Hazlerigg D, Dardente H (2018) The impact of thyroid hormone in seasonal breeding has a restricted transcriptional signature. Cell Mol Life Sci 75:905–919

Migaud M, Batailler M, Pillon D, Franceschini I, Malpaux B (2011) Seasonal changes in cell proliferation in the adult sheep brain and pars tuberalis. J Biol Rhythm 26:486–496

Milesi S, Simmoneaux V, Klosen V (2017) Down regulation of deiodinase 3 is the earliest event in photoperiod and photorefractory activation of the gonadotropic axis in seasonal hamsters. Sci Rep 7:e17739

Miranda-Angulo AL, Byerly MS, Mesa J, Wang H, Blackshaw S (2014) Rax regulates hypothalamic tanycyte differentiation and barrier function in mice. J Comp Neurol 522:876–899

Morgan PJ, Barrett P, Howell HE, Helliwell R (1994) Melatonin receptors: localization, molecular pharmacology and physiological significance. Neurochem Int 24:101–146

Muller J, Heuer H (2014) Expression pattern of thyroid hormone transporters in the postnatal mouse brain. Front Endocrinol 5:92

Mullier A, Bouret SG, Prevot V, Dehouck B (2010) differential distribution of tight junction proteins suggests a role for tanycytes in blood-hypothalamus barrier regulation in the adult mouse brain. J Comp Neurol 518:943–962

Murphy M, Jethwa PH, Warner A, Barrett P, Nilaweera KN, Brameld JM, Ebling FJP (2012) Effects of manipulating hypothalamic triiodothyronine concentrations on seasonal body weight and torpor cycles in Siberian hamsters. Endocrinology 153:101–112

Murphy M, Samms R, Warner A, Bolborea M, Fowler MJ, Brameld JM, Tsintzas K, Kharitonenkov A, Adams AC, Coskun T, Ebling FJP (2013) Increased responses to the actions of fibroblast growth factor 21 on energy balance and body weight in a seasonal model of adiposity. J Neuroendocrinol 25:180–189

Nakane Y, Ikegami K, Iigo M, Ono H, Takeda K, Takahashi D, Uesaka M, Kimijima M, Hashimoto R, Arai N, Suga T, Kosuge K, Abe T, Maeda R, Senga T, Amiya N, Azuma T, Amano M, Abe H, Yamamoto N, Yoshimura T (2013) The saccus vasculosus of fish is a sensor of seasonal changes in day length. Nat Commun 4:2108

Nakane Y, Yoshimura T (2014) Universality and diversity in the signal transduction pathway that regulates seasonal reproduction in vertebrates. Front Neurosci 8:e115

Nakao N, Takagi T, Ligo M, Tsukamoto T, Yasuo S, Masuda T, Yangisawa T, Ebihara S, Yoshimura T (2006) Possible involvement of organic anion transporting polypeptide 1c1 in the photoperiodic response of gonads in birds. Endocrinology 147:1067–1073

Nilaweera N, Herwig A, Bolborea M, Campbell G, Mayer CD, Morgan PJ, Ebling FJP, Barrett P (2011) Photoperiodic regulation of glycogen metabolism, glycolysis and glutamine synthesis in tanycytes of the Siberian hamster suggests novel roles of tanycytes in hypothalamic function. Glia 59:1695–1705

Petri I, Diedrich V, Wilson D, Fernandez-Calleja J, Herwig A, Steinlechner S, Barrett P (2016) Orchestration of gene expression across the seasons: Hypothalamic gene expression in natural photoperiod throughout the year in the Siberian hamster. Sci Rep 6:e29689

Prevot V, Croix D, Bouret S, Dutoit S, Tramu G, Sefano GB, Beauvillain JC (1999) Definitive evidence for the existence of morphological plasticity in the external zone of the median eminence during the rat estrous cycle: implication of neuro-glio-endothelial interactions in gonadotrophin-releasing hormone release. Neuroscience 94:809–819

Reppert SM, Weaver DR (2001) Molecular analysis of mammalian circadian rhythms. Annu Rev Physiol 63:647–676

Revel FG, Saboureau M, Pevet P, Mikkelsen JD, Simmoneaux V (2006) Melatonin regulates type 2 deiodinase gene expression in the Syrian hamster. Endocrinology 147:4680–4687

Roberts LM, Woodford K, Zhou M, Black DS, Haggerty JE, Tate EH, Grindstaff KK, Mengesha W, Raman C, Zerangue N (2008) Expression of the thyroid hormone transporters monocarboxylate transporter-8 (SLC16A2) and organic ion transporter-14 (SLCO1C1) at the blood-brain barrier. Endocrinology 149:6251–6261

Robins SC, Stewart I, McNay DE, Taylor V, Giachino C, Goetz M, Ninkovic J, Briancon N, Maratos-Flier E, Flier JS, Kokoeva MV, Placzek M (2013) alpha-tanycytes of the adult hypothalamic third ventricle include distinct populations of FGF-responsive neural progenitors. Nature. Communications 4:2049

Rodriguez EM, Blazquez JL, Pastor FE, Pelaex B, Pena P, Peruzzo B, Amat P (2005) Hypothalamic tanycytes: a key component of brain-endocrine interaction. Int Rev Cytol 247:89–164

Ross AW, Webster CA, Mercer JG, Moar KM, Ebling FJ, Schuhler S, Barrett P, Morgan PJ (2004) Photoperiodic regulation of hypothalamic retinoid signalling: association of retinoid X receptor γ with body weight. Endocrinology 145:13–20

Ross AW, Bell LM, Littlewood PA, Mercer JG, Barrett P, Morgan PJ (2005) Temporal changes in gene expression in the arcuate nucleus precede seasonal responses in adiposity and reproduction. Endocrinology 146:1940–1947

Ross AW, Johnson CE, Bell LM, Reilly L, Duncan JS, Barrett P, Heideman PD, Morgan PJ (2009) Divergent regulation of hypothalamic neuropeptide Y and agouti-related protein by photoperiod in F344 rats with differential food intake and growth. J Neuroendocrinol 21:610–619

Ross AW, Helfer G, Russell L, Darras VM, Morgan PJ (2011) Thyroid hormone signalling genes are regulated by photoperiod in the hypothalamus of F344 rats. PLoS One 6:e21351

Rousseau K, Atcha Z, Cagampang FRA, Le Rouzic P, Stirland AJ, Ivanov T, Ebling FJP, Klingspor M, Loudon ASI (2002) Photoperiodic regulation of leptin resistance in the seasonally breeding Siberian hamster (Phodopus sungorus). Endocrinology 143:3083–3095

Sanez de Miera C, Hanon EA, Dardente H, Birnie M, Simmoneaux V, Lincoln GA, Hazlerigg DG (2013) Circannual variation in thyroid hormone deiodinases in short-day breeder. J Neuroendocrinol 25:412–421

Shearer KD, Goodman TH, Ross AW, Reilly L, Morgan PJ, McCaffery PJ (2010) Photoperiod regulation of retinoic acid signalling in the hypothalamus. J Neurochem 112.246–257

Shearer KD, Stoney PN, Nanescu SE, Helfer G, Barrett P, Ross AW, Morgan PJ, McCaffery P (2012) Photoperiodic expression of tow RALDH enzymes and the regulation of cell proliferation by retinoic acid in the rat hypothalamus. J Neurochem 122:789–799

Sherry DF, Hoshooley JS (2010) Seasonal hippocampal plasticity in food-storing birds. Philos Trans R Soc Lond B Biol Sci 365:933–943

Stevenson TJ, Prendergast BJ (2014) Reversible DNA methylation regulates seasonal photoperiodic time measurement. Proc Natl Acad Sci USA 111:4645–4646

Tups A, Stohr S, Helwig M, Barrett P, Krol E, Schachtner J, Mercer JG, Klingspor M (2012) Seasonal leptin resistance is associated with impaired signalling via JAK2-STAT3 but not ERK, possibly mediated by reduced hypothalamic GRB2 protein. J Comp Physiol B 182:553–567

Watanabe T, Yamamura T, Watanabe M, Yasuo S, Nakao N, Dawson A, Ebihara S, Yoshimura T (2007) Hypothalamic expression of thyroid hormone-activating and –inactivating enzyme genes in relation to photorefractoriness in birds and mammals. Am J Physiol Regul Integr Comp Physiol 292:R568–R572

Wittkowski W, Muller K (1976) Untersuchungen am infundibulum des Igles. Verh Anat Ges 70: S49–S54

Wood S, Loudon ASL (2018) The pars tuberalis: the site of the circannual clock in mammals? Gen Comp Endocrinol 258:222–235

Yamamura T, Yasuo S, Hirunagi K, Ebihara S, Yoshimura T (2006) T3 implantation mimics photoperiodically reduced encasement of nerve terminals by glial processes in the median eminence of Japanese quail. Cell Tissue Res 324:175–179

Yasuo S, Watanabe M, Takagi T, Follet BK, Ebihara S, Yoshimura T (2005) The reciprocal switching of two thyroid hormone-activating and -inactivation enzyme genes is involved in the photoperiodic gonadal response of Japanese quail. Endocrinology 146:2551–2554

Yoo S, Blackshaw S (2018) Regulation and function of neurogenesis in the adult mammalian hypothalamus. Prog Neurobiol 170:53–66

Yoshimura T, Yasuo S, Watanabe M, Iigo M, Yamamura T, Hirunagi K, Ebinhara S (2003) Light-induced hormone conversion of T4 to T3 regulates photoperiodic response of gonads in birds. Nature 426:178–181

Further Recommended Reading

Dardente H, Wood S, Ebling F, Sáenz de Miera C (2019) An integrative view of mammalian seasonal neuroendocrinology. J Neuroendocrinol 31(5):e12729

Helfer G, Barrett P, Morgan PJ (2019) A unifying hypothesis for control of body weight and reproduction in seasonally breeding mammals. J Neuroendocrinol 31(3):e12680. This is an excellent review, formulating our knowledge to date on the relationship between the pars tuberalis, tanycytes and hypothalamus into a hypothesis centering around neurogenic potential of tanycytes to unify seasonal regulation in both long and short-day responsive mammals.

Prevot V, Dehouck B, Sharif A, Ciofi P, Giacobini P, Clasadonte J (2018) The versatile tanycyte: a hypothalamic integrator of reproduction and energy metabolism Endocr Rev 39(3):333–368. An excellent review providing further information on the tanycyte-blood brain barrier relationship and tanycyte plasticity.

Rodríguez E, Guerra M, Peruzzo B, Blázquez JL (2019) Tanycytes: a rich morphological history to underpin future molecular and physiological investigations. J Neuroendocrinol 31:e12690. This paper brings together a wealth of observations on tanycytes which should be taken into consideration when formulating and testing hypotheses on molecular mechanisms in the role of tanycytes at the interface between the periphery and hypothalamus.

Epigenetic Mechanisms in Developmental and Seasonal Programs

4

Tyler J. Stevenson

Abstract

Developmental epigenetic modifications generally occur during cellular embryonic differentiation and impart permanent changes that last the individual's lifespan. It is now recognized that epigenetic modifications also exhibit rhythmic patterns that impact the timing of seasonal transitions in physiology and behaviour. This chapter explores the role of epigenetic modifications during mammalian development and photoperiodic programming of seasonal rhythms, focussing on the molecular and cellular substrates in the hypothalamus that regulate seasonal timing of reproduction. The chapter draws evidence from the well-established literature on genomic imprinting and maternal programming during mammalian development to identify common genomic, molecular and cellular signalling mechanisms. One mechanism common across developmental and seasonal programs that is highlighted is the role of thyroid hormones. Recent data indicate that the epigenetic regulation of thyroid hormone deiodinase enzymes is a critical feature of developmental and seasonal programming.

Keywords

Methylation · Acetylation · Hypothalamus · Reproduction · Hormone

T. J. Stevenson (✉)
Institute of Biodiversity, Animal Health and Comparative Medicine, University of Glasgow, Glasgow, UK
e-mail: Tyler.Stevenson@glasgow.ac.uk

F. J. P. Ebling, H. D. Piggins (eds.), *Neuroendocrine Clocks and Calendars*,
Masterclass in Neuroendocrinology 10, https://doi.org/10.1007/978-3-030-55643-3_4

4.1   Introduction

The research field of epigenetics has existed for over 60 years. The predominant approach has focused on early developmental programs or the role of environment-induced modifications to germ cells that are transmitted down subsequent generations. The fundamental basis of epigenetics was originally established by embryologists that were interested in the events early in development that spanned fertilization of the zygote through to the formation of the mature organism (Felsenfeld 2014). Subsequent observations during the genetic revolution of the 1990s illustrated that epigenetic modifications could also impact the genome of an individual, resulting in a modification to the germline that was passed down the generations (Nadeau 2009). For both the developmental and transgenerational epigenetic approaches, the effectors of the modifications are large families of enzymes that include DNA methyltransferases and tet methylcytosine dioxygenases for the regulation of genome modifications; and histone acetylases, histone deacetyltransferases and histone methyltransferases enzymes for the regulation of chromatin modifications. In addition to these well-characterised families of epigenetic enzymes, there is an emerging body of evidence that has implicated additional genome modifications such as non-coding RNA (ncRNA). The central tenet of the developmental and transgenerational modifications is the permanent impact of epigenetic modifications to the genome template. A new approach to the investigation of genome modifications has examined epigenomic oscillations, also referred to as rhythmic epigenetics. Studies that have investigated the patterns of epigenetic enzyme expression and epigenetic modifications (i.e. DNA methylation) have revealed reversible changes that occur over daily, estrous and seasonal timescales (Stevenson 2018). This chapter will focus on developmental and rhythmic epigenetics in mammalian species, and will explore whether these two genome modification timescales are simply variations of a common mechanism or consist of unique adaptive specializations.

4.2   Epigenetic Enzyme Families and Mode of Action

Epigenetic modifications include a range of biochemical changes that surround the genome template and include DNA methylation, histone methylation and histone acetylation. The general pattern for each modification is to regulate the probability of transcription for a target gene in a cell- and tissue-specific manner (but see Jones 2012). DNA methylation has been identified across multiple tissues, and is driven by evolutionarily conserved enzymes: DNA methyltransferases (Dnmt) and Ten eleven translocation methylcytosine dioxygenases (Tet). To date, three Dnmt enzymes have been identified: Dnmt1 and the de novo Dnmt3a and Dnmt3b, and likewise three Tet enzymes: Tet1, Tet2 and Tet3. DNA methylation is essential for embryonic and neonatal development, and loss-of-function in enzymes is lethal. Dnmt1 functions to maintain and establish DNA methylation, while 'de novo' Dnmt3a and Dnmt3b are required for ongoing maintenance of DNA methylation (Jones 2012). Dnmt3a and

Dnmt3b catalyse the transfer of methyl groups from S-adenosyl-L-methionine to specific genomic nucleotide base pairs, predominantly cytosine paired with guanine (Klose and Bird 2006). These enzymes act to silence gene transcription by increasing the levels of DNA methylation in the promoter region of target genes. Conversely, Tet1, Tet2 and Tet3 enzymes initiate the removal of DNA methylation by the hydroxylation of DNA methyl cytosine into 5-hydroxymethlcytosine. Tet1 is highly enriched on CpG islands, and associated with promoters and distal regulatory regions, and both Tet1 and Tet3 have been identified to bind genome-wide in a diffuse manner (Wu and Zhang 2011). Conversely, the localization of Tet2 recruitment to the genome has yet to be established (Rasmussen and Helin 2016). All Dnmt and Tet enzymes are expressed in the hypothalamus and are regulated by hormonal and endogenous (i.e. circadian clock genes) signals (Stevenson 2017a).

Modifications that alter the conformation of chromatin, such as acetylation of histones, are another mechanism to induce epigenetic control over gene transcription. The addition of an acetyl group to histones induces a widening of the chromatin, and facilitates the probability of gene transcription. Multiple enzymes have been identified to acetylate histones and include the histone acetyltransferases. The removal of acetyl-groups is accomplished by histone deacetylase enzymes. Histones that lack acetyl-groups form dense clusters or condensed heterochomatin that prevents the binding of transcription factors to the genome template (Struhl 1998).

Methylation of histone proteins involved in the regulation of chromatin function can permit as well as inhibit gene transcription. Depending on the specific histone protein lysine residue, methylation can induce a euchromatic conformation and permit gene transcription or trigger a heterochromatic state and subsequently inhibit gene transcription. For example, trimethylation of histone H3 at lysine 4 increases the probability of gene transcription, whereas histone H3 and lysine 27 trimethylation is observed in the heterochromatin and results in a repressive marker linked with gene silencing (Cao et al. 2002). The general pattern for epigenetic modifications is to induce stable, long-term changes in the probability of gene transcription. For example, during development, epigenetic modifications are induced in the embryo or pre-pubertal period and remain for the lifespan of the individual. A growing body of literature has indicated that epigenetic modifications are reversible and may oscillate across multiple timescales. For brevity, this chapter will focus on DNA methylation.

4.3   Epigenetic Modifications and Developmental Programs

Most of the published research on epigenetic modifications established during development have been uncovered using mouse and human cells. In mice, epigenomic programming during development occurs during two key stages: germ cell maturation and pre-implantation. The epigenomic programs during germ cell maturation include genomic imprinting, and pre-implantation of embryos can modify the established genomic imprints. There is a substantial reduction in DNA methylation in primordial germ cells that are subsequently remethylated in prospermatogonia on embryonic day 16 in males and after birth in growing oocytes

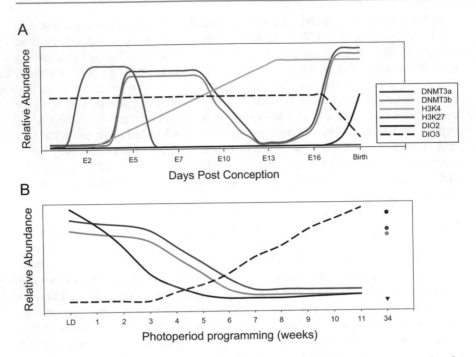

Fig. 4.1 Schematic representation of the time courses of hypothalamic gene expression for epigenetic modifiers including DNA methyltransferase 3a/3b (DNMT3a, DNMT3b) enzymes, two histone methyltransferase (H3K4, H3K27) enzymes and key regulators of development/ seasonal cyclicity such as Deiodinase Type-2 and -3 (DIO2, DIO3) enzymes in (**a**) mice and (**b**) Siberian hamsters

in females. Once the oocyte is fertilized the paternal genome undergoes demethylation, then, the maternal genome is demethylated. Shortly after implantation there is an increase in DNA methylation in the developing embryo (Seisenberger et al. 2012; Reik et al. 2001).

The change in DNA methylation levels during development is driven by the expression of Dnmt1 and de novo Dnmt3a and Dnmt3b enzymes (Fig. 4.1a). Around embryonic day 3 in the mouse (E3) there is an increase in both Dnmt3a and Dnmt3b expression that lasts until E9. The remethylation of genomic DNA is dynamic and heterogenous. During the early development period (E3–E9) there is a gradual acquisition of DNA methylation that is critical for cell differentiation. Then there is a gradual decline in expression that is increased again around E15 (Fig. 4.1a) (reviewed in Eckersley-Maslin et al. 2018). Conversely, histone trimethylation of histone protein-3 and lysine residue 4, a modification associated with an upregulation of transcript expression, is increased during development (i.e. E1–E3) (Fig. 4.1a). Subsequently, the trimethylation of lysine-27 occurs gradually during development and plateaus prior to parturition. Increased trimethylation of H4K27 acts to repress gene transcription and may act in conjunction with DNA methylation.

One critical event during embryo development involves parental-origin-specific gene expression, a process referred to as genome imprinting (Ferguson-Smith 2011). Several genomic loci have been identified to exhibit epigenetic modifications in imprinted genes, a classic example includes the gene Xist (Payer et al. 2011). In female mice, embryonic stems cells in the epiblast of the inner cell mass of the blastocyst contain two X sex chromosomes. In order to prevent X-linked gene dosage, the paternal X is preferentially inactivated by the Xist gene (Okamoto et al. 2004). The accumulation of histone trimethylation on the amino (N) terminal tail of the core histone H3 is a characteristic modification on inactive X-chromosomes (Plath et al. 2003). It is now estimated that several hundred genomic regions show parental-origin imprinting (Kelsey and Bartolomei 2012; DeVeale et al. 2012). Epigenetic modifications such as DNA methylation are pivotal for the establishment of parental imprinting of differentially methylated regions (Barlow and Bartolomei 2014). While it is generally established that genome imprinting via DNA methylation during gametogenesis is stable, there can be considerable tissue-specific variation of imprinted genes during development (Barton et al. 1991).

Another locus that has received considerable attention for the impact of genome imprinting of parent-of-origin gene expression is Dlk1-Dio3. The Dlk1-Dio3 locus contains three protein-coding genes: protein delta homolog 1 (Dlk1), retrotransposon-like 1 (Rtl1) and deiodinase type-3 (Dio3). Dlk1 is a transmembrane protein that belongs to the epidermal growth factor-like homeotic protein family and has been implicated in the differentiation of adipogenesis, haematopoiesis and neuroendocrine differentiation (Laborda 2000). Rtl1 is critical during foetal development, the maintenance of capillary endothelial cells and a low of functionality is lethal in mice (Sekita et al. 2008). Finally, the Dio3 gene is essential for the tissue- and cell-specific catabolism of thyroxine and triiodothyronine into reverse triiodo-thyronine and diiodothyronine, respectively (Bianco et al. 2002).

After fertilization and implantation, the growing embryo can be influenced by environmental factors experienced by the mother. Epigenomic effects established in utero and during early post-natal development are referred to as maternally programmed events. Maternally programmed modifications can be established by many different factors including low/high nutrient availability, exposure to abnormal levels of circulating hormones (e.g. glucocorticoids), prolonged stress and immune activation (Bilbo and Schwarz 2009; Lindsay et al. 2019). Despite genomic imprint-ing of the Dlk-Dio3 locus early in development, the hypothalamo-thyroid axis is established in mid- to late-gestation. Across humans, sheep and rats, thyrotropin-releasing hormone and thyrotropin-stimulating hormone expression are present after 10, 9 and 2 weeks, respectively (Forhead and Fowden 2014). However, maternal thyroxine and triiodothyronine can be transported through the placenta and into the fetus via thyroid hormone transporters (i.e. Mct8, Mct10). Thyroid hormone signal-ling is critical for brain development, as hypothyroidism and to a lesser extent hyperthyroidism can cause mental retardation, and congenic absence of the Mct8 transporter causes very severe neurological deficits in sensory, cognitive and motor function in humans (Friesema et al. 2004; Miranda and Sousa 2018). Given the epigenetic potential for genomic imprinting of the Dlk-Dio3 locus, and developmental programs established by thyroid hormone bioactivity, there is a strong likelihood that a similar pathway is required for seasonal programs (Saenz de Miera 2018).

4.4   Animal Models of Seasonal Rhythms

One prevailing question that researchers interested in the mechanisms of seasonal rhythms have focused much attention was 'which organisms are a suitable model'? The genetic revolution of the 1990s facilitated the generation of 'model organisms'; a few selected animals that spanned taxa and served to identify common genomic mechanisms that were involved in pathological and healthy conditions (Muller and Grossniklaus 2010). Model organisms possess many features in common, such as rapid generation times, being amenable to experimental manipulations, and some ability to translate findings into human clinical settings. Mouse models have been particularly important for developmental epigenetic research over the past 20 years (Blewitt and Whitelaw 2013). However, the artificial selection for reduced generation times has resulted in selection against those species that maintain long-term reproductive cycles, specifically seasonal breeding species. Instead, the field of seasonal biology has relied on animal species with a rich scientific literature that span decades of research. An analysis of publications in the PUBMED database using the key words 'photoperiod' or 'seasonal' produced an abundant number of studies that include a range of animals (Fig. 4.2). The most common organism identified in the publication database was 'hamster' (18%). Not surprisingly, the next organisms that were observed at a higher frequency were 'rat' (16%), 'arabidopsis' (14%) and 'mouse' (13%). Other notable animals associated with 'seasonal' were cattle (5%) and sheep (8%).

One major limitation for the lack of model organisms for seasonal rhythms has been the reliance on other animal genomes (i.e. mice). The past decade has seen an immense expansion in the availability of genomes, and future research will undoubtedly benefit from large-scale collaborations such as the Genome 10K (G10K) Consortium. The recent sequencing of seasonal rodent genomes, such as the Syrian hamster (*Mesocricetus auratus*; McCann et al. 2017) and Siberian hamster (*Phodopus sungorus*; Bao et al. 2019), has been incredibly useful for generating molecular tools to advance our understanding of the key genes involved in the control of seasonal rhythms. With the availability of a greater number of genomes from seasonal species, the field can start to advance the 'forward genetics' approach to determine the genomic basis of seasonal rhythms. Also, novel cutting-edge genome manipulation techniques, such as Cluster Regularly Interspaced Short Palindromic Repeats (CRISPR), can be used to selectively delete target genes of interest, so this permits advances in the functional analyses of genes implicated in seasonal rhythms. The Siberian hamster has been a useful model to investigate the role of epigenetic modifications for the generation and maintenance of seasonal rhythms (Stevenson 2018). There is now a growing literature and evidence to

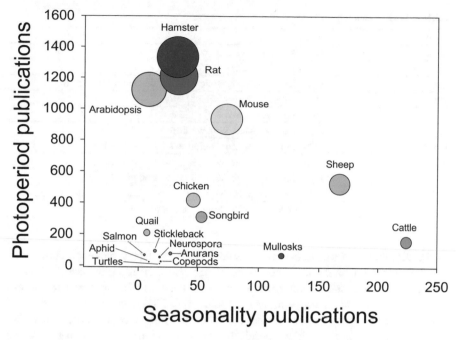

Fig. 4.2 Numbers of publications based on an analysis of the PubMed database in July 2019 using the search terms "photoperiod" or "seasonality" and species as indicated

indicate that seasonal and developmental epigenetic programs share many similarities, so these molecular markers will be discussed below.

4.5 Epigenetic Modifications and Seasonal Programs

Recent analyses of high throughput studies have revealed that epigenetic enzymes show robust circadian rhythmicity in multiple nuclei and tissues (Table 4.1). The main tissues that express rhythmic expression in epigenetic enzymes are the gonads, liver and hypothalamus. Evidence for daily rhythms in epigenetic enzyme expression indicates the modifications to the genome template are highly dynamic, robust and widespread. Here, the neuroendocrine regulation of seasonal rhythms and the potential role of epigenetic modifications as a central characteristic are presented.

Seasonal rhythms are common across taxa, yet the precise neural and mechanistic pathways that regulate annual change in peripheral physiology are not well described. Across vertebrates, the tanycyte cells bordering the 3rd ventricle are consistently implicated in the neuroendocrine control of seasonal physiology, including reproduction and energy balance (Ebling and Lewis 2018). Seasonal changes in photoperiodic information are coded by thyrotrophs in the *pars tuberalis* and subsequently signal to tanycytes via thyrotropin-stimulating hormone β subunit (Tshβ, Dupre 2011; Nakayama and Yoshimura 2018). Tanycytes are also involved

Table 4.1 Circadian rhythms in epigenetic enzymes

Enzyme	Tissue
dnmt3a	Hypothalamus, liver, lung
tet1	Brown adipose, kidney
tet2	Hypothalamus, liver, white adipose, skeletal muscle, heart
tet3	Hypothalamus, adrenal gland, lung
hdac1	Brown adipose, adrenal gland, heart
hdac3	SCN, adrenal gland, kidney, lung
hdac4	SCN, brain stem, white adipose, adrenal gland, heart, lung
hdac6	Hypothalamus, liver, white adipose, brown adipose
hdac8	Hypothalamus, brain stem, liver, adrenal gland, spleen
hdac9	SCN, brain stem, brown adipose, skeletal muscle, heart, spleen, lung
kat5	Hypothalamus, SCN, liver, skeletal muscle

in the detection and integration of internal signals in energy balance. These cells contact the cerebrospinal fluid and detect and transduce information associated with peripheral glucose concentrations to the arcuate nucleus and in turn regulate anorexigenic and orexigenic neuropeptides (Orellana et al. 2012). In addition to glucose, tanycytes can directly detect l-amino acids via the taste receptor type 1 member 1 gene, and therefore, can respond to changes in circulating nutrient levels (Lazutkaite et al. 2017). Altogether, these data highlight that tanycytes are central to the neuroendocrine integration of seasonal photoperiodic signalling and internal energy states (Bolborea and Dale 2013; Langlet 2014; Lewis and Ebling 2017).

A suite of molecular signalling pathways has been identified to reside within tanycytes that exhibit remarkable levels of plasticity across seasonal states (Petri et al. 2016). In mammals and birds, local synthesis of triiodothyronine (T_3) by tanycytes is a crucial step for the long-term morphological hypothalamic plasticity that governs annual changes in reproduction and energy balance (Yoshimura 2013; Nakane and Yoshimura 2014). Tanycyte cells express the two enzymes critical for the local synthesis of T_3, deiodinase type II (Dio2) and Dio3, as observed in quail (Yoshimura et al. 2003), songbirds (Rastogi et al. 2013; Ernst and Bentley 2016), sheep (Saenz de Miera et al. 2013) and hamsters (Stevenson and Prendergast 2013; Petri et al. 2016; Bao et al. 2019). In long-day breeding animals, summer-like long days (LD) stimulate greater T_3 hypothalamic content compared to animals exposed to winter-like short days (SD) (Yoshimura et al. 2003). Exogenous daily injections of T_3 in Siberian hamsters housed in SD are sufficient to induce testicular development (Banks et al. 2016; Freeman et al. 2007). In hamsters, LD photoperiods are associated with modest Dio2 and non-detectable levels of Dio3 expression (Petri et al. 2016). Prolonged exposure to SD (e.g. 8L:16D) results in a transient increase in Dio3 expression after 8–12 weeks, which subsequently declines to low levels of expression (Stevenson and Prendergast 2013; Petri et al. 2016). In mammals, the nocturnal duration of melatonin produced by the pineal is an internal code of photoperiod and the predominant driver of molecular signalling cascades involved in the neuroendocrine control of seasonal rhythms (Johnston and Skene 2015).

Melatonin binds to the melatonin receptor 1b located in the *pars tuberalis* and inhibits the production of Tshβ (Prendergast 2010). In LD, Tshβ expression in the *pars tuberalis* is high and stimulates the transcription of Dio2 in tanycytes (Nakao et al. 2008; Ono et al. 2008). In birds, melatonin is not necessary, nor sufficient to provide the internal physiological code for the photoperiodic regulation of seasonal rhythms (Juss et al. 1993). Instead, hypothalamic photoreceptors detect light directly and, in turn, regulate Dio2 and Dio3 tanycyte expression (Perez et al. 2019). Similar to mammals, LD photoperiods are associated with higher Dio2 and low Dio3 compared to SD conditions (Majumdar et al. 2015; Mishra et al. 2017). LD in both mammals and birds stimulates Dio2 activity, but the mechanisms that induce Dio3 in SD are not characterized. Several other genes implicated in thyroid hormone signalling and non-thyroid hormone signalling have been associated with the neuroendocrine control of seasonal rhythms in reproduction and energy balance. For example, nestin, vimentin, cellular retinol binding protein (Crbp1), the orphan G-protein coupled receptor 50 (Gpr50) and the thyroid hormone cell-membrane transporter gene (Mct8) all express complex seasonal expression profiles in tanycytes (Petri et al. 2016). These data highlight that multiple transcripts exhibit robust plasticity across seasonal timescales and are strong targets for regulation by epigenetic modifications.

Several studies have demonstrated that photoperiods experienced during development can have substantial impact on the neuroendocrine regulation of breeding (Stetson et al. 1986; Weaver and Reppert 1986). Hamsters that are gestated in LD and reared in SD conditions starting on post-natal day (PND) 18 maintain small testes and gonadal fat pad mass (Fig. 4.3a, b). Males that are gestated in LD and reared in LD were observed to increase testes mass and gonadal fat pad mass after PND21. Quantitative PCR analyses identified that hypothalamic Dio2 expression is similar across photoperiodic conditions; however, Dio3 expression was upregulated by PND21 in hamsters gestated in SD, and rapidly increased until PND32 (Fig. 4.3c). Two consecutive daily melatonin injections in PND18 hamsters housed in LD conditions prevented the increase in testes mass and stimulated Dio3 expression (Fig. 4.3d, e). These data indicate that early in post-natal development, the photoperiodic response pathway in the hypothalamus is sensitive to day length exposure, and that melatonin can rapidly inhibit reproductive development (Prendergast et al. 2013). Recent evidence indicates that the photoperiodic response in hamsters can be programmed during gestation. Male hamsters that were gestated in LD or SD and then subsequently reared in the same photoperiodic conditions were observed to have higher Tshβ and Dio2 expression in LD on PND0, and then greater Dio3 expression in SD on PND15 (Saenz de Miera et al. 2017). Altogether, the data indicate that melatonin conveys the current day length information from the maternal pineal gland across the placenta to the fetus, and via transfer in milk can facilitate adaptive photoperiodic responses after parturition.

The neuroendocrine expression of Dnmt3a in hamsters displays robust daily variation (Stevenson 2017b). In mice, Dnmt3a is expressed in the SCN, is light induced and is involved in the circadian regulation of locomotor activity (Azzi et al. 2014, 2017). Both hypothalamic Dnmt3a and Dnmt3b mRNA have been shown to

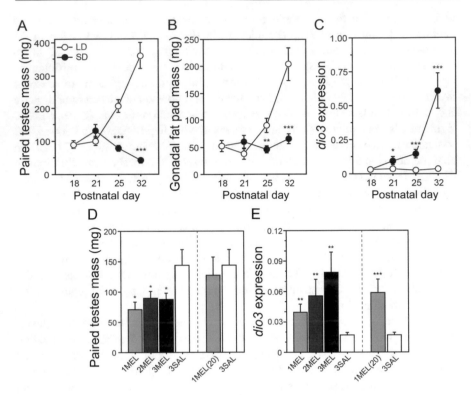

Fig. 4.3 Testes mass (**a**), gonadal fat pad mass (**b**) and hypothalamic *dio3* mRNA (**c**) on post-natal days (PND) 18–32 in male hamsters that were gestated and reared in long days (LD) and transferred to short days (SD), or kept in LD beginning on PND18. Values are mean ± SEM $^*P < 0.05$, $^{**}P < 0.01$, $^{***}P < 0.001$ vs. LD values at corresponding PND. (**d**) Testes mass and (**e**) hypothalamic *dio3* mRNA on PND21 of juvenile male hamsters housed in LD from birth and injected subcutaneously with MEL 3 h before lights-off for 1 (1MEL), 2 (2MEL) or 3 (3MEL) successive days, beginning on PND18. Control hamsters (depicted twice to facilitate comparisons) were injected with 0.1 mL of sterile SAL for 3 days beginning on PND18 (3SAL). An additional treatment group received a single bolus injection of melatonin (1MEL(20)) on postnatal day 20. $^*P < 0.05$, $^{**}P < 0.01$, $^{***}P < 0.001$ vs. 3SAL value. Data from Prendergast et al. (2013)

exhibit seasonal variation in expression in hamsters with greater levels in LD versus SD conditions (Fig. 4.1b) (Stevenson and Prendergast 2013; Stevenson 2017b), and similar seasonal changes have been observed in birds (Sharma et al. 2018). The expression of Dnmt3b immunoreactivity has been localized to the tanycytes in Siberian hamsters, and the regulation of Dio3 mRNA expression is inversely related to the levels of methylation in the Dio3 proximal promoter region (Stevenson and Prendergast 2013). In addition to the hypothalamus, Dnmt3a and Dnmt3b mRNA are expressed in the testes and uterine tissue, and are significantly upregulated in SD conditions (Lynch et al. 2016). In females, ovarian steroids provide inhibitory input to uterine Dnmt3a and Dnmt3b mRNA, and may serve to reduce fertility during the non-breeding seasons (Lynch et al. 2016). These data indicate that rhythmic patterns in DNA methylation are a key component for the neuroendocrine-gonadal control of seasonal rhythms. To date, the role of maternal programming for the regulation of Dnmt3a and Dnmt3b expression has not been identified.

Most of the research on the photoperiodic regulation of breeding has focussed on the direct experience of the animal to the prevailing light conditions. However, there is evidence that photoperiodic programming may be inherited (Prendergast et al. 2001). A series of experiments where Siberian hamsters were selected on the basis of photoresponsiveness to short days indicated that heritability ranged from $h^2 = 0.2$–0.5 (i.e. moderately strong) (Lynch et al. 1989; Kliman and Lynch 1992). In hamsters the primary trait that appears to be inherited is the period of the circadian pacemaker (Freeman and Goldman 1997a, b). In Syrian hamsters, tau-mutants will exhibit gonadal involution when housed in constant darkness or treated with exogenous melatonin (Stirland et al. 1996; Loudon et al. 1998). Selection experiments have not been conducted to determine the relative inheritable basis of photoresponsiveness, but current evidence suggests that the genetic basis must be upstream from the nocturnal melatonin signal. Altogether, it is likely that a combination of heritable, developmental and post-pubertal exposure to photoperiods is involved in programming seasonal rhythms. It follows that epigenetic modifications in key neuroendocrine substrates are critically involved. However, whether photoperiodic programs established via genetic (i.e. inherited), developmental (i.e. maternal) or post-pubertal environmental-induced programs are regulated by similar epigenetic mechanisms has not yet been established.

4.6 Variations of a Common Theme? Similarities Between Developmental and Seasonal Programs

Thyroid hormone signalling is critical for brain development and the neuroendocrine control of reproduction. It is likely that developmental and seasonal programs rely on similar epigenomic modifications and the thyroid hormone deiodinase enzymes are candidate loci. For example, genomic imprinting of the Dlk1-Dio3 is established by DNA methylation, and both hyper- and hypo-methylation of the locus can result in growth defects, severe brain malformations, muscle defects or death (Stelzer et al. 2016). Hyper-methylation of maternal alleles resulted in reduced expression of maternal-derived genes and an increase in paternal-derived genes (i.e. Dio3) compared to control parent-of-origin methylation levels. Similarly, hypo-methylation of the paternal allele repressed Dio3 expression. In the adult brain, the Dlk1-Dio3 locus includes many highly expressed genes (Perez et al. 2015). Curiously, adult neurogenic cells in the ependymal layer appear to exhibit dynamic variation in DNA methylation in the imprinted Dlk1-Dio3 region (Ferrón et al. 2011). Recent evidence suggests that the cells derived from the ependyma neurogenic niche have a remarkable degree of DNA methylation in the imprinted Dlk1-Dio3 region, and that loss of parent-of-origin epigenetic modifications induces considerable neuronal epigenomic variation (Stelzer et al. 2016). One conjecture is that developmental programs that underlie reproduction (i.e. puberty) are largely recapitulated in seasonally breeding species (Ball and Wade 2013). Indeed, there are several aspects of the neuroendo-crine control of seasonal rhythms in reproduction that are similar to development, such as neurogenesis (Hazlerigg and Lincoln 2011), epigenomic modifications (Stevenson 2017a, b; Stevenson and Lincoln 2017), physiology (Ebling 2010; Paul et al. 2018) and tanycyte morphology (Yamamura et al. 2004; Ebling 2010). Given the consistent observation for the photoperiodic regulation of Dio2 and Dio3 in adult hamsters, it is possible that photoperiodic regulation of seasonal rhythms may, in part, be influenced by mechanisms involved in genomic imprinting.

Maternal programs are a strong contributor to developmental programs involved in seasonal rhythms (Saenz de Miera 2018). Melatonin secreted from the mother can readily cross the placenta and is active in the developing human foetus (Reiter et al. 2014). Recent work in Siberian hamsters has indicated that Dio2 expression in hypothalamic tanycytes can be programmed by the photoperiod experienced by the mother during gestation. Hamsters gestated in short days were observed to express significantly lower Dio2 compared to LD control hamsters. Importantly, when animals were exposed to the converse photoperiod on post-natal day 21, tanycytes Dio2 was highly responsive to LD and elicited a rapid increase in Dio2 followed by gonadal recrudescence (Saenz de Miera 2018). Taken together, the data indicate that maternal programming of the photoperiodic response can be driven by the mother's nocturnal melatonin secretion, and that the late stages of gestation may be a sensitive period to impart long-term (epi)genomic, molecular and cellular modifications.

The primary focus here has been on the potential role of thyroid hormones to provide similar programming effects during developmental and seasonal rhythms. However, it is important to emphasize that other hormonal systems, such as sex steroids (e.g. testosterone) and adrenal hormones (e.g. glucocorticoids), are other internal signals that can impart early-life epigenomic modifications that can have lasting implications for the neuroendocrine control of adult physiology.

4.7   Summary

Epigenetic modifications have been classified into three categories: transgenerational inheritance (Daxinger and Whitelaw 2012), developmental (Feng et al. 2010) and rhythmic (Stevenson 2018). In this chapter, the genomic imprinting of Dlk-Dio3 and maternal programming of Dio2 and Dio3 were presented and compared to the photoperiodic control of seasonal rhythms by tanycyte Dio2 and Dio3 expression. The underlying conjecture is the potential similarities of epigenetic modifications for the timing of developmental and seasonal programs (Fig. 4.4). There are many unresolved questions that require further investigation, and include (1) Are seasonal programs established by genomic imprints during development? (2) Does melatonin signalling in utero establish the phase of seasonal programs? and (3) to what extent does development establish seasonal programs across vertebrate species? The major advancements afforded by mouse models and modern research

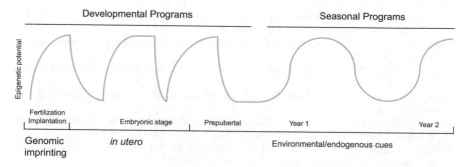

Fig. 4.4 Schematic representation of similarities of epigenetic modifications in relation to the timing of developmental and seasonal programs

techniques can now be harnessed to resolve the epi(genomic) mechanisms that govern programmed events in non-traditional animal models.

References

Azzi A, Dallman R, Casserly A, Rehraucr H, Patrignani A, Maier B, Kramer A, Brown SA (2014) Circadian behaviour is light-reprogrammed by plastic DNA methylation. Nat Neurosci 17:377–382

Azzi A, Evans JA, Leise T, Myung J, Takumi T, Davidson AJ, Brown SA (2017) Network dynamics mediate circadian clock plasticity. Neuron 93:441–450

Ball GF, Wade J (2013) The value of comparative approaches to our understanding of puberty as illustrated by investigations in birds and reptiles. Horm Behav 64:211–214

Banks R, Delibegovic M, Stevenson TJ (2016) Triiodothyronine reduces peripheral leukocytes in photo-regressed hamsters. J Biol Rhythm 31:299–307

Bao R, Onishi KG, Tolla E, Ebling FJP, Lewis JE, Barrett PJ, Prendergast BJ, Stevenson TJ (2019) Genome sequencing and transcriptome analyses of the Siberian hamster hypothalamus identify novel mechanisms for seasonal energy balance. Proc Natl Acad Sci U S A 116:13116–13121

Barlow DP, Bartolomei MS (2014) Genomic imprinting in mammals. Cold Spring Harb Perspect Biol. 6:a018382

Barton SC, Ferguson-Smith AC, Fundele R, Surani MA (1991) Influence of paternally imprinted genes on development. Development 113:679–687

Bianco AC, Salvatore D, Gereben B, Berry MJ, Larsen PR (2002) Biochemistry, cellular and molecular biology and physiological roles of the iodothyronine selenodeiodinases. Endocr Rev 23:38–89

Bilbo SD, Schwarz JM (2009) Early-life programming of later-life brain and behaviour: a critical role for the immune system. Front Behav Neurosci 3:14

Blewitt M, Whitelaw E (2013) The use of mouse models to study epigenetics. Cold Spring Harb Perspect Biol 5:a017939

Bolborea M, Dale N (2013) Hypothalamic tanycytes: potential roles in the control of feeding and energy balance. Trends Neurosci 36:91–100

Cao R, Wang L, Wang H, Xia L, Erdjument-Bromage H, Tempst P, Jones RS, Zhang Y (2002) Role of histone H3 lysine 27 methylation in Polycomb-group silencing. Science 298:1039–1043

Daxinger L, Whitelaw E (2012) Understanding transgenerational epigenetic inheritance via the gametes in mammals. Nat Rev Genet 13:153–162

DeVeale B, van der Kooy D, Babak T (2012) Critical evaluation of imprinted gene expression by RNA-seq: a new perspective. PLoS Biol 8(3):e1002600

Dupre SM (2011) Encoding and decoding photoperiod in the mammalian pars tuberalis. Neuroendocrinology 94:101–112

Ebling FJP (2010) Photoperiodic regulation of puberty in seasonal species. Mol Cell Endocrinol 324:95–101

Ebling FJP, Lewis JE (2018) Tanycytes and hypothalamic control of energy metabolism. Glia 66:1176–1184

Eckersley-Maslin MA, Alda-Catalinas C, Reik W (2018) Dynamics of the epigenetic landscape during the maternal-to-zygotic transition. Nat Rev Mol Cell Biol 19:436–450

Ernst DK, Bentley GE (2016) Neural and neuroendocrine processing of a non-photic cue in an opportunistically breeding songbird. J Exp Biol 219:783–789

Felsenfeld G (2014) A brief history of epigenetics. Cold Spring Harb Perspect Biol 6(1):a018200

Feng S, Jacobsen SE, Reik W (2010) Epigenetic reprogramming in plant and animal development. Science 330:622–627

Ferguson-Smith AC (2011) Genomic imprinting: the emergence of an epigenetic paradigm. Nat Rev Genet 12:565–575

Ferrón SR, Charalambous M, Radford E, McEwen K, Wildner H, Hind E, Morante-Redolat JM, Laborda J, Guillemot F, Bauer SR, Fariñas I, Ferguson-Smith AC (2011) Postnatal loss of Dlk1 imprinting in stem cells and niche astrocytes regulates neurogenesis. Nature 475:381–385

Forhead AJ, Fowden AL (2014) Thyroid hormones in fetal growth and prepartum maturation. J Endocrinol 221:R87–R103

Freeman DA, Goldman BD (1997a) Evidence that the circadian system mediates photoperiodic nonresponsiveness in Siberian hamsters: the effect of running wheel access on photoperiodic responsiveness. J Biol Rhythm 12:100–109

Freeman DA, Goldman BD (1997b) Photoperiod nonresponsive Siberian hamsters: effect of age on the probability of nonresponsiveness. J Biol Rhythm 12:110–121

Freeman DA, Teubner BJ, Smith CD, Prendergast BJ (2007) Exogenous T3 mimics long day lengths in Siberian hamsters. Am J Physiol Regul Integr Comp Physiol 292:R2368–R2372

Friesema ECH, Grueters A, Biebermann H, Krude H, von Moers A, Reeser M, Barrett TG, Mancilla EE, Svensson J, Kester MHA, Kuiper GGJM, Balkassmi S, Uitterlinden AG, Koehrle J, Rodien P, Halestrap AP, Visser TJ (2004) Association between mutations in a thyroid hormone transporter and severe X-linked psychomotor retardation. Lancet 364:1435–1437

Hazlerigg DG, Lincoln GA (2011) Hypothesis: cyclical histogenesis is the basis of circannual timing. J Biol Rhythm 26:471–485

Johnston JD, Skene DJ (2015) 60 years of neuroendocrinology: regulation of mammalian neuroendocrine physiology and rhythms by melatonin. J Endocrinol 226:T187–T198

Jones PA (2012) Functions of DNA methylation: islands, start sites, gene bodies and beyond. Nat Rev Genet 13:484–492

Juss TS, Meddle SL, Servant RS, King VM (1993) Melatonin and photoperiodic time measurement in Japanese quail (Coturnix japonica). Proc Bio Sci 254:21–28

Kelsey G, Bartolomei MS (2012) Imprinted genes . . . and the number is? PLoS Biol 8(3):e1002601

Kliman RM, Lynch GR (1992) Evidence for genetic variation in the occurrence of the photoresponse of the Djungarian hamster, Phodopus sungorus. J Biol Rhythm 7:161–173

Klose RJ, Bird AP (2006) Genomic DNA methylation: the mark and its mediators. Trends Biochem Sci 31:89–97

Laborda J (2000) The role of the epidermal growth-like protein dlk in cell differentiation. Histol Histopathol 15:119–129

Langlet F (2014) Tanycytes: a gateway to the metabolic hypothalamus. J Neuroendocrinol 26:753–760

Lazutkaite G, Solda A, Lossow K, Meyerhof W, Dale N (2017) Amino acid sensing in hypothalamic tanycytes via umami taste receptors. Mol Metab 6:1480–1492

Lewis JE, Ebling FJP (2017) Tanycytes as regulators of seasonal cycles in neuroendocrine function. Front Neurol 8:79

Lindsay KL, Buss C, Wadhwa PD, Entringer S (2019) The interplay between nutrition and stress in pregnancy: implications for fetal programming of brain development. Biol Psychiatry 85:135–149

Loudon AS, Ihara N, Menaker M (1998) Effects of a circadian mutation on seasonality in Syrian hamsters (Mesocricetus auratus). Proc R Soc B 265:517–521

Lynch GR, Lynch CB, Kliman RM (1989) Genetic analyses of photoresponsiveness in the Djungarian hamster, Phodopus sungorus. J Comp Physiol A 164:475–482

Lynch EWJ, Coyle CS, Lorgen M, Campbell E, Bowman A, Stevenson TJ (2016) Cyclical DNA methyltransferase 3a expression is a seasonal and oestrus timer in reproductive tissues. Endocrinology 157:2469–2478

Majumdar G, Rani S, Kumar V (2015) Hypothalamic gene switches control transitions between seasonal life history states in a night-migratory photoperiodic songbird. Mol Cell Endocrinol 399:110–121

McCann KE, Sinkiewicz DM, Norvelle A, Huhman KL (2017) De novo assembly, annotation and characterization of the whole brain transcriptome of male and female Syrian hamsters. Sci Rep 7:40472

Miranda A, Sousa N (2018) Maternal hormonal milieu influence on fetal brain development. Brain Behav 8:e00920

Mishra I, Bhardwaj SK, Malik S, Kumar V (2017) Concurrent hypothalamic gene expression under acute and chronic long days: implications for initiation and maintenance of photoperiodic response in migratory songbirds. Mol Cell Endocrinol 439:81–94

Muller B, Grossniklaus U (2010) Model organisms—a historical perspective. J Proteome 73.2054–2063

Nadeau JH (2009) Transgenerational genetic effects on phenotypic variation and disease risk. Hum Mol Genet 18:R202–R210

Nakao N, Ono H, Yamamura T, Anraku T, Takagi T, Higashi K, Yasuo S, Katou Y, Kageyama S, Uno Y, Kasukawa T, Iigo M, Sharp PJ, Iwasawa A, Suzuki Y, Sugano S, Niimi T, Mizutani M, Namikawa T, Ebihara S, Ueda HR, Yoshimura T (2008) Thyrotrophin in the pars tuberalis triggers photoperiodic response. Nature 452:317–322

Nakane Y, Yoshimura T (2014) Universality and diversity in the signal transduction pathway that regulates seasonal reproduction in vertebrates. Front Neurosci 8:115

Nakayama T, Yoshimura T (2018) Seasonal rhythms: the role of thyrotropin and thyroid hormones. Thyroid 28:4–10

Okamoto I, Otte AP, Allis CD, Reinberg D, Heard E (2004) Epigenetic dynamics of imprinted X inactivation during early mouse development. Science 303:644–649

Ono H, Hoshino Y, Yasuo S, Watanbe M, Nakane Y, Murai A, Ebihara S, Korf HW, Yoshimura T (2008) Involvement of thyrotropin in photoperiodic signal transduction in mice. Proc Natl Acad Sci 105:18238–18242

Orellana JA, Saez PJ, Cortes-Campos C, Elizondo RJ, Shoji KF, Contreras-Duarte S, Figueroa V, Velarde V, Jiang JX, Nualart F, Saez JC, Garcia MA (2012) Glucose increases intracellular free Ca(2+) in tanycytes via ATP released through connexin 43 hemichannels. Glia 60:53–68

Paul MJ, Probst CK, Brown LM, de Vries GJ (2018) Dissociation of puberty and adolescent social development in a seasonally breeding species. Curr Biol 28:1116–1123

Payer B, Lee JT, Namekawa SH (2011) X-inactivation and X-reactivation: epigenetic hallmarks of mammalian reproduction and pluripotent stem cells. Hum Genet 130:265–280

Perez JD, Rubinstein ND, Fernandez DE, Santoro SW, Needleman LA, Ho-Shing O, Choi JJ, Zirlinger M, Chen SK, Liu JS (2015) Quantitative and functional interrogation of parent-of-origin allelic expression biases in the brain. elife 4:e07860

Pérez JH, Tolla E, Dunn I, Meddle SL, Stevenson TJ (2019) A comparative perspective on extra-retinal photoreception. Trends Endocrinol Metab 30:39–53

Petri I, Diedrich V, Wilson D, Fernandez-Calleja J, Herwig A, Steinlechner S, Barrett P (2016) Orchestration of gene expression across the seasons: hypothalamic gene expression in natural photoperiod throughout the year in the Siberian hamster. Sci Rep 6:29689

Plath K, Fang J, Mlynarczyk-Evans SK, Cao R, Worringer KA, Wang H, de la Cruz CC, Otte AP, Panning B, Zhang Y (2003) Role of histone H3 lysine 27 methylation in X inactivation. Science 300:131–135

Prendergast BJ (2010) MT1 melatonin receptors mediate somatic, behavioural and reproductive neuroendocrine responses to photoperiod and melatonin in Siberian hamsters (Phodopus sungorus). Endocrinology 151:714–721

Prendergast BJ, Kriegsfeld LJ, Nelson RJ (2001) Photoperiodic polyphenisms in rodents: neuroendocrine mechanisms, costs and functions. Q Rev Biol 76:293–325

Prendergast BJ, Pyter LM, Kampf-Lassin A, Patel PN, Stevenson TJ (2013) Rapid induction of hypothalamic iodothyronine deiodinase expression by photoperiod and melatonin in juvenile Siberian hamster (Phodopus sungorus). Endocrinology 154:831–841

Rasmussen KD, Helin K (2016) Role of TET enzymes in DNA methylation, development and cancer. Genes Dev 30:733–750

Rastogi A, Kumari Y, Rani S, Kumar V (2013) Neural correlates of migration: activation of hypothalamic clocks in and out of migratory state in the blackheaded bunting (Emberiza melanocephala). PLoS One 8(10):e70065

Reik W, Dean W, Walter J (2001) Epigenetic reprogramming in mammalian development. Science 293:1089–1093

Reiter RJ, Tan DX, Korkmaz A, Rosales-Corral SA (2014) Melatonin and stable circadian rhythms optimize maternal, placental and fetal physiology. Hum Reprod Update 20:293–307

Saenz de Miera C (2018) Maternal photoperiodic programming enlightens the internal regulation of thyroid-hormone deiodinase in tanycytes. J Neuroendocrinol 31:e12679

Saenz de Miera C, Hanon EA, Dardente H, Birnie M, Simonneaux V, Lincoln GA, Hazlerigg DG (2013) Circannual variation in thyroid hormone deiodinase in a short-day breeder. J Neuroendocrinol 25:412–421

Saenz de Miera C, Bothorel B, Jaeger C, Simonneaux V, Hazlerigg D (2017) Maternal photoperiod programs hypothalamic thyroid status via the fetal pituitary gland. Proc Natl Acad Sci USA 114:8408–8413

Seisenberger S, Andrews S, Krueger F, Arand J, Walter J, Santos F, Popp C, Thienpont B, Dean W, Reik W (2012) The dynamics of genome-wide DNA methylation reprogramming in mouse primordial germ cells. Mol Cell 48:849–862

Sekita Y, Wagatsuma H, Nakamura K, Ono R, Kagami M, Wakisaka N, Hino T, Suzuki-Migishima R, Kohda T, Ogura A, Ogata T, Yokoyama M, Kaneko-Ishino T, Ishino F (2008) Role of retrotransposon-derived imprinted gene, Rtl1, in the feto-maternal interface of mouse placenta. Nat Genet 40:243–248

Sharma A, Singh D, Malik S, Gupta NJ, Rani S, Kumar V (2018) Difference in control between spring and autumn migration in birds: insight from seasonal changes in hypothalamic gene expression in captive buntings. Proc Biol Sci 285:1885

Stelzer Y, Wu H, Song Y, Shivalila CS, Markoulaki S, Jaenisch R (2016) Parent-of-origin DNA methylation dynamics during mouse development. Cell Rep 16:3167–3180

Stetson MH, Elliot JA, Goldman BD (1986) Maternal transfer of photoperiodic information influences the photoperiodic response of prepubertal Djungarian hamsters (Phodopus sungorus). Biol Reprod 34:664–669

Stevenson TJ (2017a) Environmental and hormonal regulation of neuroendocrine epigenetic enzymes. J Neuroendocrinol 29(1). https://doi.org/10.1111/jne.12471

Stevenson TJ (2017b) Circannual and circadian rhythms in hypothalamic DNA methyltransferase and histone deacetylase in Siberian hamsters (Phodopus sungorus). Gen Comp Endocrinol 243:130–137

Stevenson TJ (2018) Epigenetic regulation of biological rhythms: an evolutionary ancient molecular timer. Trends Genet 34:90–100

Stevenson TJ, Lincoln GA (2017) Epigenetic mechanisms regulating circannual rhythms, Chapter 29. In: Kumar V (ed) Biological timekeeping: clocks, rhythms and behaviour. Springer, India

Stevenson TJ, Prendergast BJ (2013) Reversible DNA methylation regulates seasonal photoperiodic time measurement. Proc Nat Acad Sci USA 110:16651–16656

Stirland JA, Mohammad YN, Loudon AS (1996) A mutation of the circadian timing system (tau gene) in the seasonally breeding Syrian hamster alters the reproductive response to photoperiod change. Proc Royal Society Lond B 263:345–350

Struhl K (1998) Histone acetylation and transcriptional regulatory mechanisms. Genes Dev 12:599–606

Weaver DR, Reppert SM (1986) Maternal melatonin communicates daylength to the fetus in Djungarian hamsters. Endocrinology 119:2861–2863

Wu H, Zhang Y (2011) Mechanisms and functions of Tet protein-mediated 5-methylcytosine oxidation. Genes Dev 25:2436–2452

Yamamura T, Hirunagi K, Ebihara S, Yoshimura T (2004) Seasonal morphological changes in the neuro-glial interaction between gonadotropin-releasing hormone nerve terminals and glial endfeet in Japanese quail. Endocrinology 145:4264–4267

Yoshimura T (2013) Thyroid hormone and seasonal regulation of reproduction. Front Neuroendocrinol 34:157–166

Yoshimura T, Yasuo S, Watanabe M, Iigo M, Yamamura T, Hirunagi K, Ebihara S (2003) Light-induced hormone conversion of T4 to T3 regulates photoperiodic response of gonads in birds. Nature 426:178–181

Recommended Further Reading

Stevenson TJ (2017) Circannual and circadian rhythms in hypothalamic DNA methyltransferase and histone deacetylase in Siberian hamsters (*Phodopus sungorus*). Gen Comp Endocrinol 243:130–137. This paper revealed that the expression levels of several epigenetic enzymes exhibit robust daily rhythms in the hypothalamus.

Stevenson TJ, Prendergast BJ (2013) Reversible DNA methylation regulates seasonal photoperiodic time measurement. Proc Natl Acad Sci USA 110:16651–16656. This paper provided the first evidence for seasonal rhythms in DNA methylation and DNA methyltransferase enzyme expression.

Plasticity of Neuroendocrine Mechanisms Regulating Seasonal Reproduction in Sheep

5

Laurence Dufourny and Isabelle Franceschini

Abstract

The sheep is not only a valuable animal model in which to investigate the mechanisms underlying seasonality, it is a commercially important species where reproduction of many breeds is profoundly seasonal. This chapter will describe how studies in sheep have revealed plasticity in the hypothalamus that likely underlies seasonal changes in neuroendocrine function. This includes changes in the kisspeptin neuronal system that provides a key drive to the gonadotrophin-releasing hormone (GnRH) secretory system, seasonal fluctuations in neurogenesis, and cell fate in the hypothalamus, morphological reorganizations as revealed by changes in polysialylated neural cell adhesion molecule immunoreactivity, and changes in permeability of the blood-brain barrier.

Keywords

Male effect · Metabolic status · Blood-brain barrier · Neuropeptides · Tanycytes

5.1 Introduction

Numerous species adapt to their constantly changing environment and its seasonal fluctuations by modulating specific physiological functions and behaviors. In sheep and many other domestic species such as goats and horses, reproduction is a seasonal function that will allow the birth of offspring at the optimal time of year for their

L. Dufourny (✉) · I. Franceschini
UMR Physiologie de la Reproduction et des Comportements, Centre INRA Val de Loire, Nouzilly, France
e-mail: laurence.dufourny@inrae.fr; Isabelle.franceschini-laurent@inrae.fr

© The Editor(s) (if applicable) and The Author(s), under exclusive license to Springer Nature Switzerland AG 2020
F. J. P. Ebling, H. D. Piggins (eds.), *Neuroendocrine Clocks and Calendars*, Masterclass in Neuroendocrinology 10, https://doi.org/10.1007/978-3-030-55643-3_5

survival, i.e., spring and early summer, when food availability is maximal and the climate temperate. In sheep, this means that gamete production and sexual behavior occur only for a few months every year in the so-called breeding season which is followed by many months of sexual quiescence ("seasonal anestrus"). This pattern of seasonal reproduction results from innate rhythmicity (Chap. 1) interacting with the perception of natural changes in day-length and its translation into a hormonal signal, the release of melatonin from pineal gland during night. Therefore, in winter, the duration of melatonin secretion is longer than that one observed in summer nights (Malpaux 2006). The melatonin signal is then read by several brain and pituitary structures, among which the *pars tuberalis* allows its transmission to hypothalamic nuclei through a mechanism involving central production of bioactive thyroid hormone (Dardente 2012;Wood et al. 2015). The cellular mechanisms induced by melatonin to synchronize the activity of gonadotrophin-releasing hormone (GnRH) neurons and the timely expression of sexual behavior are not yet fully elucidated. This chapter will summarize the recent results obtained in sheep regarding the contribution of seasonal brain plasticity to this process.

5.2   Secondary Modulators of Seasonal Reproduction

5.2.1   Social Factors

Although changes in photoperiod and thus nocturnal melatonin secretion are the primary regulators of seasonal reproduction, a phenomenon reported since the eighteenth century can result in the induction of out of season estrus cycles in small ruminants. It is called "the male effect" or colloquially as the "ram effect" and consists of introducing a sexually active male into a flock of sexually inactive females during seasonal anestrus (Fig. 5.1). This introduction of the mature male will activate multiple neuronal circuits resulting in a rapid increase of GnRH/LH pulsatile secretion, leading eventually to an LH surge triggering ovulation (Fig. 5.1). This male effect relies on the integration of multiple stimuli among which the odor of male seems to be prominent. Recent evidence pinpoints an involvement of kisspeptin (KP) neurons in this effect (Fabre-Nys et al. 2017), as the percentage of activated KP neurons increases in anestrous female sheep (ewes) exposed to sexually active males (rams) in contrast with results in anestrus females exposed to sexually active females (Fig. 5.1). This male effect method has been developed and standardized to produce hormone-free out-of-season reproduction.

5.2.2   Metabolic Status

Flushing is a method commonly used by breeders to improve reproduction in small ruminants. It consists into bringing an additional supply of energy for several consecutive weeks before and after mating in ovine species to improve ovulation rate and therefore fecundity. Not only does gonadal activity rely on metabolic status,

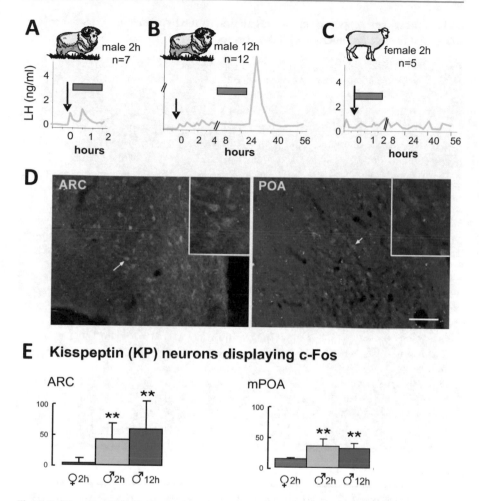

Fig. 5.1 The ram effect. Following introduction of a male (ram) in a flock of seasonally anestrus females, a rapid increase of LH pulsatile secretion is observed in females (**a**) that will eventually lead to a surge of LH (**b**). In contrast, in females exposed to females, LH levels remains stable (**c**). 12 h after exposure to a ram, numerous neurons in the arcuate nucleus (ARC) and medial preoptic area (mPOA) display c-Fos-ir, a nuclear marker for cell activation (red) in KP-ir neurons (green) (scale bar 40 μm) (**d**). significantly more dual-labelled neurons occurred within the ARC and mPOA of females exposed to rams for 2 h and 12 h than in the same regions of females exposed to females (**e**). (Adapted from Fabre-Nys et al. 2017)

but also on the duration and depth of seasonal anestrus. This was demonstrated by following two groups of ewes over consecutive years, one with a mid-high body mass index and one with a low index. Lean animals displayed longer anestrus seasons than controls with higher adiposity, and the percentage of ewes without ovulation during the breeding season was greater in lean animals (Menassol et al.

2011). These data support a role for regulation of the hypothalamo-gonadal axis by metabolic factors that interact with the seasonal status of sheep.

Box 1 Sheep as an Integrated Model of Seasonal Processes in Mammals
Sheep as experimental models have numerous advantages compared to rodents as their large size allows for long periods of frequent blood and/or cerebrospinal fluid (CSF) sampling. Moreover, this can be done on freely moving awake animals. The size of their brain also allows the accurate placement through a stereotaxic neurosurgical approach of cannula into the brain sites. This allows the infusion of experimental test compounds, tracers, and viruses into delineated regions without spreading to neighboring regions. The sheep has also been widely studied regarding its energy requirements and food intake, and the consequences of changes of nutrition on physiology are understood well. Due to the long luteal phase where ewes produce high progesterone levels, the length of the estrous cycle in the ewe relates to the length of the ovarian cycle in woman better than the ovarian cycle observed in rodents where luteal function does not develop post-ovulation in the absence of cervical stimulation and fertilization. As a consequence, information about central control of reproduction obtained in sheep may be more physiologically relevant related to humans than that obtained in models with shorter ovarian cycles. Results obtained in domestic mammals are also of economic significance for farmers. As in any other experimental model, there are also limitations for the use of sheep, as the tools such as antibodies and genetic manipulations to study the different components of the neuroendocrine system may not as be readily available as they are for laboratory rodents. The physical size of the sheep brain also requires more time for laboratory processing.

5.3   Seasonal Fluctuations of Blood Brain Barrier Permeability

5.3.1   Blood Brain Barrier

The blood-brain barrier (BBB) is made of a continuum of endothelial cells separated by tight junctions, found in brain capillaries and in choroid plexuses. Depending on their sizes and chemical nature, molecules found in the blood either diffuse freely through the BBB or are actively transported using energy-consuming cell membrane mechanisms. Passive diffusion takes place for some small and lipophilic molecules, but these attributes are not on their own predictive of the ability of a molecule to diffuse freely through the BBB. Large and hydrophilic molecules do not cross freely through the BBB; they always require specific transporters or receptors to attain entry to the cerebrospinal fluid (CSF) and/or brain parenchyma. Given that one of the key features of the BBB is its ability to give or restrain access of molecules to the brain, a key issue has been to determine whether access of molecules to the brain in sheep is modified across seasons or dependent upon photoperiodic status. This chapter will review the passage of gonadal steroids across the BBB, and then consider the seasonal variations of protein content within the CSF. The final part of this section will consider environmental endocrine disrupters such as polychlorinated biphenyls (PCBs) as these chemicals accumulate in the environment and are able to interact with steroid receptors which may affect the central control of reproduction.

5.3.2 Access of Peripheral Molecules to the Brain

Gonadal steroid feedback is modified in sheep throughout the year. During the breeding season, estrogens and progesterone are released from the ovaries and acting through both positive and negative feedback result in the occurrence of 16–18 day long ovarian cycles until pregnancy occurs. During the nonbreeding season, ovarian follicles do not develop, so estradiol levels in the plasma remain low and progesterone is not released as corpora lutea never form in the ovary. Whether or not these seasonal fluctuations in sex steroid production are associated with modulation of their passage to the brain was assessed in ovariectomized estradiol-replaced ewes treated with an intravaginal progesterone implant and exposed either to short photoperiod (16 h of dark per 24 h) or long photoperiod (8 h of dark per 24 h) Progesterone assays of extracts of brain tissue revealed a higher concentration of progesterone during long photoperiods, while progesterone metabolites were not different between groups (Thiery and Malpaux 2003). Similarly, progesterone levels within the CSF were doubled in long photoperiod compared to short photoperiod, while blood concentrations of progesterone were similar between groups, suggesting a differentiated passage across the BBB between photoperiodic conditions (Fig. 5.2). Similar results were obtained for estrogens, which seem to cross the BBB more readily during long photoperiod exposure (Thiery and Malpaux 2003) (Fig. 5.2). Of note, this modulation of BBB permeability to sex steroids is dependent upon melatonin, as pinealectomy abolished the difference between long and short photoperiod for CSF content of estrogen (Thiery et al. 2006). These results of seasonal modulation of the access of gonadal steroids into CSF have been extended by the work of Adam et al. (2006) demonstrating greater access of leptin, a protein hormone involved in food intake, to CSF in rams in long photoperiods (Adam et al. 2006). More recently, we hypothesized that CSF protein content would vary with photoperiod (Teixeira-Gomes et al. 2015). In order to test this hypothesis, CSF from ovariectomized estradiol-replaced ewes was collected from animals kept either in long photoperiod to induce seasonal anestrus, or in short photoperiod to mimic the situation encountered during breeding season. The concentrations of CSF metabolites and hormones were measured using Liquid Chromatography-Mass Spectrometry (LC-MS), allowing the identification of proteins with a mass > 10 KDa. This lead to the identification of 103 proteins in total, among which 41 differed in concentration in the CSF between short and long photoperiod: 18 were more abundant in long photoperiod and 23 in short photoperiod (Teixeira-Gomes et al.

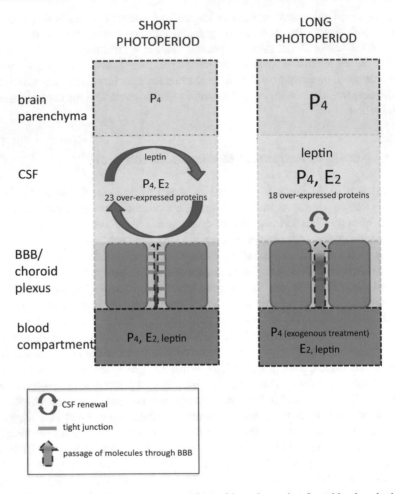

Fig. 5.2 Photoperiod regulates the passage of steroids and proteins from blood to brain, the renewal rate of cerebrospinal fluid (CSF), and the structure of tight junctions in the ovine brain. Each rectangle depicts a compartment, the size of blue rounded arrows is proportional to the rate of CSF renewal as well as the size of red arrows that represent the passage of molecules through tight junctions (represented as green bars). The size of characters is also representative of the different concentrations for molecules found in CSF and/or brain and in blood under the different photoperiods. *BBB* blood-brain barrier, *CSF* cerebrospinal fluid, *P4* progesterone, *E2* estradiol

2015). Those proteins were involved in many diverse functions including hormone transport, metabolism, angiogenesis, and immune system activity. Proteins found in CSF can originate from the circulation via filtration by the choroid plexus, or from direct synthesis within the choroid plexus, or from drainage of brain-released compounds (Strazielle et al. 2004), so the precise origin of each protein in CSF varying with photoperiodic environment and its impact on seasonal physiology remain to be determined. Understanding these fluctuations in CSF may help to decipher the intricate cells mechanisms impinging on seasonal physiology.

5.3.3 Seasonal Variation in CSF Production

CSF is produced by choroid plexus, and experiments were done to measure CSF renewal rate by removing a given volume of CSF (between 0.5 mL and 2 mL) while measuring the intraventricular pressure and the time necessary to restore the initial ventricular pressure. This experimental approach allowed a calculation of the volume of CSF produced in groups of animals placed either in short or long photoperiod. It was established that CSF production was twice as low in long photoperiod compared to short photoperiod (Thiery et al. 2009), suggesting a larger dilution of molecules during short photoperiods in CSF (Fig. 5.2).

5.3.4 Modulation of Tight Junction Composition by Photoperiod

The different concentrations of multiple proteins in CSF in ewes in long and short photoperiod led us to investigate whether the different levels of steroids and proteins found in CSF may result from a seasonal regulation of BBB permeability. Choroid plexus tissues from ewes exposed to short or long photoperiods were collected, and after protein extraction, a quantitative analysis of specific proteins found in tight junctions was performed using Western blot analyses. Four proteins were expressed at lower levels in choroid plexus during long photoperiod (zona occludens 1, zona occludens 2, afadin 6, cadherin), suggesting that the passage of molecules between epithelial cells was probably enhanced during long photoperiod (Lagaraine et al. 2011) (Fig. 5.2).

In addition to these mechanisms, it may be that a seasonal modulation of local synthesis of steroids occurs in the ovine brain as reported for songbirds (Schlinger and Remage-Healey 2012) and frogs (Santillo et al. 2017), concurring with the difference of steroids concentrations reported earlier for progesterone and estrogens within brain parenchyma.

5.3.5 Impact of Polychlorinated Biphenyls (PCBs) on BBB Permeability

PCBs that have been used widely as plasticizers are endocrine disruptors able to interact with steroid receptors that accumulate in the environment as they have a very long half-life. Their impact on choroid plexus permeability was investigated in ewes exposed either to short or long photoperiod. Animals were treated for 3 weeks with PCB153 as this is one of the most abundant congeners. As PCB153 was found to accumulate in CSF during short but not in long photoperiod, a Western blot analysis of proteins found in tight junctions in choroid plexus was carried out. In ewes in short photoperiods, PCB153 treatment induced a substantive decrease in claudin 1, afadin 6, and zona occludens 2 protein levels, while in long photoperiod animals no significant differences were observed (Szczepkowska et al. 2013). These observations suggested that seasonal regulation of the permeability of the choroid plexus was weakened by PCB153 absorption through the stomach, which could impact on animals physiology. These findings have to be considered in the light that often PCBs act as a cocktail of congeners, and the "cocktail" effect may be more powerful than the effect induced by the short-term administration of a single congener.

5.4 Plasticity of Neuropeptidergic Systems Involved in the Control of Seasonal Reproduction

5.4.1 Kisspeptin Neurons

KP is the most potent secretagogue of GnRH secretion found to date in mammals. The number of KP appositions on GnRH neurons in ewes is significantly greater during the breeding season as compared to the anestrus season (Smith et al. 2008). Several studies examined whether or not KP content in the ovine hypothalamus fluctuates with seasons (Smith et al. 2007) or photoperiod (Chalivoix et al. 2010). Two populations of KP neurons exist in the ovine diencephalon, one in the preoptic area (POA) and the other more caudally in the arcuate nucleus (ARC)-median eminence (ME) region (Franceschini et al. 2006). It appears that photoperiod alone is able to modify the content of KP within the ARC, and to a more limited extent in the POA: indeed the number of neurons displaying KP immunoreactivity is significantly lower in animals in long photoperiod with an inactivated gonadotroph axis than in animals in short photoperiods with an activated gonadotroph axis (Chalivoix et al. 2010). The factors responsible for this decrease in long photoperiod remain to be fully established, but good candidates are neurokinin B and dynorphin both co-expressed with KP neurons of the ARC (Goodman et al. 2007) that could exert a paracrine/autocrine regulation. It was recently demonstrated that neurokinin B content also decreased in the hypothalamus during the anestrus season (Weems et al. 2017), and that KP/neurokinin B content may be affected by the increase of dopaminergic appositions originating from the retrochiasmatic area in anestrus season (Weems et al. 2017). However, other factors may also influence the content of KP neurons, for example neuromodulators involved in food intake, as it was demonstrated in sheep that the depth of anestrus and its duration is directly linked to metabolic status (Menassol et al. 2011). Moreover, KP expression is correlated with metabolic status, as evidenced by lean sheep showing lower KP expression than well-fed animals (Backholer et al. 2010).

5.4.2 Neurons Involved in Food Intake

Two major systems driving food intake in sheep are located within the ARC. One system is orexigenic and is constituted of neurons synthesizing both neuropeptide Y and Agouti-Related Protein (AgRP), while the second is anorexigenic and comprized neurons expressing both pro-opiomelanocortin (POMC) and cocaine- and amphetamine-regulated transcript (CART). Both systems interact with each other and also with KP neurons, and are the recipient of peripheral hormone signals such as leptin produced by fat tissue and ghrelin from the stomach in sheep (Backholer et al. 2010). The action of neuropeptide Y on KP synthesis is more complex than the simple neuropeptide Y-induced stimulation of KP expression reported in vitro (Luque et al. 2007), as in vivo work demonstrated that NPY/KP regulation is dependent on metabolic status, since leptin inhibits NPY but stimulates KP expression (De Bond and Smith 2014). CART may stimulate KP neurons and therefore help translate the energetic status to the reproductive axis (True et al. 2013). Melanocortin, a POMC-derived peptide, appears to have a dual action on KP expression depending on the site of action: being inhibitory in the ARC but stimulatory in the POA (Backholer et al. 2009). We investigated whether seasonal fluctuations of the interactions between KP and NPY neurons and between KP and POMC neurons occurred in ewes exposed either to short or long photoperiod treatment. We found similar numbers of NPY appositions on KP neurons in the ARC of ewes regardless of the photoperiod that they had been exposed to. In contrast, the appositions of β-endorphin, a peptide cleaved from the POMC precursor, on KP neurons were doubled in ewes having an activated gonadotroph axis as compared to ewes exposed to long photoperiod (Hellier and Dufourny, unpublished data). An intracerebroventricular infusion of β-endorphin (5 µg) in ewes having high LH levels evoked an increase of the percentage of activated KP neurons within the ARC 2 h later, as inferred from the number of KP neurons colocalizing c-Fos (Hellier and Dufourny, unpublished data). These observations suggest that β-endorphin modulates KP neuron activity and therefore influences the central control of reproduction.

5.5 Plasticity Mechanisms Involved in Seasonal Reproduction in Sheep

5.5.1 Morphological Reorganizations

Immunohistochemical analysis in sheep of polysialylated neural cell adhesion molecule (PSA-NCAM), a marker for brain synaptic plasticity, revealed that morphological reorganizations occurred in close proximity to GnRH neurons between the breeding season and anestrus season (Xiong et al. 1997; Viguie et al. 2001) (Fig. 5.3a). Further studies demonstrated that not only was the number of appositions on GnRH neurons greater during the breeding season (Xiong et al. 1997), but also the chemical nature of these appositions was different (Jansen et al. 2003; Sergeeva and Jansen 2009; Smith et al. 2008). These morphological reorganizations also occurred elsewhere, for example in the retrochiasmatic area, where dopaminergic neurons (A15) relaying estrogen negative feedback receive two times more appositions on their dendrites and display an increased dendritic length during anestrus (Adams et al. 2006). This latter phenomenon is dependent on the presence of thyroid hormones (Adams et al. 2006).

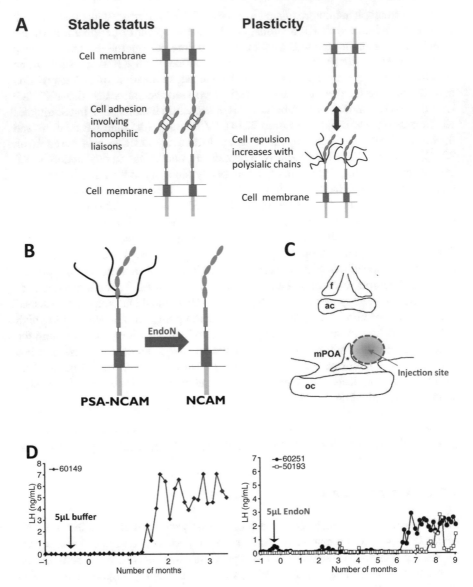

Fig. 5.3 Polysialylated neural cell adhesion molecule (PSA-NCAM) and morphological rearrangements at the membrane level. In a stable status, cells develop interactions through homophilic liaisons between proteins anchored in cytoplasmic membrane (**a**). When polysialic acid (PSA) chains are added on NCAM protein chain, it results in cell plasticity stemming from repulsion between membranes (**a**). In order to evaluate the physiological importance of PSA-NCAM for seasonal reproduction, we used an enzyme that cleaves PSA residues from NCAM (**b**): endoneuraminidase N (EndoN). We injected it at the level of the preoptic area (POA) where most GnRH neurons are observed in ewes (**c**), and transferred the animals to a short photoperiod. A delay in the LH rise in short photoperiod occurred in two-thirds of treated animals (**d**), suggesting that morphological plasticity involving PSA-NCAM is an important mechanism for the synchronization of seasonal reproduction. Adapted from the work of Chalivoix et al. (2013)

These data strongly suggest that morphological rearrangements are essential for the central control of reproduction, we therefore chose to investigate morphological reorganizations induced by photoperiod in the ewe diencephalon (Chalivoix et al. 2013). For that, ovariectomized estradiol-replaced (OVX + E2) ewes exposed to either short or long photoperiod were switched to the alternate photoperiods. Blood samples were collected every 2 weeks until circulating LH levels reached the expected concentrations (0 ng/mL after a switch to long photoperiod and LH > 1 ng/mL for at least two consecutives blood sampling after a switch to short photoperiod). PSA-NCAM levels were then quantified through Western blot analysis of microdissected hypothalamic areas. Following a transition to short photoperiod, as early as day 15, a sharp decrease of PSA-NCAM occurred in the organum vasculosum of lamina terminalis-POA region known to host most GnRH neuronal cell bodies in sheep. Later decreases in PSA-NCAM levels were observed in more caudal areas, for example, the ARC. Following the transition to long photoperiod, the rate of PSA-NCAM increased transiently in the same regions where decreases were reported following exposure to short photoperiod, including the ARC and POA. Of note, only one area displayed a decrease of PSA-NCAM subsequent to a transition to long photoperiod: the premammillary nucleus (Chalivoix et al. 2013).

In a second experiment (Chalivoix et al. 2013), endoneuraminidase N, an enzyme that cleaves polysialic acid chains from NCAM (Fig. 5.3b), was injected within the POA (the region encompassing most GnRH somas in sheep, Fig. 5.3c) before a transition to short photoperiod, and the time necessary to observe a rise in LH levels was measured in treated animals and controls (Fig. 5.3d). Two-thirds of treated animals showed delays three times longer than control ewes to develop an increase in their LH levels indicative of transition to the breeding state (>250 days vs 84 days). These data suggest that specific kinetics of morphological rearrangements take place depending on photoperiod and on the hypothalamic region examined. This plasticity may be a key component for the timing of seasonal reproduction.

In a parallel study (Chalivoix et al. 2010), the association between GnRH neurons and PSA-NCAM in groups of OVX + E2 ewes submitted to a transition from long to short photoperiod was quantified. The association of GnRH with PSA-NCAM in animals with an activated gonadotrope axis after a transition to short photoperiod was five times greater than in animals with an inactive axis. However, the numbers of synapses per GnRH neuron was not modified with photoperiodic status. This may reflect the fact that the morphological rearrangements suggested by PSA-NCAM variations on GnRH neurons consist of a change in the phenotype of inputs, rather than an overall increase or decrease in a specific input.

Cellular morphological rearrangements have also been described in the sheep *pars tuberalis* where the highest density of melatonin binding sites is found (Wood et al. 2015). Subsets of *pars tuberalis* cells producing thyroid-stimulating hormone (TSH) are more numerous in summer, increase their junctional contacts and increase their rough endoplasmic reticulum compared to winter where those thyrotroph cells are separated from each other by folliculostellate cells (Wood et al. 2015). This plastic phenomenon may be a key factor for the transduction of melatonin signal to hypothalamic neurons for the synchronization of seasonal functions throughout year.

5.5.2   Seasonal Fluctuations of Neurogenesis and Cell Fate

Recent work performed by the team led by Martine Migaud used uptake of the thymidine analog bromodeoxyuridine (BrdU) infused into the CSF to demonstrate that new cells emerge in the adult ovine brain (Fig. 5.4), most specifically in the thalamic and hypothalamic compartments. These newborn cells are more numerous when the BrdU injection is carried out in sheep exposed to short photoperiod, suggesting that cell neogenesis may be enhanced by the long duration of melatonin secretion under this photoperiod (Migaud et al. 2011). Cell neogenesis also occurs in several brain areas in rams, including the hippocampus, where cell proliferation is greater in long photoperiod in feral sheep of the Soay breed (Hazlerigg et al. 2013). In this study, hypothalamic cell proliferation and survival at 28 days post BrdU infusion was dependent on season, with a higher survival of new cells during short photoperiods (Hazlerigg et al. 2013). In ewes, as highlighted by immunostaining for doublecortin, a marker for neuroblasts, immature neurons were found in the ARC and ME (Batailler et al. 2014). Regarding the fate of hypothalamic newborn cells, further studies demonstrated that a substantial proportion mature into glial cells, while only a restricted portion becomes neurons (Fig. 5.4) (Butruille et al. 2018). Interestingly, immunostaining for markers associated with glial cells (GFAP, Iba1,

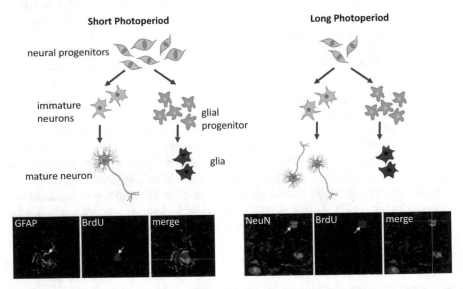

Fig. 5.4 Neurogenesis in ovine hypothalamus depends on photoperiod. Top: in short photoperiod, the number of neural progenitors is greater than in long photoperiod. These progenitors differentiate into glial progenitors and into a limited number of immature neurons but similar levels of both populations appeared under each photoperiod. In contrast, the markers associated with mature neurons and more specifically with neural plasticity were more abundant in long photoperiod than in short photoperiod. Below: examples of new hypothalamic cells having incorporated BrdU and expressing either a glial marker (GFAP) or a neuronal marker (NeuN) as shown (adapted from Migaud et al. 2011)

CNPase, Olig2) did not vary significantly between short and long photoperiods, while the density of a neuronal marker (PSA-NCAM) was greater in short photoperiods (Butruille et al. 2018) in the ARC-ME area. This could suggest that emergence of new neurons is more abundant in short photoperiods in the mediobasal hypothalamus, independent of estradiol fluctuations as suggested initially (Migaud et al. 2011). The most recent findings demonstrated that infusion of the antimitotic drug AraC into the third ventricle resulted in a decrease of neurogenesis associated with an impaired timing of seasonal reproduction, specifically an earlier termination of the breeding season in treated animals (Batailler et al. 2018). Overall these data suggest that seasonal fluctuations of neurogenesis may play a significant role in the integration of melatonin signals and timing of seasonal reproduction.

5.6   Perspectives

Many questions remain regarding the functional consequences of seasonal morphological rearrangements on the start and termination of breeding season in sheep. For example, is the fluctuation of CSF content a consequence or a component of the modifications that occur in the brain parenchyma throughout the year? What is the fate of newborn cells? Do they migrate and if they do, into which brain regions, and what are their peptidergic and/or monoaminergic phenotypes? How will these new cells integrate into existing networks and interact with others populations involved in the central control of reproduction, namely GnRH and KP neurons? Future studies will also focus on studying the different genetic, endocrine, metabolic, and social factors responsible for the induction of plastic phenomenon in line with the seasonal regulation of reproduction.

References

Adam CL, Findlay PA, Miller DW (2006) Blood-brain leptin transport and appetite and reproductive neuroendocrine responses to intracerebroventricular leptin injection in sheep: influence of photoperiod. Endocrinology 147:4589–4598

Adams VL, Goodman RL, Salm AK, Coolen LM, Karsch FJ, Lehman MN (2006) Morphological plasticity in the neural circuitry responsible for seasonal breeding in the ewe. Endocrinology 147:4843–4851

Backholer K, Smith J, Clarke IJ (2009) Melanocortins may stimulate reproduction by activating orexin neurons in the dorsomedial hypothalamus and kisspeptin neurons in the preoptic area of the ewe. Endocrinology 150:5488–5497

Backholer K, Smith JT, Rao A, Pereira A, Iqbal J, Ogawa S, Li Q, Clarke IJ (2010) Kisspeptin cells in the ewe brain respond to leptin and communicate with neuropeptide Y and proopiomelanocortin cells. Endocrinology 151:2233–2243

Batailler M, Chesneau D, Derouet L, Butruille L, Segura S, Cognie J, Dupont J, Pillon D, Migaud M (2018) Pineal-dependent increase of hypothalamic neurogenesis contributes to the timing of seasonal reproduction in sheep. Sci Rep 8:6188

Batailler M, Droguerre M, Baroncini M, Fontaine C, Prevot V, Migaud M (2014) DCX-expressing cells in the vicinity of the hypothalamic neurogenic niche: a comparative study between mouse, sheep, and human tissues. J Comp Neurol 522:1966–1985

Butruille L, Batailler M, Mazur D, Prevot V, Migaud M (2018) Seasonal reorganization of hypothalamic neurogenic niche in adult sheep. Brain Struct Funct 223:91–109

Chalivoix S, Bagnolini A, Caraty A, Cognie J, Malpaux B, Dufourny L (2010) Effects of photoperiod on kisspeptin neuronal populations of the ewe diencephalon in connection with reproductive function. J Neuroendocrinol 22:110–118

Chalivoix S, Guillaume D, Cognie J, Thiery JC, Malpaux B, Dufourny L (2013) Photoperiodic variations of the polysialylated form of neural cell adhesion molecule within the hypothalamus and related reproductive output in the ewe. Cell Tissue Res 352:387–399

Chalivoix S, Malpaux B, Dufourny L (2010) Relationship between polysialylated neural cell adhesion molecule and beta-endorphin- or gonadotropin releasing hormone-containing neurons during activation of the gonadotrope axis in short daylength in the ewe. Neuroscience 169:1326–1336

Dardente H (2012) Melatonin-dependent timing of seasonal reproduction by the *pars tuberalis*: pivotal roles for long daylengths and thyroid hormones. J Neuroendocrinol 24:249–266

De Bond JA, Smith JT (2014) Kisspeptin and energy balance in reproduction. Reproduction 147: R53–R63

Fabre-Nys C, Cognie J, Dufourny L, Ghenim M, Martinet S, Lasserre O, Lomet D, Millar RP, Ohkura S, Suetomi Y (2017) The two populations of Kisspeptin neurons are involved in the ram-induced LH pulsatile secretion and LH surge in anestrous ewes. Endocrinology 158:3914–3928

Franceschini I, Lomet D, Cateau M, Delsol G, Tillet Y, Caraty A (2006) Kisspeptin immunoreactive cells of the ovine preoptic area and arcuate nucleus co-express estrogen receptor alpha. Neurosci Lett 401:225–230

Goodman RL, Lehman MN, Smith JT, Coolen LM, de Oliveira CV, Jafarzadehshirazi MR, Pereira A, Iqbal J, Caraty A, Ciofi P, Clarke IJ (2007) Kisspeptin neurons in the arcuate nucleus of the ewe express both dynorphin A and neurokinin B. Endocrinology 148:5752–5760

Hazlerigg DG, Wyse CA, Dardente H, Hanon EA, Lincoln GA (2013) Photoperiodic variation in CD45-positive cells and cell proliferation in the mediobasal hypothalamus of the Soay sheep. Chronobiol Int 30:548–558

Jansen HT, Cutter C, Hardy S, Lehman MN, Goodman RL (2003) Seasonal plasticity within the gonadotropin-releasing hormone (GnRH) system of the ewe: changes in identified GnRH inputs and glial association. Endocrinology 144:3663–3676

Lagaraine C, Skipor J, Szczepkowska A, Dufourny L, Thiery JC (2011) Tight junction proteins vary in the choroid plexus of ewes according to photoperiod. Brain Res 1393:44–51

Luque RM, Kineman RD, Tena-Sempere M (2007) Regulation of hypothalamic expression of KiSS-1 and GPR54 genes by metabolic factors: analyses using mouse models and a cell line. Endocrinology 148:4601–4611

Malpaux B (2006) Seasonal regulation of reproduction in mammals. In: Neill JD (ed) Knobil and Neill's physiology of reproduction, 3rd edn. Elsevier, New York, pp 2231–2281

Menassol JB, Collet A, Chesneau D, Malpaux B, Scaramuzzi RJ (2011) The interaction between photoperiod and nutrition and its effects on seasonal rhythms of reproduction in the ewe. Biol Reprod 86:52

Migaud M, Batailler M, Pillon D, Franceschini I, Malpaux B (2011) Seasonal changes in cell proliferation in the adult sheep brain and *pars tuberalis*. J Biol Rhythm 26:486–496

Santillo A, Falvo S, Di Fiore MM, ChieffiBaccari G (2017) Seasonal changes and sexual dimorphism in gene expression of StAR protein, steroidogenic enzymes and sex hormone receptors in the frog brain. Gen Comp Endocrinol 246:226–232

Schlinger BA, Remage-Healey L (2012) Neurosteroidogenesis: insights from studies of songbirds. J Neuroendocrinol 24:16–21

Sergeeva A, Jansen HT (2009) Neuroanatomical plasticity in the gonadotropin-releasing hormone system of the ewe: seasonal variation in glutamatergic and gamma-aminobutyricacidergic afferents. J Comp Neurol 515:615–628

Smith JT, Clay CM, Caraty A, Clarke IJ (2007) KiSS-1 messenger ribonucleic acid expression in the hypothalamus of the ewe is regulated by sex steroids and season. Endocrinology 148:1150–1157

Smith JT, Coolen LM, Kriegsfeld LJ, Sari IP, Jaafarzadehshirazi MR, Maltby M, Bateman K, Goodman RL, Tilbrook AJ, Ubuka T, Bentley GE, Clarke IJ, Lehman MN (2008) Variation in kisspeptin and RFamide-related peptide (RFRP) expression and terminal connections to gonadotropin-releasing hormone neurons in the brain: a novel medium for seasonal breeding in the sheep. Endocrinology 149:5770–5782

Strazielle N, Khuth ST, Ghersi-Egea JF (2004) Detoxification systems, passive and specific transport for drugs at the blood-CSF barrier in normal and pathological situations. Adv Drug Deliv Rev 56:1717–1740

Szczepkowska A, Lagaraine C, Robert V, Dufourny L, Thiery JC, Skipor J (2013) Effect of a two-week treatment with a low dose of 2,2′4,4′,5,5′-hexachlorobiphenyl (PCB153) on tight junction protein expression in ovine choroid plexus during long and short photoperiods. Neurotoxicol Teratol 37:63–67

Teixeira-Gomes AP, Harichaux G, Gennetay D, Skipor J, Thiery JC, Labas V, Dufourny L (2015) Photoperiod affects the cerebrospinal fluid proteome: a comparison between short day- and long day-treated ewes. Domest Anim Endocrinol 53:1–8

Thiery JC, Lomet D, Bougoin S, Malpaux B (2009) Turnover rate of cerebrospinal fluid in female sheep: changes related to different light-dark cycles. Cerebrospinal Fluid Res 6:9

Thiery JC, Lomet D, Schumacher M, Liere P, Tricoire H, Locatelli A, Delagrange P, Malpaux B (2006) Concentrations of estradiol in ewe cerebrospinal fluid are modulated by photoperiod through pineal-dependent mechanisms. J Pineal Res 41:306–312

Thiery JC, Malpaux B (2003) Seasonal regulation of reproductive activity in sheep: modulation of access of sex steroids to the brain. Ann N Y Acad Sci 1007;169–175

True C, Verma S, Grove KL, Smith MS (2013) Cocaine- and amphetamine-regulated transcript is a potent stimulator of GnRH and Kisspeptin cells and may contribute to negative energy balance-induced reproductive inhibition in females. Endocrinology 154(8):2821–2832

Viguie C, Jansen HT, Glass JD, Watanabe M, Billings HJ, Coolen L, Lehman MN, Karsch FJ (2001) Potential for polysialylated form of neural cell adhesion molecule-mediated neuroplasticity within the gonadotropin-releasing hormone neurosecretory system of the ewe. Endocrinology 142:1317–1324

Weems P, Smith J, Clarke IJ, Coolen LM, Goodman RL, Lehman MN (2017) Effects of season and estradiol on KNDy neuron peptides, Colocalization with D2 dopamine receptors, and dopaminergic inputs in the ewe. Endocrinology 158:831–841

Wood SH, Christian HC, Miedzinska K, Saer BR, Johnson M, Paton B, Yu L, McNeilly J, Davis JR, McNeilly AS, Burt DW, Loudon AS (2015) Binary switching of calendar cells in the pituitary defines the phase of the circannual cycle in mammals. Curr Biol 25:2651–2662

Xiong JJ, Karsch FJ, Lehman MN (1997) Evidence for seasonal plasticity in the gonadotropin-releasing hormone (GnRH) system of the ewe: changes in synaptic inputs onto GnRH neurons. Endocrinology 138:1240–1250

Recommended Further Reading

Lévy F, Batailler M, Meurisse M, Migaud M (2017) Adult neurogenesis in sheep: characterization and contribution to Reproduction and Behavior. Front Neurosci 11:570
Neurogenesis is not only observed in the hypothalamus but also in other brains areas in sheep and this review summarizes recent data about neurogenesis potential involvement in several physiological functions and behaviors.

Dardente H, Wood S, Ebling F, Saenz de Miera C (2019) An integrative view of mammalian seasonal neuroendocrinology. J. Neuroendocrinol. 31:e12729
This review summarizes the most recent data on molecular pathways involved in the translation of photoperiod to the hypothalamus and also expand the discussion by addressing the possible involvement of RFRP-3 neurons in the central control of reproduction.

Clocks and Calendars in Birds

6

Barbara Helm

Abstract

Among research on biological rhythms, avian studies stand out through their embedding of neuroendocrinology in evolutionary and ecological contexts. Birds differ from mammals by generally being diurnal, by using input pathways of photic information to daily and annual timing that may not require the eyes, and by an interconnected multiple pacemaker system in the brain. Although there are considerable differences among avian species, the pineal gland and retina can function as complete mini-clocks featuring photoreception, sustained rhythm generation, and output generation. Melatonin is produced mainly in the pineal gland and, in many avian species, plays an important role in circadian rhythmicity, but not in annual cyclicity. The avian suprachiasmatic nucleus (SCN) is less critical for rhythmicity than in mammals, although most clock functions are available within its two paired nuclei. Possibly facilitated by the multiple pacemaker system, avian circadian clocks are remarkably plastic, especially during migration seasons when many species spontaneously assume nocturnal activity. The annual cycles of birds are underpinned by an interaction of circannual rhythms with strong photoperiodism. It is unclear how these ancient timing mechanisms will cope with rapidly changing temporal environments as circadian disruption by artificial light at night and annual cycle shifts in response to global warming become ever more evident.

Keywords

Multiple pacemaker · Circannual · Diurnal · Global change · Migration

B. Helm (✉)
GELIFES - Groningen Institute for Evolutionary Life Sciences, University of Groningen, Groningen, The Netherlands
e-mail: B.Helm@rug.nl

© The Editor(s) (if applicable) and The Author(s), under exclusive license to
Springer Nature Switzerland AG 2020
F. J. P. Ebling, H. D. Piggins (eds.), *Neuroendocrine Clocks and Calendars*,
Masterclass in Neuroendocrinology 10, https://doi.org/10.1007/978-3-030-55643-3_6

6.1   Introduction

Humans have long valued birds as conspicuous timekeepers, from the crow of the rooster waking the village to the arrival of migrants announcing spring. Daily and annual cycles of physiology and behavior commonly persist in wild birds in captivity, paving the way to early experimentation, so birds have a long history as important model organisms for chronobiological research. For example, song production shows daily and annual rhythms, and in parallel to night flights of free-living conspecifics, caged migratory birds display periodic nocturnal activity (i.e., migratory restlessness). Many seminal studies of the formal properties of circadian (Aschoff 1967) and circannual rhythms (Gwinner 1986) used birds as their subject. Contributions of avian studies to mechanistic advances in chronobiology were less frequent because fewer molecular and genetic tools were available for birds than for mammals or fruit flies, but outstanding examples exist, such as the characterization of a multiple photoreceptor-pacemaker system (Menaker and Underwood 1976).

Perhaps the greatest ongoing contribution of avian chronobiology is its explicit behavioral, evolutionary, and ecological contexts. Examples include the first demonstrations of entrainment to social *zeitgebers* (Menaker and Eskin 1966; Gwinner 1966) and deciphering of time-compensated sun-compass orientation in captive and wild birds (Kramer 1957; Padget et al. 2018). Studies in birds also point to the many factors that shape the output of the circadian and circannual systems in the real world, from polar to equatorial environments (Visser et al. 2010; Helm et al. 2017). The current development of comparative genomic resources, combined with sophisticated satellite tracking tools, is poised to uncover links between timekeeping mechanisms underlying rhythmicity and behavior in the wild. In this present phase of chronobiology, when extensive molecular insights are integrated at an organismic level, avian studies are likely to lead to future breakthroughs.

This chapter provides an introduction to endogenous avian clocks and calendars, summarizing the main mechanisms while emphasizing the above strengths of studies in birds. Conceptually, the avian clock-and-calendar system can be partitioned into input pathways, by which external time information is perceived; the clock system, consisting of central pacemakers and peripheral clocks, which keep internal time; and effector systems, which produce behavioral and physiological outputs from clock time and environmental modifiers (Helm et al. 2017). Figure 6.1 illustrates this system for circadian clocks.

This chapter will first explain avian light input pathways, followed by an overview of the circadian system and the role of melatonin. It will then introduce circannual rhythms and photoperiodism, emphasizing plasticity and diversity of timekeeping based on the broad avian taxonomic approach. Finally, it will apply insights from birds to address the impact of anthropogenic environmental change on biological rhythms.

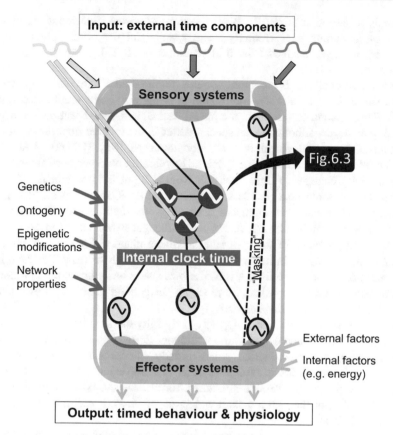

Fig. 6.1 Schematic of the avian circadian system (blue) within the organism (green). Input from multiple environmental factors (yellow: light; grey: other) reaches central and peripheral clocks (indicated by sine waves) directly or via sensory systems that sometimes contain clocks. External synchronizing cues (*zeitgebers*) can entrain internal time of the central clock system (pale-red central circle), which contains three pacemakers (red; see Fig. 6.3 for details), of which two are photoreceptive. The central clock interacts with peripheral clocks and acts on effector systems via neuronal or other (e.g., humoral, thermal) pathways that produce behavioral and physiological output; masking is indicated by dashed lines. Left blue arrows: mechanisms that shape plasticity of the circadian system; right green arrows: environmental modifiers acting on effector systems. Based on (Helm et al. 2017)

6.2   Light Input Pathways in Birds

The avian clock-and-calendar system is receptive to a wide range of stimuli, including photic, social, thermal, and metabolic factors (Helfer et al. 2019; Caro et al. 2013; Gwinner 1966; Menaker and Eskin 1966). As in mammals, light has by far the greatest effects on the circadian and circannual system of birds. However, light input pathways for timekeeping differ substantially between birds and mammals (Cassone et al. 2017). Birds receive non-visual light input via multiple structures, including eyes (retina), pineal gland, and deep-brain photoreceptors mostly in the hypothalamus (Fig. 6.2) (Kuenzel et al. 2015; Davies et al. 2012; Nakane et al. 2014).

Unlike mammals, birds commonly do not require ocular light input to entrain to daily changes in light intensity and to annual changes in daylength (Cassone et al. 2017). For circadian entrainment, the pineal, retina, and deep-brain photoreceptors may all play a role, although avian species differ in the relative importance of these structures. The pineal constitutes a major input pathway (Okano et al. 1994; Menaker et al. 1997), but in some species, deep-brain photoreceptors are sufficient to detect daily changes in light intensity. Retinal input is important for circadian entrainment of some taxa, but less so for songbirds (Cassone et al. 2017). The redundancy of ocular light input has been elegantly demonstrated by a series of experiments on songbirds by Menaker and colleagues (Menaker and Underwood 1976). Briefly, removal of the eyes and the pineal gland did not disrupt circadian entrainment, as long as light levels were intense enough to reach the deep-brain photoreceptors. Under low light levels, the birds were arrhythmic, but entrainment was re-instated and re-abolished, by plucking feathers on the birds' crown and by darkening it by injecting ink, respectively.

On an annual timescale, birds appear to rely fully on deep-brain photoreceptors for circannual entrainment and photoperiodism. That eyes are not necessary for photoinduction of reproduction was already demonstrated by enucleation experiments in the 1930s (Cassone et al. 2017). Subsequent studies investigated more closely the photoreceptive structures, as well as the wavelength-dependent penetration of light through the skull and brain of birds (Foster and Follett 1985; Nakane et al. 2014).

Recent years have seen great efforts at identifying the photopigments, the neuro-anatomical locations, and the molecular transduction of avian light input pathways. Although no consensus has been established, it is clear that birds use several types of opsins as sensors for timekeeping. These include pinopsin, iodopsin (opn1), rhodopsin (opn2), melanopsin (opn4), neuropsin (opn5), and Vertebrate Ancient opsin (VAopsin) (Okano et al. 1994; Davies et al. 2012; Nakane et al. 2014; Kuenzel et al. 2015). Several of these can colocalize and potentially act in conjunction, for example, to broaden spectral sensitivity.

6.3   Avian Circadian System

A second major difference from mammals is the much greater structural diversity of the avian circadian system. A multiple pacemaker system, as described below for birds, is common among higher organisms, making mammals an apparent exception. However, centralization of the mammalian circadian system may have been overrated, given the increasing evidence of complex interactions between central and peripheral pacemakers (Menaker et al. 1997; Van der Veen et al. 2017).

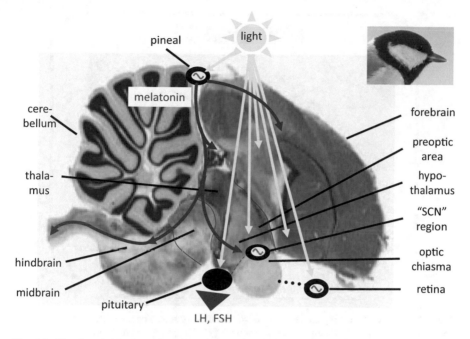

Fig. 6.2 Timekeeping in the avian brain and associated structures. Sagittal section of the brain of a great tit (*Parus major;* thionin-stained slide by Davide Dominoni) and approximated locations of pineal, pituitary, and retina. Light input pathways are indicated by yellow arrows; pacemakers are indicated by sine waves; and major daily (melatonin) and annual (LH, luteinizing hormone; FSH, follicle-stimulating hormone) endocrine outputs are shown in red. Inlay for orientation: male great tit, Luc Viatour, Belgium, wikimedia.org

Birds have at least three structures that function as central pacemakers (Fig. 6.2), of which two, the pineal and retina, are photoreceptive. The third pacemaker structure is two paired nuclei in the mediobasal hypothalamus, above the optic chiasm. These are arguably functionally and phylogenetically homologous to the mammalian suprachiasmatic nucleus (SCN) and are hence often named "SCN." It is possible that additional but as yet unidentified pacemakers exist, because individual birds can show several rhythmic components that differ from each other in free-running period length (see below). The three identified pacemakers are autonomous and can produce sustained periodic output, which in turn regulates downstream rhythmicity. They are nonetheless interconnected and communicate through endocrine and neuronal pathways (Gwinner and Brandstätter 2001; Kumar et al. 2004) (see below; Fig. 6.3). The relative importance of the pacemakers in this system differs between species. An important circadian role falls to the indoleamine hormone melatonin, which in birds is rhythmically synthesized and secreted by the pineal gland and sometimes by the retina. As photoreceptive pacemakers that also secrete melatonin, the pineal and retina are functional miniature clocks that offer intriguing research opportunities at tissue and cellular levels.

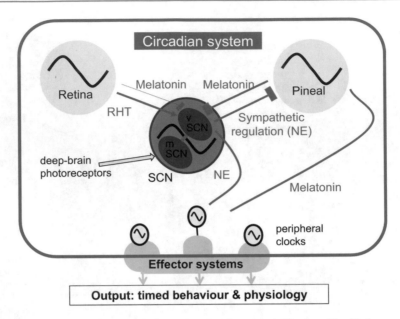

Fig. 6.3 Schematic working model of the avian circadian system. The three identified pacemakers are indicated by large circles containing sine waves; light receptive structures are shown in yellow. Interactions between circadian pacemakers are shown by blue connectors (arrows: activational; rectangles: inhibitory; open-ended: connectivity). Peripheral clocks are shown in grey, effectors in green; NE, norepinephrine; vSCN, visual SCN; mSCN, medial SCN; RHT, retinohypothalamic tract; based on (Cassone 2014); see Fig. 6.1 for context

The avian pineal gland is a strong pacemaker, whose rhythmicity persists in tissue culture and even in isolated pinealocytes (Cassone et al. 2017; Gwinner and Brandstätter 2001). In songbirds, pinealectomy almost completely abolishes circulating melatonin concentrations and thereby often, but not always, abolishes free-running rhythms. In pinealectomized house sparrows (*Passer domesticus*), rhythmicity was restored by implanting a pineal from a donor bird into the anterior chamber of the eye. The receiving bird then displayed overt rhythms with period length and phase of the donor (Zimmerman and Menaker 1979). In some other species, pinealectomy abolishes free-running rhythmicity only partly, or not at all. For example, in European starlings (*Sturnus vulgaris*), rhythms of locomotor activity were diminished after pinealectomy, whereas feeding remained rhythmic (Gänshirt et al. 1984).

The role of the retina in the circadian system differs between species. In contrast to songbird studies, in feral pigeon (*Columba livia*) and quail (*Coturnix coturnix*), only joint removal of eyes and pineal rendered birds arrhythmic (Oshima et al. 1989). The retinas of pigeons and quail produce large amounts of rhythmic melatonin and release it into the bloodstream, and in quail, this rhythmic production also persists in tissue culture (Nakane and Yoshimura 2019).

The most complex pacemaker is the SCN, which consists of the visual vSCN (sometimes called lateral, lSCN) and the medial mSCN (Yoshimura et al. 2001;

Cassone et al. 2017) (Fig. 6.3). Although both nuclei are involved in the circadian system, they display functional division, and their features differ between species. Studies of two galliform species (quail; chicken *Gallus gallus*), one columbiform species (pigeon), and one passeriform species (Java sparrow, *Padda oryzivora*) found that clock genes (*per2*) were expressed rhythmically in the mSCN but not in the vSCN (Yoshimura et al. 2001), whereas in house sparrow, rhythmic expression was described in both nuclei (Abraham et al. 2002). Conversely, other studies report rhythmic electrical activity, with daytime peaks, in the vSCN but not in the mSCN (Cassone et al. 2017).

Simultaneous analysis of gene expression patterns of SCN, pineal, and retina within individuals clarifies the phase relationships between the three pacemakers. For example, tree sparrows (*Passer montanus*) showed robust rhythmic expression of clock genes in hypothalamus, pineal, and retina. The temporal aspects of these profiles of expression were nearly identical for most clock genes, with potentially important exceptions (i.e., *per2*) (Renthlei et al. 2019).

Pathways of interaction between the pacemakers are only partly understood (Fig. 6.3). Melatonin is generally the key circadian hormone, binding to many sites in the avian brain (Fusani and Gahr 2015; viviD and Bentley 2018). Melatonin reaches the retina and SCN via high-affinity Mel1A (MT1) and other receptors, where it exerts an inhibitory action. In support of functional division within the SCN, high-affinity Mel1A receptors have been detected only in the vSCN and not in the mSCN (Yoshimura et al. 2001; Cassone 2014). The role of other hormones in the avian circadian system is less clear. For example, although many birds rhythmically secrete corticosterone (the main avian corticosteroid) (Rich and Romero 2001), effects of this hormone on the circadian system are not evident. Important neuromodulators include dopamine (Besharse and McMahon 2016) and norepinephrine (NE).

Neuronal connections between the pacemakers include a polysynaptic sympathetic pathway from the SCN to the pineal gland. The vSCN regulates rhythmic NE drive to targets including the pineal, where increased NE inhibits melatonin production during daytime (Kumar et al. 2004; Cassone 2014). The SCN receives rhythmic input also from the retina via the retinohypothalamic tract (RHT), although it is debated whether projections are received only by the vSCN or also by the mSCN (Yoshimura et al. 2001; Cassone 2014). Fig. 6.3 summarizes how the pacemakers may interact with each other in a neuroendocrine loop (Cassone et al. 2017). Melatonin secreted from the pineal binds to receptors in the vSCN and thereby inhibits activity of the mSCN via neuronal connections. When pineal melatonin secretion decreases, SCN activity resumes, inhibiting the pineal via NE neurotransmission (Cassone 2014). Light can reinforce this rhythm and affect its phase by activating the SCN while suppressing melatonin synthesis.

The observation that experimental impairment of either the pineal or the SCN weakens the rhythm of the other shows that the interacting pacemakers stabilize and amplify each other. Their interaction strengthens the circadian system through internal resonance, providing birds with highly self-sustained overt rhythmicity (Gwinner and Brandstätter 2001; Cassone 2014).

Functionally, the high structural diversity of the avian compared to the mammalian circadian system provides many nuts and bolts for adjustment, through both evolutionary change and phenotypic plasticity. For example, reducing the amplitude of the circadian system through down-tuning a contributing pacemaker is thought to increase plasticity because weakly self-sustained rhythms are more responsive to environmental cues (*zeitgebers*). The circadian system could then be easily adjusted to the environment, for example, to entrain to subtle photic change in polar regions, or to shifting light conditions during migration (Gwinner and Brandstätter 2001).

On a molecular level, the genes that are known to be involved in the circadian clock largely resemble those in mammals (i.e., *period, cryptochrome, clock, bmal;* see Chap. 11), although *per1* is not expressed in birds. Between avian species, these genes appear to be highly conserved, except for polymorphism in repeat numbers of trinucleotides that may be functionally important (Johnsen et al. 2007). The interplay between the neuroendocrine and the molecular rhythm generation is beginning to be understood, for example, by reported interactions between the protein product of the clock gene *bmal1* and melatonin (Cassone et al. 2017).

6.4 The Role of Melatonin

The importance of melatonin cycles for circadian rhythms has been clearly shown, for example, by reinstating rhythmicity of pinealectomized birds through periodic application of melatonin (Gwinner and Brandstätter 2001). However, in various species, daily rhythmicity of melatonin is weak or absent under natural and simulated light–dark cycles, for example, among waders (Charadriiformes) and owls (Strigiformes). Owls have a rudimentary pineal gland and very low plasma melatonin amplitudes even during darkness, despite clear behavioral rhythmicity (Gwinner and Brandstätter 2001). Furthermore, in polar birds, exposure to continuous light in summer, may suppress melatonin, although some species maintain surprisingly robust melatonin cycles (Ashley et al. 2014). It is unclear whether in species with no apparent melatonin cycles, its circadian function is redundant, or whether melatonin continues in its function at low levels, perhaps from sources other than the pineal (viviD and Bentley 2018).

In species with pronounced rhythmic secretion of pineal melatonin, the melatonin profile reflects photoperiod. Fig. 6.4 shows melatonin profiles of captive European blackbirds (*Turdus merula*) in winter and summer (Dominoni et al. 2013a). During winter, duration of elevated melatonin is extended, just as it is in mammals (viviD and Bentley 2018). However, unlike mammals, birds also show strong seasonal modulation of the melatonin amplitude, with higher levels during short summer nights than during long winter nights. In house sparrows, these differences persisted under continuous darkness and were retained in vitro. Cultured pineal glands continued to secrete higher amounts of melatonin at night in summer, but for shorter duration, than during winter (Gwinner and Brandstätter 2001).

The observations that the pattern of melatonin secretion changes across the seasons could indicate a role in regulating seasonal cycles, as clearly demonstrated

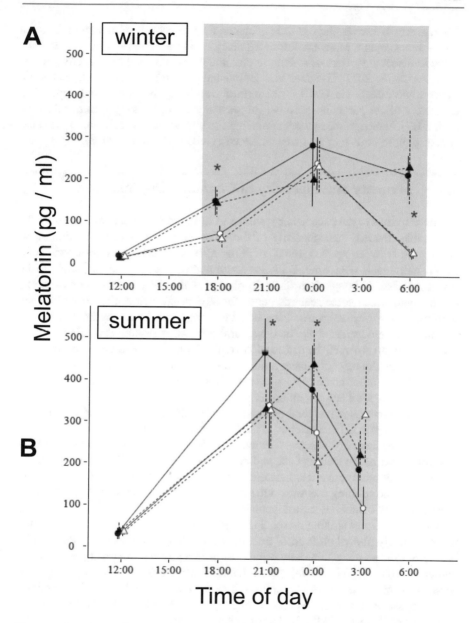

Fig. 6.4 Variation in plasma melatonin profiles depending on season and nocturnal illumination. Captive European blackbirds (*Turdus merula*), originating either from urban (triangle) or forest (circle) habitats, were held under simulated winter (**a**) and summer (**b**) photoperiods (night shown in grey), either under dark (black symbols) or dimly lit nights (0.3 lx; white symbols). Melatonin (mean ± SEM) was measured at mid-night and mid-day in both seasons. Morning and evening sampling differed between the seasons (winter 6:00 and 18:00; summer at 3:00 and 21:00 h), to keep the interval to the respective twilights equal. Red asterisks indicate significant effects of light treatment (Dominoni et al. 2013a)

in mammals. However, there is little evidence for a direct role of melatonin in avian annual timekeeping. Many studies using designs similar to those used in mammals failed to detect any effect of melatonin on annual or circannual reproductive cycles (Cassone et al. 2017; Gwinner and Brandstätter 2001). Nonetheless, melatonin exerts some effects via GnIH (gonadotropin-inhibitory hormone) and appears to selectively affect particular seasonal processes, that is, the song system (Cassone et al. 2017). Hence, some authors argue that the importance of melatonin for annual timekeeping in birds may be underestimated (viviD and Bentley 2018).

6.5   Diversity and Plasticity of Circadian Organization

The descriptions of the pacemaker system and of the role of melatonin illustrate the remarkable diversity and plasticity of the avian circadian system. In addition to differences between species, birds' rhythms also vary greatly within species and within individuals over time. Daily behavioral rhythmicity generally tends to be strong in birds, although taxa differ in clarity of the daily pattern. For example, geese, waders, and some seabirds generally have weaker day–night rhythms than songbirds. Nevertheless, across taxa, behavioral rhythmicity can be finely adjusted depending on environment and on behavioral context. A striking example is vocalization, where in roosters, the period of the endogenous circadian crowing rhythm is determined by the most dominant individual (Shimmura et al. 2015). Likewise, the timing of locomotor activities can change dramatically with annual cycle phases such as reproduction and migration (Fig. 6.5a).

Seasonal changes in temporal behavior may involve modification of the underlying circadian system. For example, in starlings, the phase of reproductive activation affected circadian rhythmicity (Gwinner 1974). When tested under constant conditions, European starlings showed conspicuous splitting of locomotor activity during reproductive activation, indicating the decoupling of at least two underlying oscillators. The splitting was shown to be causally linked to the seasonal increase in testosterone by combining castration and injections.

The perhaps most striking seasonal change in avian circadian organization occurs when normally diurnal birds show nocturnal migratory restlessness ("zugunruhe"). Figure 6.5 shows change in daily organization in a strongly migratory species, the garden warbler (*Sylvia borin*) (Bartell and Gwinner 2005). During migration seasons, in birds kept under natural daylength, a component of daytime activity ("A") disassociates and moves into the night (Fig. 6.5a). This nocturnal component, migratory restlessness ("M"), is characterized by flight-like behaviors which can be clearly distinguished from daytime activities. Such restless nights in migratory birds can continue for many weeks, lasting as long as the migration seasons, and sometimes longer (Akesson et al. 2017). That daytime and nocturnal activities are driven by separate oscillators has been elegantly shown also in garden warblers (Fig. 6.5b (Bartell and Gwinner 2005)). Birds were entrained to a skeleton photoperiod that provides a weak *zeitgeber*. Upon release to constant conditions, the two activity components dissociated and free-ran with different period lengths.

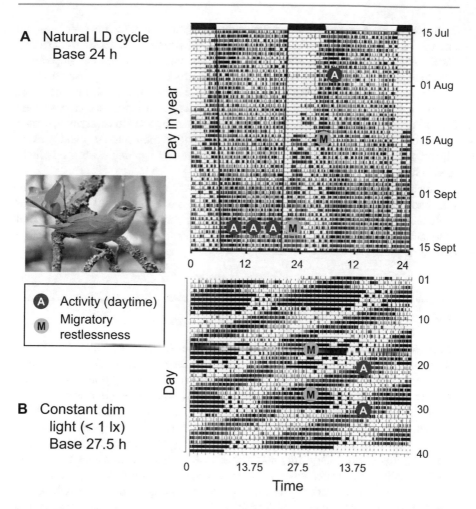

Fig. 6.5 Seasonal plasticity of the circadian system of garden warblers (*Sylvia borin*). (**a**) Double-plotted actograms showing seasonal development of migratory restlessness (green M) under simulated natural photoperiod. The light-dark bars above the actogram show initial LD cycles. In August, a bout of daytime activity (red A) progressed into the night to eventually assume a new phase relationship with the remaining daytime activity. Video analysis showed that this nocturnal activity consisted almost exclusively of migratory restlessness, as indicated by migration-type behavior (green M). (**b**) Dissociation of daytime activity (red A) and migratory restlessness (green M) under constant dim light. The solid dark bouts of activity represent migratory restless-ness, as confirmed by video recordings. Because the two activity types have different period lengths, the traces for daytime activity and migratory restlessness cross; when the oscillators driving these two activities were in antiphase, migratory restlessness was most intense. The daytime oscillator had a period length of 23.2 h, whereas the nocturnal oscillator had a period length of 27.7 h. Activity is plotted on a 27.5 h scale to facilitate viewing of the two rhythms; for details, see (Bartell and Gwinner 2005). (**a**) reproduced with kind permission of *Journal of Biological Rhythms*; (**b**) courtesy of Paul Bartell. Inlay: image of garden warbler from Billyboy, Sweden, wikimedia.org

Switches to, and out of, nocturnal activity occur not only through seasonal change, but also in response to metabolic state (Gwinner et al. 1988; Helfer et al. 2019). Wild migratory birds alternate night flights with several days of stopover to feed to regain their energy reserves. At sites with ample food, they pause nocturnal activity until body mass has sufficiently increased. However, if food is scarce, birds resume nocturnal activity regardless of their body mass, until they reach a rewarding food source. This metabolically sensitive behavior can be used in captivity to switch birds from diurnal to additional nocturnal activity (by food removal) and back to diurnal activity (by food return), as shown, for example, in garden warbler (Gwinner et al. 1988).

Much more can be learned from the extraordinary temporal plasticity of migratory birds than can be summarized in this chapter (Akesson et al. 2017). Molecular tools are rapidly generating exciting new findings, such as insights in temporal reorganization in the brain associated with switches to nocturnal activity (Rastogi et al. 2011).

6.6   Circannual Rhythms

Birds were long suspected to possess long-term internal timekeepers to enable their spectacular, precisely timed annual movements (Akesson et al. 2017). In particular, the return of migrants for breeding was thought to require endogenous timekeeping because environmental conditions in the winter quarters can be poor or misleading predictors for conditions on the breeding grounds (see Text Box 1). Photoperiod and ambient temperature, which provide seasonal information for resident species, change with location and are therefore shaped by the birds' movements. For example, cross-hemispheric migrants experience long days in winter that would normally induce local breeding. However, instead of winter breeding, these birds delay reproductive activation until the approach of spring at their remote breeding grounds, when austral daylength decreases. A second group of birds predicted to possess strong endogenous rhythms were those living near the equator, where despite almost constant daylength, many show clear annual cycles. In both groups of birds, particularly clear circannual rhythms have indeed been demonstrated experimentally (Gwinner 1986; Gwinner 1996; Helm et al. 2013).

Box 1. Effects of Migration on Experienced Daylength
The annual change in daylength (photoperiod) depends on geographic location on Earth (see inlay figure). At the equator, daylength is continuously very close to 12 h (purple line), although subtle annual changes exist. With increasing distance away from the equator (i.e., increasing latitude), daylength increasingly changes over the year, such that it is maximal during summer solstice and minimal during winter solstice (red and blue curves). Because the

(continued)

Box 1 (continued)

annual change in daylength (i.e., the photoperiodic amplitude) increases with distance away from the equator, the rate of daylength change over consecutive days also increases with higher latitude: In spring, daylength increases faster, and in autumn, it decreases faster, with greater distance away from the equator. The solstices are inverted between the northern and southern hemispheres: On the northern hemisphere (blue curve), longest days occur during the June solstice, whereas on the southern hemisphere (red curve), they occur during the December solstice. Only twice a year, during the equinoxes in March and September, is daylength identical across Earth (measuring 12 h).

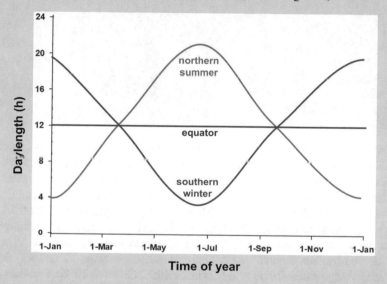

The specificity of daylength on a given date to location has major implications for organisms that migrate. By migratory change in latitude, daylength will increase or decrease and so will the rate of change in daylength. Thus, migratory birds experience two, confounded, sources of change in photoperiod: those arising from time of year (Earth's rotation around its axis) and those induced by their own movement. As a consequence, for a migratory bird, phases of the annual cycle may be spent under nearly unchanging daylength, or days may be long, rather than short, in winter. Very complicated patterns can arise, depending on the specific time and location of a bird's migration in a given year. For example, a bird breeding in the northern hemisphere, but wintering on the equator, will experience an extended phase of unchanging daylength and thus minimal calendaric information (after the blue curve switches to the purple line). A bird that crosses the equator will experience long days during breeding, followed by decreasing daylength in

(continued)

Box 1 (continued)
late summer, and then again long days during winter (switching between blue curve and red curve). The latitudinal changes are often also associated with changes in thermoperiod, so that the bird may experience warming, not cooling, in autumn. In addition, with reference to time of sunrise and sunset, migration also results in time-shifts if carried out in east–west direction (i.e., across longitudes), equivalent to crossing of time zones.

Because migration changes the annual photoperiod, migratory birds need to be highly discriminatory in the use of photoperiodic cues. This is achieved through an endogenous circannual rhythm that regulates birds' responses to daylength in a phase-dependent way. For example, cross-hemispheric migrants do not respond to long days with reproductive activation in winter, but do so in spring, during migration. Consequently, austral colonization events are rare. Where they occur, they probably required delayed migration departure from the wintering site, which enabled entrainment to local conditions. This interpretation is supported by evidence of a fully phase-inverted annual cycle (Winkler et al. 2017).

Just like for circadian rhythms, demonstrating the endogenous nature of circannual rhythms involved evidence that periodically recurring processes free-run under constant environmental conditions. The most commonly used light regimes were constant 12 h days (LD 12:12 h), but free-running circannual rhythms were also shown under constant dim light and under constant daylengths from 10 to 18 h (Rani and Kumar 2013; Helm et al. 2013). Circannual rhythms were documented for a range of behavioral and physiological processes. The first avian demonstrations showed that migratory restlessness (e.g., Figure 6.5) free-ran with period lengths of 9–10 months (Gwinner 1986; Gwinner 1996). Parallel studies under constant conditions and in the field confirmed that circannual rhythms triggered the onset of spring migratory behavior roughly at the time when overwintering birds prepared to leave their African winter quarters. Subsequent research showed that processes associated with migration such as fat deposition, choice of compass direction, and molt and reproductive cycles, were also under circannual control (Fig. 6.6) (Gwinner 1986; Gwinner 1996). For example, under constant conditions, garden warblers spontaneously transitioned from low to high hypothalamic GnRH (gonadotropin-releasing hormone) production in early spring (Bluhm et al. 1991). Circannual rhythms were also documented in species that remained in equatorial habitats throughout the year and in other non-migratory species. For example, African stonechats (*Saxicola torquata*) showed persistent gonadal and molt cycles that lasted for over 10 years within individuals and that developed innately in juveniles that never experienced changing daylength (Gwinner 1996).

Circannual cycles of different seasonal activities are not always coupled: In some species, either molt or reproductive cycles, but not both, were observed to persist under constant conditions, while in other species, the relative timing of activities

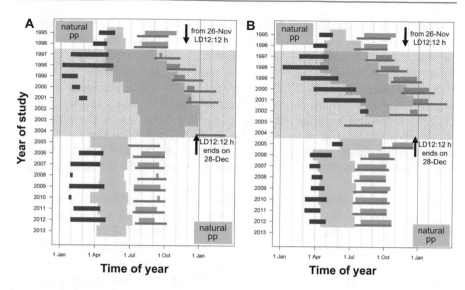

Fig. 6.6 Entrained, free-running, and re-entrained seasonal activities of red knots (*Calidris canutus*). The depicted two waders (**a, b**) were initially kept under a simulated, natural photoperiod, then exposed to constant LD 12:12 h from November 26, 1996, to December 28, 2004 (shaded area; shifts shown by arrows), and then transferred back to natural photoperiod. The birds' seasonal phases are indicated by different colors: light blue: elevated body mass; bright purple: molt to breeding plumage; pale purple: molt to non-breeding plumage; steel blue: wing molt; based on (Karagicheva et al. 2016)

changed over time. These observations suggest a modular organization of the circannual system. Fig. 6.6 shows annual and circannual cycles of a charadriiform bird, the red knot (*Calidris canutus*, based on (Karagicheva et al. 2016)). Birds were entrained for 2 years to local photoperiod in the Netherlands, followed by 8 years of 12 h days, and then re-entrainment. In the two exemplary birds, annual cycles free-ran with period lengths of approximately 15 months, but the constituent behaviors differed in persistence and temporal characteristics.

The example of red knots (Fig. 6.6) illustrates further properties of circannual rhythms. Most tested bird species are strongly photoperiodic and readily entrain to simulated natural daylength cycles in a phase-specific way (see below). Entrainment is often instantaneous (Fig. 6.6a), but transients have also been reported (Fig. 6.6b) (Gwinner 1986).

Generally, circannual rhythms appear to be less strongly self-sustained than circadian rhythms. An extreme example is European starlings, where some birds entrained to T-cycles (i.e., artificial photoperiodic cycles with period lengths differing from 1 year) of less than 2 months (Gwinner 1986). Other species show more robust rhythms. For example, the reproductive system of migratory Garden warblers kept on a constant 12.8 h days failed to respond to usually inductive 15 h days in November, but regained reproductive responsiveness in late winter (Gwinner 1996).

Differences in robustness of circannual rhythms are evident from the range of conditions under which they are expressed. At one extreme are species like the subtropical spotted munia (*Lonchura punctulata*), whose circannual rhythms persist even under dim constant light of approximately 95 lux (Agarwal et al. 2017; Chandola-Saklani et al. 2015). Other species, for example, European starlings, express circannual rhythms only under a narrow range of photoperiods, or require an obligatory advance by photoperiod at certain phases to continue the rhythm (Gwinner 1986; Helm et al. 2013; Helm et al. 2009). Several lines of evidence suggest that differences are at least partly related to a species' life history. For example, in some closely related taxa circannual systems differ according to migration strategy.

The mechanistic basis of circannual rhythm generation is still largely unknown. Experimental studies in many taxa including birds clearly refute simple counting of days or of circadian cycles (i.e., frequency demultiplication). Among the lines of evidence are independence of circannual rhythms from manipulated number of days (e.g., via T-cycles). Circannual rhythms also persisted in birds whose circadian system had been made arrhythmic, for example, by bright light or pinealectomy (Agarwal et al. 2017; Rani and Kumar 2013). Causation simply through sequence of interconnected stages is equally unlikely because the various annual cycle stages can differ from each other in their persistence and period length under constant conditions, in contrast to their apparent interconnection under naturally changing photoperiod (Fig. 6.6).

Instead, it is more likely that circannual cycles are generated by interactions between tissue-level processes and systemic control (Stevenson and Lincoln 2017). Support for these ideas comes from mammalian studies that have exploited knowledge of photoperiodic input pathways to tentatively locate a circannual pacemaker in the *pars tuberalis* of the pituitary gland. Several studies on birds corroborate the importance of thyroid pathways for circannual rhythms, potentially through epigenetic mechanisms (Chandola-Saklani et al. 2015; Stevenson and Lincoln 2017; Nakane and Yoshimura 2019; Rani and Kumar 2013).

6.7   Photoperiodism and Neuroendocrine Annual Regulators

Photoperiod is the strongest *zeitgeber* for the entrainment of circannual rhythms in birds and affects many aspects of their life-cycles, including migration, molt, and reproduction. Phase specificity of photoperiodic responses has been widely demonstrated, although no formal circannual phase-response curves exist for birds (Gwinner 1996; Helm et al. 2009). Most species advance their annual cycle in response to long days during the pre-breeding phase and in response to short days during the post-breeding phase. Shortening summer daylength also accelerates developmental processes and post-juvenile molt in young birds. The mechanism of photoperiodic action is best understood for its stimulation of the HPG (hypothalamic–pituitary–gonadal) axis by long days. Photoperiodic input pathways differ between birds and mammals (see above), but converge by affecting TSH (thyrotropin) secretion in the *pars tuberalis* (Nakane and Yoshimura 2019). Mechanistic details of the ensuing steps are described in greater detail elsewhere in this volume.

In birds, deep-brain photoreception is sufficient for triggering photoperiodic responses (Fig. 6.2), and circadian reference time is locally available in the hypothalamus (Nakane et al. 2014). This perception mechanism is acutely sensitive to daylength. For example, differences in light intensity simulating cloud cover, and daylength increases of 17 min, were both sufficient to stimulate reproductive development (Hau et al. 1998). Involvement of the circadian clock for photoperiodic time measurement has been demonstrated by experimental evidence that light must be timed to a photoinducible window to be stimulatory (see Text Box 2).

Box 2. Evidence of Circadian Involvement in Photoperiodic Timekeeping

It has been long known that plants, invertebrates, and vertebrates use daylength to time or entrain their annual cycles (Foster and Kreitzman 2009), although caveats exist (see Text Box 1). In principle, daylength information can be used for annual timing in two ways: An organism can use the duration of light in the environment directly, for example, by *accumulating* a light-induced substance that disintegrates during darkness. Thereby, if daylength, for example, becomes long enough in spring, the amount of this substance could exceed a threshold and trigger a cascade of mechanistic events, such as reproductive activation. This mechanism is referred to as hourglass. Alternatively, the organism could *measure* the duration of daylength using its circadian clock. This would imply that it matters when, rather than for how long, light is perceived. In this scenario, light has a dual function: It firstly entrains a circadian oscillator which drives a circadian rhythm of light sensitivity. Secondly, when daylength is sufficiently long, light received during the photosensitive phase will trigger a photoperiodic cascade.

The two processes can be experimentally distinguished by elegant protocols that have been used to also study avian photoperiodism (i.e., Nanda–Hamner protocol, Buensing protocol, night interruption protocol; Foster and Kreitzman 2009). Briefly, the Nanda–Hamner protocol provides a block of light (often 6 h) which entrains the circadian clock, but is too short to start a photoperiodic induction. Then, after a dark phase of varying length, a second block of light is provided, which if falling onto the photosensitive phase will trigger a photoperiodic induction. Systematic tests of different durations of darkness showed that photoperiodic induction was triggered only when the inductive second light block occurred within intervals of 24 h or multiples thereof. Only then, the second light block coincided with the photosensitive phase, proving that circadian entrainment is required. Night

---

(continued)

Box 2 (continued)
interruption protocols follow similar logic. Here, a block of light (often 6 h) entrains the circadian clock every day. Every day, a short light pulse disrupts darkness at a specific time of night for a group of birds. The birds interpret this short pulse as marking the end of the day, and if it generates a sufficiently long day, a photoperiodic reaction follows. In this protocol, all animals receive the same amount of light, but only those which are photoinduced receive the short pulse at the right time.

Hence, in birds, as in mammals and many other taxa, experimental evidence clearly supports circadian involvement in photoperiodic timing.

Long-day stimulation can increase LH (luteinizing hormone) within a day. The sequence of responses has been best characterized in quail (Nakane et al. 2014). Long-day stimulation of opsin-containing deep-brain photoreceptors increases TSHβ locally in the *pars tuberalis*, which in turn induces expression of the *dio2* (type 2 deiodinase) gene in the mediobasal hypothalamus. The enzyme encoded by it, DIO2, converts T4 (thyroxine) to its bioactive form T3 (triiodothyronine). Conversely, short days up-regulate expression of *dio3* (type 3 deiodinase), which encodes the thyroid-inactivating enzyme DIO3. The photoperiodic switch between these enzymes achieves substantial local changes of active thyroid hormones. High local levels of T3 in the mediobasal hypothalamus induce growth of the testes by activating GnRH secretion into the portal capillaries, which in turn triggers gonadotropin secretion from the pituitary gland.

Stimulation of the HPG axis integrates daylength with other environmental factors, for example, ambient temperature and social factors. The mechanistic integration of these effects is only beginning to be understood (Perfito et al. 2015; Caro et al. 2013). For example, in female starlings, the DIO2/DIO3 switch described above is sensitive to availability of a mate. Information on ambient temperature from skin receptors is thought to be processed in the preoptic area (Fig. 6.2), which in birds also contains photoreceptors. How this information may affect reproductive timing is unclear (Caro et al. 2013). There is, however, some indication for differences between the sexes at various levels of regulation, from circannual rhythms to environmental responsiveness (Ball and Ketterson 2008; Rani and Kumar 2013).

In contrast to detailed insights on photostimulation, less is known about the mechanisms that terminate reproductive state. Among the proposed mechanisms for regression are effects of locally activated T3 in the periphery which are opposite to its stimulatory effects in the mediobasal hypothalamus. This mechanism is short-day induced and is responsive to temperature and food (Nakane and Yoshimura 2019). Additionally, GnIH appears to interact with melatonin and to counteract reproductive activation (viviD and Bentley 2018).

The mechanisms of photostimulation explained above are largely based on experiments with quail, but just as with the circadian system, the photoperiodic

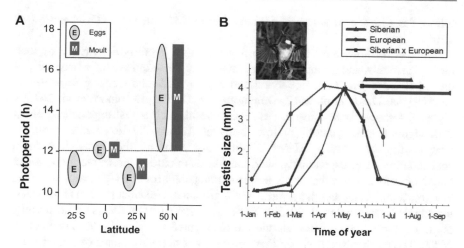

Fig. 6.7 Diverse, inherited breeding, and molt timing in stonechats (*Saxicola* spp.). (**a**) Photoperiods under which wild populations within the *Saxicola* group breed and molt at their respective native latitudes. The photoperiodic range for egg-laying is indicated by yellow oval shapes and that of molt by green rectangles; based on (Helm 2009). (**b**) Testicular and molt cycle (curves) and molt (horizontal bars) (mean ± SEM) of male stonechats from two locations (Siberian stonechats from Kazakhstan (red triangles), European stonechats from Austria (blue dots)), and of their F1-hybrids (purple). Birds were studied in captivity under identical, natural photoperiod; cycles for females were similar; based on (Helm et al. 2009)

system appears to vary between species. An example of different inherited reproductive responses to identical photoperiods comes from closely related stonechats (Fig. 6.7). Across their extensive breeding range, stonechats naturally breed and molt under a wide range of daylengths (Fig. 6.7a) (Helm 2009). However, migratory populations maintain distinct timing (Fig. 6.7b), as shown for Siberian long-distance migrants and European short-distance migrants, who differed in reproductive responses to identical, simulated daylength. Reproductive competence in both sexes (Helm et al. 2009) was regained earlier and maintained for longer in European than Siberian stonechats. F1 hybrids showed intermediate timing of reproductive activation, but regressed their gonads simultaneously with the Siberian parents. Molt timing differed in similar ways.

6.8 Clocks and Calendars in a Changing World

The ancient, diverse timers of birds are confronted with rapid changes to temporal environments. By flooding darkness with artificial light at night (ALAN), human activity erodes the difference (amplitude) between night and day (Falchi et al. 2016). The relationship between daylength and seasonality is also changing, as a consequence of climate warming. Spring-like conditions occur progressively earlier in the year, whereas autumn-like conditions occur progressively later. Most organisms follow the advance of spring conditions, but at different rates (Thackeray et al. 2016).

Whether, or how, birds respond to these changes is partly determined by their biological clocks and calendars. As expected from the exquisite light sensitivity of the avian brain (Fig. 6.2), free-living and captive birds show strong responses to ALAN (Van Doren et al. 2017; Dominoni et al. 2013a, Dominoni et al. 2013b). Figure 6.4 shows melatonin profiles of captive blackbirds that experienced either dark nights (black symbols) or low levels of ALAN (0.3 lux; white symbols). Despite the low level, ALAN significantly reduced the birds' melatonin concentrations. Correspondingly, wild blackbirds in cities were active for a greater length of time each day than those in surrounding, dark forests. Upon capture, urban blackbirds had faster and more weakly self-sustained, circadian rhythms than forest blackbirds (Dominoni et al. 2013b). Even more dramatic are effects on nocturnally migrating birds that collide with and are disoriented by ALAN (Van Doren et al. 2017). The mechanistic basis for these problems is currently unknown, but there is indication that cryptochromes play a role (Cassone 2014). Even less is known about how the birds' circadian system responds to a warming climate.

Annual cycles are also affected by ALAN. Advanced reproductive activation in illuminated areas has long been reported in wild birds (Rowan 1937) and has been experimentally confirmed even for subtle ALAN. For example, blackbirds that were exposed to ALAN described above (Fig. 6.4) initially accelerated breeding state but subsequently paused testicular regrowth in their second year. Behavioral data suggest that the birds interpreted the low light levels (0.3 lux) as long days (Dominoni et al. 2013c). Climate warming is also clearly affecting avian annual cycles. The well-documented shifts appear to be insufficient for keeping up with shifting seasonality (Visser and Gienapp 2019), although some scope for evolutionary change in the circannual program has recently been reported (Helm et al. 2017).

It can be expected that changes to the temporal environment will occur at progressively faster rates and might stretch the limits of plasticity and of evolutionary potential of biological timekeeping. To predict and understand the challenge and to possibly mitigate against the consequences, it is important to gain a better understanding of the mechanisms that drive and regulate birds' biological rhythms.

Acknowledgments The author thanks Julia Karagicheva, Paul Bartell, Davide Dominoni, Takashi Yoshimura, and Michiel Vellema for kindly sharing materials, insights, and thoughtful discussions.

References

Abraham U, Albrecht U, Gwinner E, Brandstatter R (2002) Spatial and temporal variation of passer Per2 gene expression in two distinct cell groups of the suprachiasmatic hypothalamus in the house sparrow (Passer domesticus). Eur J Neurosci 16:429–436
Agarwal N, Mishra I, Komal R, Rani S, Kumar V (2017) Circannual testis and moult cycles persist under photoperiods that disrupt circadian activity and clock gene cycles in spotted munia. J Exp Biol 220:4162–4168

Akesson S, Ilieva M, Karagicheva J, Rakhimberdiev E, Tomotani B, Helm B (2017) Timing avian long-distance migration: from internal clock mechanisms to global flights. Philos Trans R Soc Lond Ser B Biol Sci 372

Aschoff J (1967) Circadian rhythms in birds. Proc. XIVth Intern. Orn. Congr, Oxford

Ashley NT, Ubuka T, Schwabl I, Goymann W, Salli BM, Bentley GE, Buck CL (2014) Revealing a circadian clock in captive arctic-breeding songbirds, Lapland longspurs (Calcarius lapponicus), under constant illumination. J Biol Rhythm 29:456–469

Ball GF, Ketterson ED (2008) Sex differences in the response to environmental cues regulating seasonal reproduction in birds. Philosophical Transactions of the Royal Society B: Biological Sciences 363:231–246

Bartell PA, Gwinner E (2005) A separate circadian oscillator controls nocturnal migratory restlessness in the songbird Sylvia borin. J Biol Rhythm 20:538–549

Besharse JC, Mcmahon DG (2016) The retina and other light-sensitive ocular clocks. J Biol Rhythm 31:223–243

Bluhm CK, Schwabl H, Schwabl I, Perera A, Follett BK, Goldsmith AR, Gwinner E (1991) Variation in hypothalamic gonadotrophin-releasing hormone content, plasma and pituitary LH, and in-vitro testosterone release in a long-distance migratory bird, the garden warbler (Sylvia borin), under constant photoperiods. J Endocrinol 128:339–345

Caro SP, Schaper SV, Hut RA, Ball GF, Visser ME (2013) The case of the missing mechanism: how does temperature influence seasonal timing in endotherms? PLoS Biol 11:e1001517

Cassone VM (2014) Avian circadian organization: a chorus of clocks. Front Neuroendocrinol 35:76–88

Cassone VM, Paulose JK, Harpole CE, Li Y, Whitfield-Rucker M (2017) Avian circadian organization. In: Kumar V (ed) Biological timekeeping: clocks, rhythms and behavior. New Delhi, Springer India

Chandola-Saklani A, Negi K, Kathait A (2015) A brief exposure to thyroxine synchronizes the circannual testicular cycle and associated molt in the subtropical spotted munia (Lonchura punctulata). J Ornithol 156:453–461

Davies WIL, Turton M, Peirson SN, Follett BK, Halford S, Garcia-Fernandez JM, Sharp PJ, Hankins MW, Foster RG (2012) Vertebrate ancient opsin photopigment spectra and the avian photoperiodic response. Biol Lett 8:291–294

Dominoni D, Goymann W, Helm B, Partecke J (2013a) Urban-like night illumination reduces melatonin release in European blackbirds (Turdus merula): implications of city life for biological time-keeping of songbirds. Front Zool 10:60

Dominoni DM, Helm B, Lehmann M, Dowse HB, Partecke J (2013b) Clocks for the city: circadian differences between forest and city songbirds. Proc Biol Sci 280:20130593

Dominoni DM, Quetting M, Partecke J (2013c) Long-term effects of chronic light pollution on seasonal functions of European blackbirds (Turdus merula). PLoS One 8:e85069

Falchi F, Cinzano P, Duriscoe D, Kyba CCM, Elvidge CD, Baugh K, Portnov BA, Rybnikova NA, Furgoni R (2016) The new world atlas of artificial night sky brightness. Sci Adv 2

Foster RG, Follett BK (1985) The involvement of a rhodopsin-like photopigment in the photoperiodic response of the Japanese quail. J Comp Physiol A 157:519–528

Foster RG, Kreitzman L (2009) Seasons of life: The biological rhythms that enable living things to thrive and survive. Yale University Press, New Haven, CT

Fusani L, Gahr M (2015) Differential expression of melatonin receptor subtypes MelIa, MelIb and MelIc in relation to melatonin binding in the male songbird brain. Brain Behav Evol 85:4–14

Gänshirt G, Daan S, Gerkema MP (1984) Arrhythmic perch hopping and rhythmic feeding of starlings in constant light: separate circadian oscillators? J Comp Physiol A 154:669–674

Gwinner E (1966) Entrainment of a circadian rhythm in birds by species-specific song cycles (Aves, Fringillidae: Carduelis spinus, Serinus serinus). Experientia (Basel) 22:765

Gwinner E (1974) Testosterone induces "splitting" of circadian Locomotor activity rhythms in birds. Science 185:72–74

Gwinner E (1986) Circannual rhythms. Berlin, Springer, Heidelberg

Gwinner E (1996) Circadian and circannual programmes in avian migration. J Exp Biol 199:39–48

Gwinner E, Brandstätter R (2001) Complex bird clocks. Philos Trans R Soc Lond B 356:1801–1810

Gwinner E, Schwabl H, Schwabl-Benzinger I (1988) Effects of food-deprivation on migratory restlessness and diurnal activity in the garden warbler *Sylvia borin*. Oecologia 77:321–326

Hau M, Wikelski M, Wingfield JC (1998) A neotropical forest bird can measure the slight changes in tropical photoperiod. Proceedings of the Royal Society of London Series B- Biological Sciences 265:89–95

Helfer G, Barrett P, Morgan PJ (2019) A unifying hypothesis for control of body weight and reproduction in seasonally breeding mammals. J Neuroendocrinol 31:e12680

Helm B (2009) Geographically distinct reproductive schedules in a changing world: costly implications in captive stonechats. Integr Comp Biol 49:563–579

Helm B, Ben-Shlomo R, Sheriff MJ, Hut RA, Foster R, Barnes BM, Dominoni D (2013) Annual rhythms that underlie phenology: biological time-keeping meets environmental change. Biological Sciences, Proceedings of the Royal Society B, p 280

Helm B, Schwabl I, Gwinner E (2009) Circannual basis of geographically distinct bird schedules. J Exp Biol 212:1259–1269

Helm B, Visser ME, Schwartz W, Kronfeld-Schor N, Gerkema M, Piersma T, Bloch G (2017) Two sides of a coin: ecological and chronobiological perspectives of timing in the wild. Philosophical Transactions of the Royal Society B: Biological Sciences 372:1734

Johnsen A, Fidler AE, Kuhn S, Carter KL, Hoffmann A, Barr IR, Biard C, Charmantier A, Eens M, Korsten P, Siitari H, Tomiuk J, Kempenaers B (2007) Avian clock gene polymorphism: evidence for a latitudinal cline in allele frequencies. Mol Ecol 16:4867–4880

Karagicheva J, Rakhimberdiev E, Dekinga A, Brugge M, Koolhaas A, Ten Horn J, Piersma T (2016) Seasonal time keeping in a long-distance migrating shorebird. J Biol Rhythm 31:509–521

Kramer G (1957) Experiments on bird orientation and their interpretation. Ibis 99:196–227

Kuenzel WJ, Kang SW, Zhou ZJ (2015) Exploring avian deep-brain photoreceptors and their role in activating the neuroendocrine regulation of gonadal development1. Poult Sci 94:786–798

Kumar V, Singh BP, Rani S (2004) The bird clock: a complex, multi-oscillatory and highly diversified system. Biol Rhythm Res 35:121–144

Menaker M, Eskin A (1966) Entrainment of circadian rhythms by sound in Passer domesticus. Science 154:1579–1581

Menaker M, Moreira LF, Tosini G (1997) Evolution of circadian organization in vertebrates. Braz J Med Biol Res 30:305–313

Menaker M, Underwood H (1976) Extraretinal photoreception in birds. Photochem Photobiol 23:299–306

Nakane Y, Shimmura T, Abe H, Yoshimura T (2014) Intrinsic photosensitivity of a deep brain photoreceptor. Curr Biol 24:R596–R597

Nakane Y, Yoshimura T (2019) Photoperiodic regulation of reproduction in vertebrates. Annual Review of Animal Biosciences 7:173–194

Okano T, Yoshizawa T, Fukada Y (1994) Pinopsin is a chicken pineal photoreceptive molecule. Nature 372:94–97

Oshima I, Yamada H, Goto M, Sato K, Ebihara S (1989) Pineal and retinal melatonin is involved in the control of circadian locomotor activity and body temperature rhythms in the pigeon. J Comp Physiol A 166:217–226

Padget O, Bond SL, Kavelaars MM, Van Loon E, Bolton M, Fayet AL, Syposz M, Roberts S, Guilford T (2018) In situ clock shift reveals that the sun compass contributes to orientation in a pelagic seabird. Curr Biol 28:275–279. e2

Perfito N, Guardado D, Williams TD, Bentley GE (2015) Social cues regulate reciprocal switching of hypothalamic Dio2/Dio3 and the transition into final follicle maturation in European starlings (Sturnus vulgaris). Endocrinology 156:694–706

Rani S, Kumar V (2013) Avian circannual systems: persistence and sex differences. Gen Comp Endocrinol 190:61–67

Rastogi A, Kumari Y, Rani S, Kumar V (2011) Phase inversion of neural activity in the olfactory and visual systems of a night-migratory bird during migration. Eur J Neurosci 34:99–109

Renthlei Z, Gurumayum T, Borah BK, Trivedi AK (2019) Daily expression of clock genes in central and peripheral tissues of tree sparrow (Passer montanus). Chronobiol Int 36:110–121

Rich EL, Romero LM (2001) Daily and photoperiod variations of basal and stress-induced corticosterone concentrations in house sparrows (Passer domesticus). J Comp Physiol B 171:543–547

Rowan W (1937) Effects of traffic disturbance and light illumination on London starlings. Nature 139:668–669

Shimmura T, Ohashi S, Yoshimura T (2015) The highest-ranking rooster has priority to announce the break of dawn. Sci Rep 5:11683

Stevenson TJ, Lincoln GA (2017) Epigenetic mechanisms regulating Circannual rhythms. In: Kumar V (ed) Biological timekeeping: clocks, rhythms and behavior. Springer India, New Delhi

Thackeray SJ, Henrys PA, Hemming D, Bell JR, Botham MS, Burthe S, Helaouet P, Johns DG, Jones ID, Leech DI, Mackay EB, Massimino D, Atkinson S, Bacon PJ, Brereton TM, Carvalho L, Clutton-Brock TH, Duck C, Edwards M, Elliott JM, HALL SJ, Harrington R, Pearce-Higgins JW, Hoye TT, Kruuk LE, Pemberton JM, Sparks TH, Thompson PM, White I, Winfield IJ, Wanless S (2016) Phenological sensitivity to climate across taxa and trophic levels. Nature 535:241–245

Van der Veen DR, Riede SJ, Heideman PD, Hau M, Van der Vinne V, Hut RA (2017) flexible clock systems: adjusting the temporal programme. Philos Trans R Soc Lond Ser B Biol Sci 372:1734

Van Doren BM, Horton KG, Dokter AM, Klinck H, Elbin SB, Farnsworth A (2017) High-intensity urban light installation dramatically alters nocturnal bird migration. Proc Natl Acad Sci 114:11175–11180

Visser ME, Caro SP, Van Oers K, Schaper SV, Helm B (2010) Phenology, seasonal timing and circannual rhythms: towards a unified framework. Philosophical Transactions of the Royal Society B: Biological Sciences 365:3113–3127

Visser ME, Gienapp P (2019) Evolutionary and demographic consequences of phenological mismatches. Nature Ecology & Evolution 3:879–885

Vivid D, Bentley G (2018) Seasonal reproduction in vertebrates: melatonin synthesis, binding, and functionality using Tinbergen's four questions. Molecules 23:652

Winkler DW, Gandoy FA, Areta JI, Iliff MJ, Rakhimberdiev E, Kardynal KJ, Hobson KA (2017) Long-distance range expansion and rapid adjustment of migration in a newly established population of barn swallows breeding in Argentina. Curr Biol 27:1080–1084

Yoshimura T, Yasuo S, Suzuki Y, Makino E, Yokota Y, Ebihara S (2001) Identification of the suprachiasmatic nucleus in birds. Am J Physiol Regul Integr Comp Physiol 280:R1185–R1189

Zimmerman NH, Menaker M (1979) The pineal gland: a pacemaker within the circadian system of the house sparrow. Proc Natl Acad Sci U S A 76:999–1003

Further Recommended Reading

Akesson S, Ilieva M, Karagicheva J, Rakhimberdiev E, Tomotani B, Helm B (2017) Timing avian long-distance migration: from internal clock mechanisms to global flights. Philos Trans R Soc Lond B Biol Sci 372, pii: 20160252.
This article highlights the importance of clocks and calendars for real-world processes, by combining mechanistic overview and case studies of migration in the wild.

Cassone VM (2014) Avian Circadian Organization: A Chorus of Clocks. Frontiers in neuroendocrinology 35:76–88
Succinct overview of mechanistic studies into avian circadian rhythms, which leads to important literature.

Gwinner E (1996) Circadian and circannual programmes in avian migration. Journal of Experimental Biology 199:39–48
Classic, nutshell review of key experiments and evidence for circadian and circannual regulation of migration.
Nakane Y, Yoshimura T (2019) Photoperiodic Regulation of Reproduction in Vertebrates. Annual Review of Animal Biosciences 7:173–194
This article reviews mechanistic insight into photoperiodism of birds in direct comparison with other vertebrates.

Calendar Timing in Teleost Fish

7

Alexander C. West, David G. Hazlerigg, and Gabrielle Grenier

Abstract

Teleosts are the largest and most diverse group of vertebrates. Although a complex variety of environmental cues influence and time their behaviour and physiology, seasonality is prevalent in many groups and has been particularly studied in salmonids where photoperiodic effects on juvenile development (smoltification) and reproductive physiology (c.g. spawning) are well characterized. This chapter considers evidence for processing of photoperiodic information via local regulation of thyroid hormone availability in the saccus vasculosus, a circumventricular organ located on the ventral side of the brain behind the pituitary gland. As this structure is not present in all photoperiodic teleosts, the chapter also discusses the role of the optic tectum, as this region expresses photoreceptors and melatonin receptors. Unlike mammals, fish (like birds) display decentralized control of photoperiodic responses, as multiple tissues may possess the cellular machinery to respond independently.

Keywords

Teleost · Photoperiod · Circannual · Saccus vasculosus · Smoltification

A. C. West (✉) · D. G. Hazlerigg
Arctic chronobiology and physiology research group, Department of Arctic and Marine Biology, The Arctic University of Norway, Tromsø, Norway
e-mail: alexander.west@uit.no; david.hazlerigg@uit.no

G. Grenier
Freshwater Ecology Group, Department of Arctic and Marine Biology, Faculty of Biosciences, The Arctic University of Norway, Tromsø, Norway
e-mail: gabrielle.grenier@uit.no

F. J. P. Ebling, H. D. Piggins (eds.), *Neuroendocrine Clocks and Calendars*, Masterclass in Neuroendocrinology 10, https://doi.org/10.1007/978-3-030-55643-3_7

7.1   Introduction

Life first evolved in water, indeed the first 150–200 million years of chordate evolution took place exclusively in aquatic environments. The legacy of this is still clear today with over half of all vertebrate species inhabiting rivers, lakes, and oceans. This chapter will consider the teleostei clade (hereafter teleosts), by far the largest phylogenetic group in the vertebrate lineage boasting nearly 30,000 species (Fig. 7.1) (Ravi and Byrappa 2018). Teleosts are remarkably diverse in morphology, physiology, and behaviour and have become resilient to widely different water properties, from the sub-zero Arctic seas and to the hot springs of El Pandeño de los Pandos in Mexico whose water temperatures peak at a stifling 46 °C.

Almost all terrestrial habitats experience large fluctuations in light and/or temperature, variables which are primarily driven on daily, lunar, and annual cycles due to the interaction between the earth, sun, and moon (Fig. 7.2a). Marine and aquatic environments are additionally characterized in terms of rhythmic changes in salinity, turbidity, tide, current, flow, and transience. As a consequence, there is a strong evolutionary adaptive value in the ability to predict these rhythmic environmental changes through endogenous biological timers (West and Bechtold 2015). Daily and

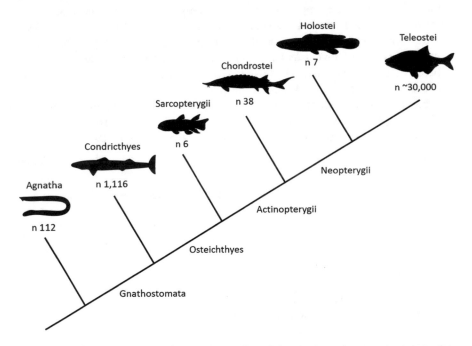

Fig. 7.1 Phylogenetic relationships of extant fishes. Number of species in each clade is given beneath each group, and data were retrieved from the IUCN Red List (IUCN 2019). Common names for each clade include lamprey and hagfish (*Agnatha*); sharks, skates, and rays (*Chondrichthyes*); coelacanth and lungfishes (*Sarcopterygii*); sturgeons and paddle fishes (*Chondrostei*); bowfin and gars (*Holostei*); and teleosts (*Teleostei*)

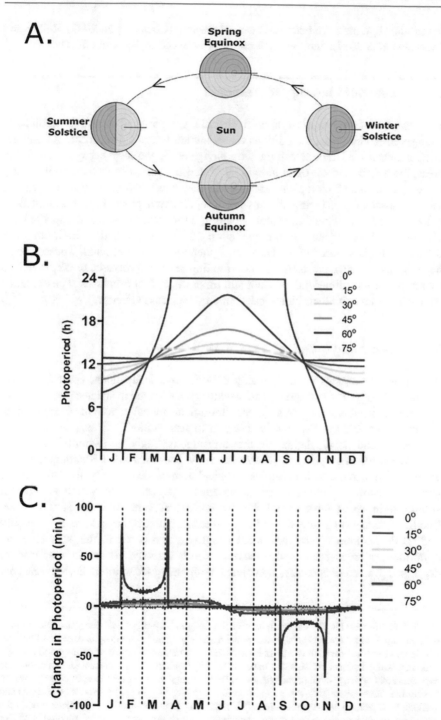

Fig. 7.2 Seasonal photoperiods. (**a**) Annual changes in day-length are generated through the altered relationship between the earth and sun. The earth, drawn here from above the orbital plane, is tilted on its axis by 23.5°. As it travels along its orbit, the direction of this axis changes,

lunar/tidal rhythms have been reviewed elsewhere (Cowan et al. 2017; Raible and Tessmar-raible 2017); here, we will consider seasonal rhythms in teleosts.

7.2 Seasonal Biology in Teleosts

Seasonal variation describes how a specific geographical location predictably changes in environmental conditions on an annual basis. This enforces a temporal environmental landscape which must be navigated by the local ecosystem. In such areas, the genetic success of an individual organism is often dependant on its ability to compartmentalize biological processes to their most opportune time of year. In teleosts, seasonally changing phenotypes in reproductive physiology, pigmentation, colour perception, migration, osmoregulation, dormancy, growth, and appetite have all been characterized. Experimentation under controlled conditions has demonstrated how seasonal variation and phenotype are connected. These studies have revealed that the mechanisms underpinning seasonal processes break down into two major groups: timer-independent and timer-dependent processes. The evidence for each of these and their biological context are discussed below.

7.2.1 Timer-Independent Seasonal Biology

Several teleost species unambiguously exhibit timer-independent control of their seasonal biology. These responses are usually characterized in species which inhabit unstable seasonal environments; where although an annual pattern in environmental conditions persists, there is considerable year to year variability in the precise timing. Timer-independent regulation of the reproductive axis is exemplified in the electrosensitive mormyrid fish (*Mormyrus rume proboscirostris* Boulanger, 1898), which is native to the African tropics. Tropical regions are typically divided into wet and dry seasons, where the climate produces cyclical floods which generate a significant influx of nutrients and alter the ecological niche structure. However, the flooding seasons are greatly dependant on weather patterns that change considerably with both the time of year and local geography. As a result, this species is an opportunistic breeder and only becomes reproductively mature in response to decreased water conductivity, associated with increased rainfall during seasonal

Fig. 7.2 (continued) thereby changing relative day-length. Day-lengths are longest at the summer solstice, shortest at the winter solstice and equal at the spring and autumn equinoxes. (**b**) Photoperiod length over the year in the northern hemisphere. The range and profile of photoperiod changes with increasing latitude. At latitudes beyond the Arctic circle (75°), constant photoperiods are experienced in both the summer and winter. (**c**) Daily change in photoperiod length over the year in the northern hemisphere. Below the Arctic circle (0-60°), change in photoperiod is continuous and gradual. However, above the Arctic circle (75°), the change in photoperiod is dramatic around the equinoxes and falls to zero in the summer and winter. There is no photoperiod information at 75° for over 6 months of the year

flooding events (Schugardt and Kirschbaum 2004). Significantly, gonadal maturation and regression can be manipulated on multiple successive occasions in the mormyrid, revealing a lack of post-breeding refractoriness. This demonstrates that the seasonal patterns of reproduction in this fish are entirely dependent upon the seasonal cycles in rainfall rather than having an obligatory endogenous seasonal component to their reproductive physiology.

Another example of a timer-independent seasonal phenotype is observed in the Japanese medaka (*Oryzias latipes* Temminck & Schlegel, 1846). This organism has evolved a seasonal-associated change in body pigmentation essential for courtship known as nuptial coloration. However, this phenotypic transformation, which is accompanied by the expression of a photopigment necessary to detect the new body coloration, is acutely induced by warm, summer-like water temperatures. Significantly, this warm-water induction persists even when experienced in opposition to winter-like light-dark (LD) cycles (Shimmura et al. 2017). These results demonstrate the dominance of a less reliable seasonal indicator (temperature) over that of a consistent seasonal indicator (light-dark cycle, photoperiod). Such a feature is characteristic of short-lived, fast-breeding, robust organisms where significant gains in genetic fitness may be realized though opportunistic reproductive strategies. Furthermore, these examples demonstrate the need to experimentally establish precisely how the phenotype of a seasonal organism interacts with the environment. Specifically, they highlight how observations of seasonal cycles under natural conditions do not necessarily indicate the presence of a biological seasonal timing mechanism.

7.2.2 Timer-Dependent Seasonal Biology: Anticipation of Seasonal Change

Many biological processes associated with seasonality require significant morphological and/or physiological remodelling which can take weeks or months to complete. Therefore, many seasonal fishes rely on indicative environmental cues to anticipate seasonal change. Daily light duration (photoperiod) is the most reliable proximate factor indicating time of year. Photoperiods increase and decrease symmetrically around the winter and summer solstices meaning that a single day does not provide sufficient information to identify the time of year (Fig. 7.2b). Therefore, photoperiod must be interpreted relative to its recent history, with extending photoperiods indicating progression towards summer and contracting photoperiods signifying the oncoming of winter (West and Wood 2018).

Photoperiodic change has been shown to influence the reproductive physiology of several teleost groups. One of the best studied families are the salmonids. Salmonids are total spawners, meaning they have a single reproductive event each year, which usually takes place during the late autumn to early winter (See Box 1). However, the initial stimulation of the reproductive axis, which ultimately culminates in the spawning event, is initiated months earlier in the spring. Rainbow trout (*Oncorhynchus mykiss* Walbaum, 1792) maintained under short photoperiods (SP, winter-like photoperiods) for a year will spontaneously mature, indicating the presence of an internal calendar mechanism. However, it has been demonstrated that rainbow trout can be reproductively stimulated by abrupt changes in the anticipated photoperiod. The premature extension of the photoperiod during the spring and reduction in photoperiod during the autumn act independently to advance the spawning phase by up to 4 months (Randall and Bromage 1998; Taranger et al. 1998). These experiments can be interpreted as evidence for photoperiod entraining the internal calendar mechanism, suggesting that the fish perceive these photoperiodic advancements as evidence that their internal clock is running slow, and therefore make compensatory efforts to adjust it.

Text Box 1 The Anadromous Life Cycle of the Atlantic Salmon

Anadromy describes a migratory life cycle where fish spawn and develop in freshwater habitats but then migrate to seawater environments for the majority of their adult life. Atlantic salmon eggs hatch into alevin in the early spring, and they seek shelter in the gravel until the yolk sac is absorbed (A). After 3–6 weeks, the fish emerge from the substrate as fry (B). Fry quickly develop into the parr, a largely benthic fish which lives in freshwater streams and rivers for 1–5 years (C). Once a critical size threshold is reached the parr become sensitive to photoperiod. After exposure to winter photoperiods, the extending photoperiods of spring and summer stimulate the development of the freshwater-adapted parr into the seawater-adapted smolt (D, see Fig. 7.3 for details). Smolts develop for 2–3 years in marine environments where they reach adult proportions (E). The adults then return to their natal stream (F) where the salmon spawn and fertilize eggs which are then buried in the gravel where they slowly develop over the winter (G). Figure by Jayme van Dalum.

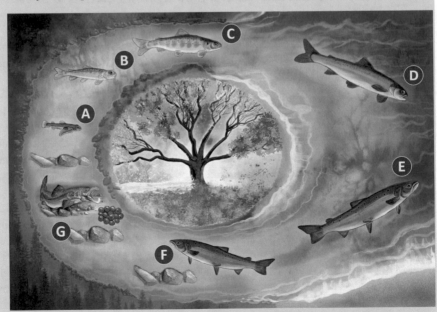

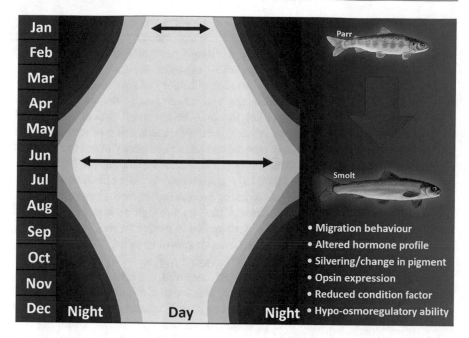

Jan
Feb
Mar
Apr
May
Jun
Jul
Aug
Sep
Oct
Nov
Dec

Parr

Smolt

Night Day Night

• Migration behaviour
• Altered hormone profile
• Silvering/change in pigment
• Opsin expression
• Reduced condition factor
• Hypo-osmoregulatory ability

Fig. 7.3 Smoltification of the Atlantic salmon. Parr-smolt transformation or smoltification describes a profound change in physiology and behaviour exhibited in many salmonid groups. Freshwater-adapted parr are characterized by their cryptic parr markings, hyper-osmoregulatory activity of the gills, stout body, territorial behaviour, and rheotaxis. Conversely, the seawater-adapted smolts are defined in terms of their silvery appearance, hypo-osmoregulatory activity of the gills, slim body profile, and loss of rheotaxis swimming. In laboratory conditions, photoperiod exposure to winter-like conditions for 6 weeks, then transferal to summer-like conditions for 6 weeks, is sufficient to drive a profound change in the endocrine profile of parr animals. The lengthening days decrease circulating plasma concentration of prolactin and increase concentration of growth hormone, cortisol, thyroid hormone, and insulin-like growth factor I (IGF-I) (McCormick et al. 2011a). These circulating hormones then act in concert to deliver the parr-smolt transformation. Figure by Jayme van Dalum

Juvenile development in salmon is also subjected to seasonal timing (Fig. 7.3). The process, known as smoltification, consists of several independent but coordinated changes in pigmentation, silvering, expression of visual pigments, metabolism, behaviour, and osmoregulation. Smoltification is an essential life-history progression, required for successful seaward migration and subsequent marine survival. Most research on smoltification has focused on the Atlantic salmon (*Salmo salar* Linneaus, 1758), which usually migrate during the spring months. The smoltification process is stimulated by changing photoperiod. In lab conditions, Atlantic salmon parr (freshwater juveniles) must experience winter-like (short) photoperiod (SP) for 6–8 weeks before being exposed to summer-like (long) photoperiod (LP) for another 6–8 weeks. These data support a conceptualization of smoltification whereby SP exposure drives the salmon into a photosensitive state which is then stimulated by LP. The mechanistic basis for the development of photosensitivity is, at present, not understood. However, it is clearly a progressive process, as shorter periods of time under SP are insufficient to deliver a full smolt phenotype, demonstrating that the salmon has long-term timekeeping mechanism by which it is able to determine the 'dosage' of its exposure to SP.

Salmonids are further characterized by the sufficiency of photoperiod to regulate their seasonal biology. That is not to say that other factors do not play a role. Temperature, for example, determines the permissive range and developmental rate of reproductive and smolt phenotypes. However, modulation of temperature is not necessary for a seasonal trait to emerge and does not directly affect the seasonal timer (Jobling et al. 1995; Pankhurst et al. 1996; Taranger et al. 1998; McCormick et al. 2011b; Handeland et al. 2013). The importance of such modulatory effects appears to vary widely among teleosts. Many groups including the percid, moronid, and gadid families regulate their seasonal biology through both photoperiod and temperature cues. Fishes from these groups spawn in the late winter to early spring, and similar to the salmonids, engage in a single spawning event. For most species, the shortening photoperiod is necessary for synchronization of the reproductive phase; however, it is not sufficient by itself, requiring an additional reduction in temperature to fully realize the phenotype. Although the absolute values differ between species, this chilling phase must last several months in order to achieve gametogenesis and spawning. Temperature reduction is also necessary for the progression of egg yolk development, known as vitellogenesis, as shown in the sea bass (*Dicentrarchus labrax* Linnaeus, 1758). Vitellogenesis is inhibited by high temperatures in sea bass (Prat et al. 1999), as is gonadal recrudescence, as demonstrated in the striped bass (*Morone saxatilis* Walbaum, 1792) (Clark et al. 2005) and yellow perch (*Perca flavescens* Mitchill, 1814) (Shewmon 2007).

Within these groups, the animals must first be within a receptive photoperiod in order to respond to changing water temperatures, indicating that changing temperature, although essential for reproduction, is acting as a secondary proximate cue to allow for a nuanced response to the environment. Whether temperature itself plays a role in the timing process is unclear, as to date it has not been rigorously tested.

7.2.3   Timer-Dependent Seasonal Biology: Circannual Rhythms

As discussed in the previous section, there are several examples where long-term timing mechanisms are employed to anticipate the changing environment, thereby favourably aligning variable phenotypes to the time of year. There is now significant evidence that some of these long-term timers may persist in constant conditions for several years and so generate a circannual (about a year) rhythm in changing physiology or behaviour. Typically, circannual rhythms are identified in organisms that have reduced exposure to seasonal indicators, thereby necessitating an endogenous way of tracking seasonal time. In teleosts, this applies to species which live at high polar latitudes (>66°N or S) which experience rapid changes in photoperiod around the equinoxes, climaxing in constant light in the summer and an absence of day-break in the winter (Fig. 7.2c). Circannual rhythms also help to limit the phase of metabolically expensive seasonal phenotypes, particularly reproductive activation. This helps to isolate the breeding season to the phase when the survival of the offspring has the highest ratio to the investment of energy. Consequently, reproductive seasons tend to be more defined at higher latitudes where resources are restricted (Wootton and Smith 2015).

The circannual rhythm has been identified in the regulation of several seasonal traits. The first evidence for teleost circannual rhythms was demonstrated in the white sucker (*Carostomus commersoni* Lacépède, 1803), which displays ~10-month cycles in behavioural thermoregulation under constant 12-L:12-D conditions (Kavaliers 1982). Reproductive circannual rhythms have also been demonstrated in SP-housed rainbow trout and sea bass (*Dicentrarchus labrax* Linneaus, 1758), which persist with a frequency of 10–12 months for 4 years (Duston and Bromage 1991; Prat et al. 1999). Elements of smoltification also appear to be under the control of a circannual mechanism. Whereas technically, full smoltification is a unidirectional life-history transition which requires transfer to seawater to develop, pre-migratory elements may develop and regress depending on the environmental conditions. This is because the opportunity for the completion of parr-smolt transformation, known as the smolt-window, is finite (Soivio and Muona 1988; Kurokawa 1990; Stefansson et al. 1998). If the smolt-window elapses, the salmon undergo a process of desmoltification, whereby the changing endocrinology and a number of preparatory adaptations to marine life are reversed, including silvering, body composition, hypo-osmoregulatory ability, and loss of rheotaxis. In the Atlantic salmon, condition factor and body coloration fluctuate with a ~ 10-month period under 12-L:12-D conditions, indicating a role of endogenous timing for at least some components of smolt phenotype development (Eriksson and Lundqvist 1982).

Feeding behaviour also follows strong seasonal patterns in many teleosts. Most fishes consume little in the winter and feed actively in the spring and summer months, a trait which is often punctuated by the spawning period at which point feeding is halted (Lall and Tibbetts 2009). This behaviour is particularly exaggerated in the Arctic charr (*Salvelinus alpinus* Linneaus, 1758), which is characterized by profound seasonal changes in food intake, growth rate, and adiposity. Most interestingly, the annual cycles of the Arctic charr are persistent under constant photoperiods, temperature, and ad libitum food, revealing the fundamental endogenous process which underpins the drive (Sæther et al. 1996).

7.2.4 Timer Properties

In animals, the underlying mechanisms which govern long-term timers and circannual rhythms are poorly understood. However, there are clues to its component parts. For example, the current literature, outlined above, strongly indicates that timer-dependent seasonal biology is consistently coupled to photoperiodic sensing. It is therefore reasonable to assume that the molecular components involved in photoperiodism are an integral part of a functioning biological calendar.

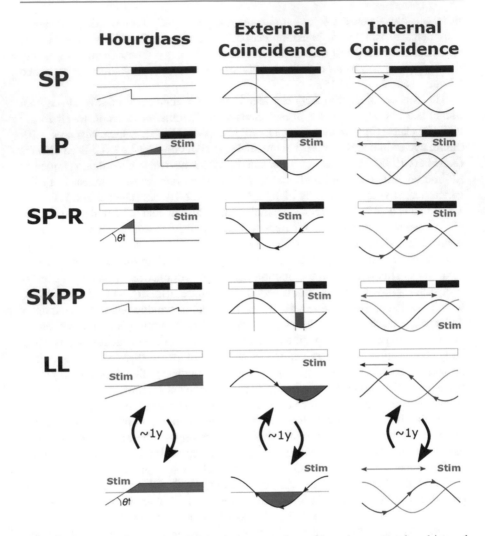

Fig. 7.4 Photoperiodism models. Schematic representations of hourglass, external, and internal coincidence models of photoperiodic sensitivity. The responses of these models to SP (short photoperiod), LP (long photoperiod), SP-R (short photoperiod refractory), SkPP (skeleton photoperiod), and LL (constant light) are shown. Hourglass model: a substance is accumulated during the light phase and is degraded in the dark phase (black line). SP does not allow the substance to accumulate beyond a threshold (red line), which can only be reached when the light phase is extended beyond a critical day-length (light-dark bars), as seen under LP. The model can be further adapted to accommodate a circannual rhythm by assuming that there is spontaneous change in the rate of accumulation (θ) of the stimulating factor which may be able to develop and suppress the summer phenotype under constant photoperiods (see SP-R). External Coincidence: The endogenous circadian clock used to provide an internal timing framework which is subdivided into a light-insensitive phase and a light-sensitive phase. SP only exposes light to the insensitive phase and so does not stimulate summer phenotypes. LP exposes light to the light-sensitive phase which stimulates the development of summer phenotypes. This model assumes a fixed phase of the circadian rhythm. However, if a spontaneous change in phase is allowed that advances in the 'endogenous summer' and delays in the 'endogenous winter', then a circannual timer can be adapted into this framework (see SP-R). Internal Coincidence: a circadian clock is used to tether

7.3   Photoperiodism in Teleosts

Sensitivity to photoperiod is a crucial feature of the seasonal biology of many other organisms, particularly birds and mammals. Within this literature, three main conceptualizations of how photoperiodic sensitivity occurs have been suggested (Fig. 7.4): one which is independent of circadian time (the hourglass mechanism), and two which rely on an endogenous circadian oscillator (external and internal coincidence models). For ease of explanation, we will assume that the seasonal traits that we discuss are typically suppressed under SP and stimulated under LP. The models may be simply adapted to account for traits which are expressed at other times of year.

- The hourglass model relies on an accumulation of a stimulating factor under the light phase. Under SP, the concentration of the stimulating factor does not reach a critical threshold needed to develop a summer-type phenotype. Only when days are extended does enough time elapse for a threshold level to be reached.
- The external coincidence model depends on the co-occurrence between light and a specific phase of a circadian oscillation. Under SP, the photosensitive phase of this circadian rhythm does not coincide with light exposure and so the summer phenotype is not developed. However, under LP, the endogenous light-sensitive phase overlaps with light exposure and the summer phenotype is permitted.
- The internal coincidence model relies on light-dark cycles to entrain circadian rhythms without light being necessary to directly stimulate a seasonal phenotype. Under this framework, the peak of each rhythm is associated with either dusk or dawn, as the photoperiod changes throughout the year, the phase relationship between these two rhythms is stretched or compressed, thereby changing their ability to interact with each other and modulate seasonal changes in physiology or behaviour.

Each of these models can be adapted to accommodate photorefractoriness or circannual rhythms (Fig. 7.4). However, to date, the mechanism which generates these long-term timing processes is totally unknown. Despite this, these models help develop the problem to the level at which it is partly understood through the data and so are still useful contributions to our understanding of the system as a whole. Several experimental procedures have been devised in an attempt to differentiate between the three models, including skeleton photoperiods and constant light procedures (Fig. 7.4). Indeed, these procedures have been used in other non-fish

Fig. 7.4 (continued) specific processes to either dawn or dusk. Change in photoperiod alters the phase relationship between the dawn and dusk oscillators and alters their interaction, precipitating alterations in seasonal phenotype. Under constant conditions, the phase relationship between these two factors could spontaneously change generating a circannual rhythm in seasonal phenotype (see LL). Stimulation of the seasonal axis in each case is represented by 'Stim'

animals to support the existence of each of the photosensitivity models. In teleosts, the consensus indicates that timekeeping occurs through a rhythm-based method. Research efforts have used skeleton photoperiods and resonance paradigms to stimulate the reproductive axes of sticklebacks (*Gasterosteus aculeatus* Linneaus, 1758), damselfish (*Chrysiptera cyanea* Quoy & Gaimard, 1825), catfish (*Heteropneustes fossilis* Bloch, 1794), bitterling (*Rhodeus ocellatus ocellatus* Kner, 1866), mosquitofish (*Gambusia affinia affinia* Baird & Girard, 1853), and rainbow trout (Baggerman 1972; Nishi 1979; Duston and Bromage 1986; Sundararaj and Vasal 2011; Takeuchi et al. 2015). These studies demonstrate that it is not the number of hours of light which is important for regulation of the reproductive axis, but rather whether the light falls within an endogenously driven photostimulatory phase.

However, skeleton photoperiods and resonance experiments are unable to distinguish between the external and internal coincidence models. This can only really be done through the use of long-term constant light experiments which would only be expected to be able to drive circannual rhythms under an internal coincidence framework. Few studies have used these conditions for multi-year investigations in teleosts, and those which have reported some unexpected effects. The best characterized is the rainbow trout, which when maintained under constant illumination (LL) for several years undergo spawning bouts every 5–6 month, in stark contrast to those maintained under SP which spawn with a regular 12-month intervals (Duston and Bromage 1986). Whereas this is certainly evidence for an endogenous long-term timer, the adaptive value of such an oscillator is hard to see. One interpretation of the data suggests that the rainbow trout only develops an extended post-breeding refractory phase under SP, which may be indicative of the adaptive value of the circannual mechanism for the spontaneous development of the reproductive axis when photoperiodic cues are limited. Hence, both SP and LL reproductive rhythms are evidence of a circannual clock, but the LL group shows the extent to which the rhythm can be compressed through the exposure of the animals to ectopic light.

It is possible that different species have evolved different timer mechanisms, or even that different timer mechanisms have evolved more than once in the same organism. For example, the SP exposure required for salmonids to smoltify acts as an hourglass, with length of winter being critical for full smolt development, although admittedly this in itself could be based on an upstream circadian framework. Interestingly, the long-day extension required for smoltification following SP exposure is longer for those fish kept on shorter SPs (Berge et al. 1995; McCormick et al. 1995; Strand et al. 2018). Furthermore, although smolt phenotypes can be stimulated through skeleton photoperiods, they are not as developed as the control LP groups (Thorarensen and Clarke 1989). Collectively, these data indicate a long-day induction mechanism which sits somewhere between the hourglass and external coincidence models, where the rate at which a summer phenotype is induced is dependent on when the light is experienced.

7.4   The Teleost Circadian Clock

One pertinent topic which has not yet been discussed is the state of the circadian system in fish. The molecular structure of the core clock appears to be conserved in fish with homologues to the core mammalian clock genes playing key roles in the generation of circadian rhythms. Unlike the mammalian system, the teleost clock is not as robust in constant conditions, with constant light (LL) pausing the clock in zebrafish (*Danio rerio* Hamilton, 1822) (Tamai et al. 2007). This effect appears to be the same in salmonids whose molecular rhythms are lost in extended LL, and whose pineal cultures tonically express melatonin under DD (Ligo et al. 2007; Huang et al. 2010). Although these data point towards a weak circadian framework, especially in salmonids, characterization of the molecular clock is made more difficult by the increased number of clock gene paralogues which are present in teleosts due to multiple whole-genome gene duplication events. Without a systematic characterization of the clock network in rhythmic and constant conditions in multiple tissues, it remains possible that the clock persists in these un-examined paralogues.

7.5   Seasonal Neuroendocrine Cascade in Teleosts

Downstream of the photoperiodic timing mechanism is the signal transduction cascade. In mammals, this has been well defined, see Chap. 2. Briefly, environmental photoperiod is reflected in the secretion profile of endogenous melatonin from the pineal gland. The duration of the melatonin signal is detected by the *pars tuberalis* (PT, a specialized pituitary tissue; expressing high levels of melatonin receptors) which integrates the information and controls both the release of prolactin from the anterior pituitary, and the regulation of the thyroid hormone (TH) metabolizing enzyme deiodinase 2 (DIO2) thorough retrograde signalling of the thyroid synthesizing hormone (TSH) to the hypothalamus. The resulting control of TH metabolism is pivotal for the execution of downstream seasonal circuits including reproduction.

The narrative of photoperiodic signal transduction is much less well defined in teleosts (Fig. 7.5, Migaud et al. 2010). As with mammals, circulating melatonin concentrations fluctuate with the light-dark cycle and are phase aligned with the dark period. Light pulses suppress production and secretion of melatonin; however, in contrast to mammals, this is locally controlled by the intrinsic photosensitivity of pineal cells (Falcón et al. 2011). There is also evidence that 24-h rhythms of circulating melatonin persist in constant darkness, highlighting the circadian clock-driven nature of the production of this hormone. However, this is not a general feature of teleosts; for example, salmonids exhibit no endogenous rhythm in melatonin concentrations in the circulation (Ligo et al. 2007). Such evidence may indicate a lack of endogenous rhythmicity within the pineal gland or may simply show that melatonin production has been decoupled from the clock. Circulating melatonin concentrations are also sensitive to a number of external factors, including the spectral quality of light exposure, light exposure history, and salinity. In particular,

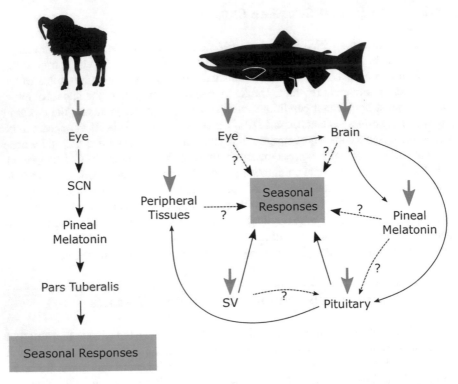

Fig. 7.5 Comparative photoperiodic systems of mammals and fish. In mammals, light (orange arrow) is detected by the eye alone. Information of irradiance is transmitted to the SCN (suprachiasmatic nucleus), the master circadian clock in mammals. The SCN then controls the pineal gland through an indirect neural pathway to secrete melatonin to inversely reflect the environmental photoperiod. The melatonin duration is detected by the *pars tuberalis* of the pituitary which then directs seasonal responses through anterograde and retrograde signalling. In fish, the neuroendocrine regulation is less well characterized and appears to be a much more decentralized system. In contrast to mammals, light (orange arrows) is detected directly in many central and peripheral tissues of fish and the role of melatonin is unclear. Seasonal regulation of thyroid hormone metabolism is linked to photoperiod in several tissues, and this may indicate that many seasonal responses are conserved but may be intrinsic to local tissues

pineal melatonin secretion is sensitive to temperature that positively drives the activity of AANAT2, the rate-limiting enzyme in pineal melatonin production in fishes (Falcón et al. 1996). This presents the possibility that the melatonin signal is able to encode both photoperiodic and temperature information, which could be used to unambiguously indicate the time of year. However, attempts to functionally link melatonin to photoperiodic processes have failed to provide a clear picture of the hormone's influence on seasonal circuits. Exogenous melatonin administration in fish has led to neutral-, pro- ,and anti-gonadal effects, with outcome specific to species, sex, season, dose, and route of administration (Falcón et al. 2011). Furthermore, the putative site of seasonal timekeeping and major target of photoperiodic

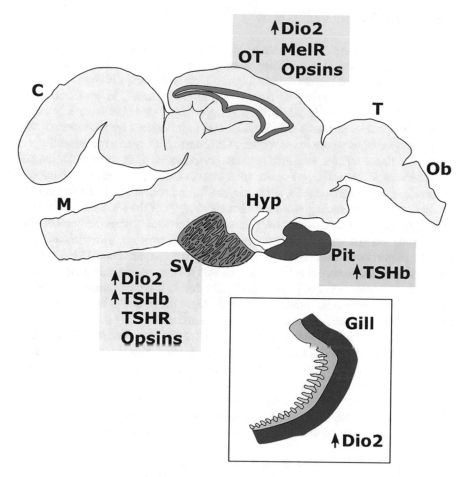

Fig. 7.6 Photoperiodic metabolism of thyroid hormone in teleosts. Multiple tissues including the gill exhibit photoperiodic control of some of the key regulators in the thyroid hormone pathway suggesting that the impact of seasonal thyroid hormone metabolism may be acting locally. *OT* optic tectum, *SV* saccus vasculosus, *Pit* pituitary, *Hyp* hypothalamus, *Ob* olfactory bulb, *T* telencephalon, *C* cerebellum, *M* mesencephalon, *Dio2* deiodinase type 2, *TSHb* thyroid-stimulating hormone beta subunit, *TSHR* thyroid-stimulating hormone receptor, *MelR* melatonin receptors

melatonin action in mammals, the PT, is present only in tetrapods, thereby eliminating this tissue as a central processor of seasonal biology in fish.

Similarly to mammals, there is good evidence that thyroid hormone remains a key regulator of seasonal processes in teleosts (Cyr et al. 1988). Serum thyroid hormone concentrations correlate strongly with reproductive status in the rainbow trout and other salmonids. However, little is known of the mechanistic basis for this interaction (summarized in Fig. 7.6). This is in part due to the complex regulation of thyroid hormone, and the interactions that the hormone has with other key seasonally controlled endocrine factors including growth hormone, cortisol, and prolactin.

7.6   The Saccus Vasculosus

Recent studies into the seasonal role of the saccus vasculosus (SV) have shed light on the upstream mechanisms linking photoperiod to seasonal changes in thyroid hormone metabolism. The SV is a fish-specific circumventricular organ located on the ventral side of the brain posterior to the pituitary gland. It is not found in any other vertebrate groups. In adult masu salmon (*Oncorhynchus masou* Brevoort, 1856), SV tissue expresses TSH receptors and is influenced by photoperiod, with long photoperiod exposure inducing both *Dio2* and *TSHβ* gene expression. Impressively, SV tissue remains sensitive to photoperiod ex vivo, likely through intrinsic expression of SWS1 and Opn4 opsins (Nakane et al. 2013). The organ is composed of three cell types: coronet cells, supporting cells, and cerebrospinal fluid-contacting bipolar neurons. Interestingly, further characterization of the SV identified that the entire thyroid hormone metabolism pathway is expressed within the coronet cells. These cells are distinctively crowned on the apical membrane with globule tipped primary (non-motile) cilia. The cilia express the photopigments and TSHβ, whereas DIO2 is compartmentalized to the main cell body. Thus, the coronet cells of the SV demonstrate conservation of photoperiodically driven thyroid hormone metabolism all within a single cell type (Nakane et al. 2013). This evidence had made coronet cells a compelling candidate for the integration and control of photoperiodic information in fishes. Indeed, surgical excision of the SV removes the photoperiodic response of the gonads and the adult SV shares expression of a number of pituitary associated transcription factors, hinting perhaps at its analogous role to the *pars tuberalis* (Nakane et al. 2013; Maeda et al. 2015). However, the SV is not a ubiquitous feature of teleosts; notable exceptions include the highly seasonal pike (*Esox lucius* Linnaeus, 1758) and Japanese medaka. Hence, photoperiodic timekeeping may not be restricted to the SV, and in some species, it must necessarily occur in other tissues.

At present, little is known about the internal mechanisms controlling timing of migration through photoperiodic sensitivity. No evidence has yet been provided of a role of the SV; however, its involvement cannot be ruled out. A study in the Atlantic salmon has reported the seasonal expression of a *TSHβ* paralogue in a sub-portion of the pituitary gland anatomically reminiscent of the mammalian *pars tuberalis* (Fleming et al. 2019). The peak of mRNA abundance in the pituitary coincides with downstream migration, although a functional association between these processes has yet to be established. A separate investigation showed that the optic tectum, a brain area typically associated with processing visual information, displays photoperiodic stimulation of *Dio2* expression (Lorgen et al. 2015). The induction of *Dio2* occurs locally in areas of cell proliferation within the brain that may be functionally linked to thyroid hormone-dependent neurogenesis known to be essential for the development of important smolt characteristics including olfactory imprinting and adrenocorticotrophic stimulation. Contrasting with the SV system, photoperiod-dependent *Dio2* expression in the optic tectum is regionally distinct from TSH expression, suggesting that a distinct upstream pathway may be responsible. Compellingly, the optic tectum expresses a suite of photoreceptors and a very high density of melatonin receptors; these characteristics represent potential input pathways for photoperiodic information. Interestingly, research into biological timing in zebrafish has shown that both nervous and non-nervous tissues exhibit strong circadian rhythms that can be directly re-entrained by light during explant culture (Sassone-Corsi et al. 2000). This is radically different to the centralized organization observed in mammals, and credits the possibility for decentralized control of photoperiodic responses where tissues may possess the machinery to respond independently. Indeed, summer-like photoperiods are able to increase *Dio2* expression in the gill of Atlantic salmon (Lorgen et al. 2015). However, whether this response represents a local tissue effect has yet to be determined.

7.7   Conclusions

The seasonal biology of teleosts is widespread. However, it is clear that only a subsection of examples which develop seasonal traits do so under the guidance of a timer mechanism. This demonstrates that the adaptive value of timer mechanisms is not universal as is often assumed, but is rather specific to ecological context. Where timers are important, evidence suggests that they rely heavily on photoperiodic cues to maintain synchronicity with the annual cycle. However, in contrast to mammals and birds, little is known of the mechanisms responsible for the detection of the environment, input pathways or the nature of the timekeeping system which integrates this information and facilitates an adaptive output. With the advent of improved genetic tools and CrispR technology, some of these significant knowledge gaps can now be properly addressed. The positive implications of this research are clear for fish research and the aquaculture industry. However, progress in this area will also provide a valuable dataset relevant to all vertebrate seasonal research. The economy, robustness, and easy scalability of many fish make them ideal research models. Whereas in the past, fish researchers have often relied heavily on mammalian characterizations to guide their research; henceforth, this balance may tilt the other way, with the improved understanding of fish permitting valuable insight into the conservation of vertebrate mechanisms.

References

Baggerman B (1972) Photoperiodic responses in the stickleback and their control by a daily rhythm of photosensitivity. Gen Comp Endocrinol 3:466–476. https://doi.org/10.1016/0016-6480(72)90177-3

Berge ÅI, Berg A, Barnung T, Hansen T, Fyhn HJ, Stefansson SO (1995) Development of salinity tolerance in underyearling smolts of Atlantic salmon (*Salmo salar*) reared under different photoperiods. Can J Fish Aquat Sci 52(2):243–251. https://doi.org/10.1139/f95-024

Clark RW, Henderson-Arzapalo A, Sullivan CV (2005) Disparate effects of constant and annually-cycling daylength and water temperature on reproductive maturation of striped bass (*Morone saxatilis*). Aquaculture 249:497–513. https://doi.org/10.1016/j.aquaculture.2005.04.001

Cowan M, Azpeleta C, López-Olmeda JF (2017) Rhythms in the endocrine system of fish: a review. J Comp Physiol B 187:1057–1089. Springer Berlin Heidelberg. https://doi.org/10.1007/s00360-017-1094-5

Cyr DG, Bromage NR, Duston J, Eales JG (1988) Seasonal patterns in serum levels of thyroid hormones and sex steroids in relation to photoperiod-induced changes in spawning time in rainbow trout, *Salmo gairdneri*. Gen Comp Endocrinol 69:217–225. https://doi.org/10.1016/0016-6480(88)90008-1

Duston J, Bromage N (1986) Photoperiodic mechanisms and rhythms of reproduction in the female rainbow trout. Fish Physiol Biochem 2:35–51

Duston J, Bromage N (1991) Circannual rhythms of gonadal maturation in female rainbow trout (*Oncorhynchus mykiss*). J Biol Rhythm 6(1):49–53

Eriksson L-O, Lundqvist H (1982) Cirannual rhythms and photoperiod regulation of growth and smolting in Baltic salmon (Salmo salar L.). Aquaculture 28:113–121

Falcón J, Besseau L, Magnanou E, Herrero MJ, Nagai M, Boeuf G (2011) Melatonin, the time keeper: biosynthesis and effects in fish. Cybium 35(1):3–18. http://www.yies.pref.yamanashi.jp/env-phy/gyouseki/59.pdf\npapers3://publication/uuid/9D60D6E4-9E07-4B47-BD1A-7CC3EFEDEAB5

Falcón J, Bolliet V, Collin JP (1996) Partial characterization of serotonin N-acetyltransferases from northern pike (Esox lucius, L.) pineal organ and retina: effects of temperature. Pflugers Arch Eur J Physiol 432(3):386–393. https://doi.org/10.1007/s004240050149

Fleming MS, Maugars G, Lafont A-G, Rancon J, Fontaine R, Nourizadeh-Lillabadi R, Weltzien F-A, Yebra-Pimentel ES, Dirks R, McCormick SD, Rousseau K, Martin P, Dufour S (2019) Functional divergence of thyrotropin beta-subunit paralogs gives new insights into salmon smoltification metamorphosis. Sci Rep 9(4561):1–15. https://doi.org/10.1038/s41598-019-40019-5

Handeland SO, Imsland AK, Björnsson BT, Stefansson SO (2013) Long-term effects of photoperiod, temperature and their interaction on growth, gill Na^+, K^+-ATPase activity, seawater tolerance and plasma growth-hormone levels in Atlantic salmon *Salmo salar*. J Fish Biol 83:1197–1209. https://doi.org/10.1111/jfb.12215

Huang TS, Ruoff P, Fjelldal PG (2010) Effects of continuous light on daily levels of plasma melatonin and cortisol and expression of clock genes in pineal gland, brain, and liver in Atlantic salmon postsmolts. Chronobiol Int 27(9–10):1715–1734. https://doi.org/10.3109/07420528.2010.521272

IUCN (2019) The IUCN red list of threatened species 2019–2

Jobling M, Johnsen HK, Pettersen GW, Henderson RJ (1995) Effect of temperature on reproductive development in Arctic charr, *Salvelinus alpinus* (L.). J Therm Biol 20(1):157–165. https://doi.org/10.1016/0306-4565(94)00044-J

Kavaliers M (1982) Seasonal and Circannual rhythms in behavioral thermoregulation and their modifications by Pinealectomy in the white sucker, Catostomus commersoni. J Comp Physiol 146:235–243

Kurokawa T (1990) Influence of the date and body size at smoltification and subsequent growth rate and photoperiod on desmoltification in underyearling masu salmon (Oncorhynchus masou). Aquaculture 86:209–218

Lall SP, Tibbetts SM (2009) Nutrition, feeding, and behavior of fish. Vet Clin North Am - Exot Anim Pract 12(2):361–372. Elsevier Ltd. https://doi.org/10.1016/j.cvex.2009.01.005

Ligo M, Abe T, Kambayashi S, Oikawa K, Masuda T, Mizusawa K, Kitamura S, Azuma T, Takagi Y, Aida K, Yanagisawa T (2007) Lack of circadian regulation of in vitro melatonin release from the pineal organ of salmonid teleosts. Gen Comp Endocrinol 154:91–97. https://doi.org/10.1016/j.ygcen.2007.06.013

Lorgen M, Casadei E, Król E, Douglas A, Birnie MJ, Ebbesson LOE, Nilsen TO, Jordan WC, Jørgensen EH, Dardente H, Hazlerigg DG, Martin SAM (2015) Functional divergence of type 2 Deiodinase Paralogs in the Atlantic Salmon. Curr Biol 25:936–941. https://doi.org/10.1016/j.cub.2015.01.074

Maeda R, Shimo T, Nakane Y, Nakao N, Yoshimura T (2015) Ontogeny of the saccus vasculosus, a seasonal sensor in fish. Endocrinology 156(11):4238–4243. https://doi.org/10.1210/en.2015-1415

McCormick SD, Björnsson BT, Sheridan M, Eilerlson C, Carey JB, O'Dea M (1995) Increased daylength stimulates plasma growth hormone and gill Na⁺, K⁺- ATPase in Atlantic salmon (*Salmo salar*). J Comp Physiol B 165:245–254. https://doi.org/10.1007/BF00367308

McCormick SD, Hansen LP, Quinn TP, Saunders RL (2011a) Movement, migration, and smolting of Atlantic salmon (Salmo salar). Can J Fish Aquat Sci 55(S1):77–92. https://doi.org/10.1139/d98-011

McCormick SD, Shrimpton JM, Zydlewski JD (2011b) Temperature effects on osmoregulatory physiology of juvenile anadromous fish. Global Warming Cambridge University Press. https://doi.org/10.1017/cbo9780511983375.012

Migaud H, Davie A, Taylor JF (2010) Current knowledge on the photoneuroendocrine regulation of reproduction in temperate fish species. J Fish Biol 76(1):27–68. https://doi.org/10.1111/j.1095-8649.2009.02500.x

Nakane Y, Ikegami K, Iigo M, Ono H, Takeda K, Takahashi D, Uesaka M, Kimijima M, Hashimoto R, Arai N, Suga T, Kosuge K, Abe T, Maeda R, Senga T, Amiya N, Azuma T, Amano M, Abe H, Yamamoto N, Yoshimura T (2013) The saccus vasculosus of fish is a sensor of seasonal changes in day length. Nat Commun 4:1–7. https://doi.org/10.1038/ncomms3108

Nishi K (1979) A daily rhythm in the photosensitive development of the ovary in the bitterling, Rhodeus ocellatus ocellatus. Bull Fac Fish Hokkaido Univ 30(2):109–115

Pankhurst NW, Purser GJ, Van Der Kraak G, Thomas PM, Forteath GNR (1996) Effect of holding temperature on ovulation, egg fertily, plasma levels of reproductive hormones and in vitro ovarian steroidogenesis in the rainbow trout *Oncorhynchus mykiss*. Aquaculture 146:277–290. https://doi.org/10.1016/S0044-8486(96)01374-9

Prat F, Zanuy S, Bromage N, Carrillo M (1999) Effects of constant short and long photoperiod regimes on the spawning performance and sex steroid levels of female and male sea bass. J Fish Biol 54:125–137

Raible F, Tessmar-raible K (2017) An overview of monthly rhythms and clocks. Front Neurol 8 (May):1–14. https://doi.org/10.3389/fneur.2017.00189

Randall CF, Bromage NR (1998) Photoperiodic history determines the reproductive response of rainbow trout to changes in daylength. J Comp Physiol - A Sensory, Neural, Behav Physiol 183 (5):651–660. https://doi.org/10.1007/s003590050288

Ravi V, Byrappa V (2018) The divergent genomes of Teleosts. Annu Rev Anim Biosci 6:47–68

Sæther B-S, Johnsen HK, Jobling M (1996) Seasonal changes in food consumption and growth of Arctic charr exposed to either simulated natural or a 12: 12 LD photoperiod at constant water temperature. J Fish Biol 48:1113–1122. https://doi.org/10.1006/jfbi.1996.0114

Sassone-Corsi P, Whitmore D, Foulkes NS (2000) Light acts directly on organs and cells in culture to set the vertebrate circadian clock. Nature 404(6773):87–91. https://doi.org/10.1038/35003589

Schugardt C, Kirschbaum F (2004) Control of gonadal maturation and regression by experimental variation of environmental factors in the mormyrid fish, Mormyrus rume proboscirostris. Environ Biol Fish 70:227–233

Shewmon (2007) Environmental manipulation of growth and sexual maturation in yellow perch. Perca flavescens 38(3):383–394

Shimmura T, Nakayama T, Shinomiya A, Fukamachi S, Yasugi M, Watanabe E, Shimo T, Senga T, Nishimura T, Tanaka M, Kamei Y, Naruse K, Yoshimura T (2017) Dynamic plasticity in phototransduction regulates seasonal changes in color perception. Nat Commun 8(1):1–7. Springer US. https://doi.org/10.1038/s41467-017-00432-8

Soivio A, Muona M (1988) Desmoltification of heat-accelerated Baltic Salmon (Salmo salar) in brackish water. Aquaculture 71:89–97

Stefansson SO, Berge ÅI, Gunnarsson GS (1998) Changes in seawater tolerance and gill Na$^+$,K$^+$-ATPase activity during desmoltification in Atlantic salmon kept in freshwater at different temperatures. Aquaculture 168:271–277. https://doi.org/10.1016/S0044-8486(98)00354-8

Strand JET, Hazlerigg D, Jørgensen EH (2018) Photoperiod revisited: is there a critical day length for triggering a complete parr – smolt transformation in Atlantic salmon Salmo salar? J Fish Biol 93:440–448. https://doi.org/10.1111/jfb.13760

Sundararaj BI, Vasal S (2011) Photoperiod and temperature control in the regulation of reproduction in the female catfish *Heteropneustes fossilis*. J Fish Res Board Canada 33(4):959–973. https://doi.org/10.1139/f76-123

Takeuchi Y, Hada N, Imamura S, Hur S, Bouchekioua S, Takemura A (2015) Existence of a photoinducible phase for ovarian development and photoperiod-related alteration of clock gene expression in a damsel fish. Comp Biochem Physiol Part A 188:32–39. https://doi.org/10.1016/j.cbpa.2015.06.010

Tamai TK, Young LC, Whitmore D (2007) Light signaling to the zebrafish circadian clock by Cryptochrome 1a. PNAS 104(37):14712–14717

Taranger GL, Haux C, Stefansson SO, Hansen T, Bjornsson T (1998) Abrupt changes in photoperiod affect age at maturity, timing of ovulation and plasma testosterone and oestradiol-17 b profiles in Atlantic salmon, Salmo salar. Aquaculture 162:85–98

Thorarensen H, Clarke WC (1989) Smoltification induced by a "skeleton" photoperiod in underyearling coho salmon (*Oncorhynchus kisutch*). Fish Physiol Biochem 6(1):11–18. https://doi.org/10.1007/BF01875600

West AC, Bechtold D (2015) The cost of circadian desynchrony: evidence, insights and open questions. BioEssays:777–788. https://doi.org/10.1002/bies.201400173

West AC, Wood SH (2018) Science direct seasonal physiology: making the future a thing of the past. Curr Opin Psychol 5:1–8. https://doi.org/10.1016/j.cophys.2018.04.006

Wootton RJ, Smith C (2015) Reproductive biology of teleost fishes. Wiley

Further Recommended Reading

Nakane Y, Ikegami K, Iigo M, Ono H, Takeda K, Takahashi D, Uesaka M, Kimijima M, Hashimoto R, Arai N, Suga T, Kosuge K, Abe T, Maeda R, Senga T, Amiya N, Azuma T, Amano M, Abe H, Yamamoto N, Yoshimura T (2013) The saccus vasculosus of fish is a sensor of seasonal changes in day length. Nat. Commun. 4:1–7

Research paper identifying the saccus vasculosus as a key transducer of photoperiod in some species of teleosts, a structure not found in higher vertebrates.

Saha S, Singh KM, Gupta BBP (2019) Melatonin synthesis and clock gene regulation in the pineal organ of teleost fish compared to mammals: Similarities and differences. General and Comparative Endocrinology 279:27–34

Detailed review of the control of melatonin production by photoperiod and temperature.

Action of Light on the Neuroendocrine Axis

8

Jens Hannibal

Abstract

Photoentrainment of the circadian clock located in the hypothalamic suprachiasmatic nucleus (SCN) is fundamental for the stable regulation of neuroendocrine function underlying physiological functions such as metabolism, sleep, immune responses, and reproduction. Masking by light directly suppresses melatonin secretion independent of the circadian system, with impact on several neuroendocrine axes. This chapter describes recent findings in anatomy and physiology on how light mediates its effects on SCN-regulated timing of the neuroendocrine system, including the hypothalamic-pituitary-adrenal (HPA) axis, the hypothalamic-pituitary-thyroid (HPT) axis, the hypothalamic-pituitary-gonadal (HPG) axis, and melatonin and arginine-vasopressin (AVP) secretion. In modern societies, artificial light at night (ALAN) seems to affect circadian and neuroendocrine systems, and should be considered in the understanding the health problems of the industrialized human population.

Keywords

Photoreceptors · Neurotransmitters · Neuroendocrine · Circadian · Seasonal

J. Hannibal (✉)
Department of Clinical Biochemistry, Bispebjerg Frederiksberg Hospital, University of Copenhagen, Copenhagen, Denmark
e-mail: j.hannibal@dadlnet.dk

F. J. P. Ebling, H. D. Piggins (eds.), *Neuroendocrine Clocks and Calendars*,
Masterclass in Neuroendocrinology 10, https://doi.org/10.1007/978-3-030-55643-3_8

8.1   Introduction

Life on Earth has adapted to the daily changes in light and darkness caused by the planet's rotation on its own axis during the 24-h astronomical cycle and seasonal changes in the northern and southern hemispheres due to the 23° tilt in the Earth's axis. In temperate regions, day-length (photoperiod) varies markedly during the seasons, providing the most predictable indicator of the time of the year. The ability to anticipate the changes in environmental conditions is a clear selective advantage for survival and is ensured by an internal timing system found in almost all living organisms, a system capable of synchronization with the light/dark cycle (Daan and Aschoff 2001). In mammals, light perceived by the retina is the strongest signal used by the internal circadian and circannual timing systems to stay synchronized (entrained) with the solar cycle (Golombek and Rosenstein 2010). The circadian system consists of a network of endogenous clocks in the brain and peripheral tissues coupled by hormonal signals and by the autonomic nervous system, all conducted by the brain master clock, located in the hypothalamic suprachiasmatic nucleus (SCN) (Klein et al. 1991). The SCN produces coherent output rhythms driving circadian changes in physiology and behavior, and controls multiple neuroendocrine axes that regulate metabolism and seasonal reproduction, for example, fat storage in preparation for hibernation (Klein et al. 1991). Due to slight deviation of endogenous rhythms from the astronomical day of 24 h, the SCN needs daily resetting by environmental light, which makes SCN-controlled physiological processes under indirect retinal control. This process, known as photoentrainment (Golombek and Rosenstein 2010), is dependent on retinal photopigments, located on classical photoreceptor cells (rods and cones) in the outer retina, and on a recently identified system of retinal ganglion cells, which are intrinsically photosensitive due to the expression of the photopigment melanopsin (Do and Yau 2010). The melanopsin-containing retinal ganglion cells (mRGCs) constitute a non-image-forming (NIF) light perception system, which reaches the SCN as a monosynaptic neuronal pathway, known as the retinohypothalamic tract (RHT) (Do and Yau 2010; Hannibal 2002). Photoentrainment of SCN rhythmicity ensures stable oscillation of temporal niches for sleep/wake, food intake, activity, core body temperature, and regulation of many hormones, including neuroendocrine axis as the hypothalamic-pituitary-adrenal (HPA) axis, the hypothalamic-pituitary-thyroidal (HPT) axis, the hypothalamic-pituitary-gonadotropic (HPG) axis, and melatonin and arginine-vasopressin (AVP) secretion. In mammals, the circannual rhythms (e.g., self-sustained rhythms with a period typically less than 1 year) are influenced by the SCN and melatonin secreted from the pineal gland. Melatonin is a nocturnally secreted hormone that provides a neurochemical representation of the night length to the SCN and other neuroendocrine tissues, and is therefore an important seasonal indicator, ultimately regulating the function of many areas of the brain and body involved in seasonal reproduction and physiology (Pevet and Challet 2011).

The present chapter considers the effects of ambient light on the circadian regulation of neuroendocrine hormone secretion. It focuses on the photoentrainment process and the possible role of artificial light at night (ALAN), an increasing problem in industrialized parts of the world, which may have great impact on health and wellbeing of all living organisms.

8.2 The Neuroendocrine Axis

The neuroendocrine axis can be defined as "the structural and functional basis for interactions between brain, hormones, and glands that allow an organism to respond to external stimuli with complex, sometimes long-lasting physiological changes, such as during stress or reproduction" (Binder et al. 2009). The classical pathway involves hypothalamic neurons releasing hypophysiotropic factor/neuromediators/ neurotransmitters into the hypophyseal portal circulation, which transport the releasing factor to the anterior pituitary. Here, they bind to specific receptors on subpopulations of pituitary cells causing the release of pituitary hormones to the blood targeting endocrine glands. Feedback inhibition from secreted hormones occurs in both the brain and pituitary.

Figure 8.1 illustrates three major neuroendocrine axes that are regulated by the circadian-timing system. (1) The HPA axis in which corticotropin-releasing hormone (CRH) is released from axon terminals of the parvocellular neurons of the hypothalamic paraventricular nucleus (PVN) reaches the portal capillaries and stimulates the release of adrenocorticotropin (ACTH), causing the release of corticosterone/cortisol from the adrenal cortex. (2) The HPT axis, driven by the release of thyrotropin-releasing hormone (TRH), is secreted mainly from the TRH-expressing neurons of the PVN, from which neurosecretory axon terminals release it into the portal circulation, binding to thyroid-stimulating hormone (TSH) expressing pituitary cells. Circulating TSH stimulates the release of the thyroid hormones (TH; thyroxine (T4) and triiodothyronine (T3)) via the TSH receptor located in the thyroid gland. (3) The HPG axis controlling the release of gonadotropin-luteinizing hormone (LH) and follicle stimulation hormone (FSH) from gonadotropic pituitary cells by gonadotropin-releasing hormone (GnRH) produced in neurons located in the basal forebrain and released in the median eminence into the portal capillaries (Kalsbeek and Buijs 2002).

Prolactin secreted by the pituitary and released upon secretion of releasing factors in the hypothalamus can also be considered as part of the neuroendocrine axis. Despite its name and function primary as promoting lactation upon breast-sucking stimulation, prolactin has a broad range of functions (Grattan 2015). In contrast to the aforementioned endocrine axis, the secretion of prolactin has no specific endocrine target, which feedbacks to the brain and pituitary (Grattan 2015). Regulation from the hypothalamus also differs being primarily inhibitory via specific dopaminergic neurons located in the arcuate nucleus/pars tuberalis, the so-called TIDA neurons (Grattan 2015). Circadian prolactin secretion is dependent on estradiol and involves signals from the SCN to oxytocinergic PVN neurons (Kennett et al. 2008), whereas circannual secretion of prolactin involves a pituitary-based timing mechanism (Lincoln et al. 2006) (see also Chaps. 1 and 2). The hypothalamo-neurohypophysial system (HNS) also belongs to the neuroendocrine axis. The

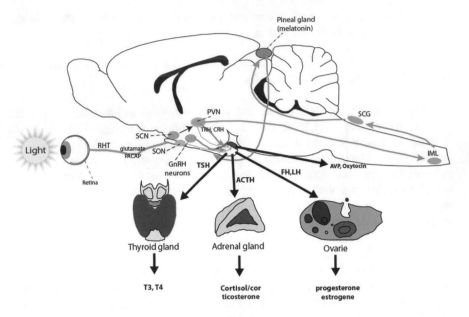

Fig. 8.1 Photic regulation of the neuroendocrine system. Light is perceived by rod, cone, and melanopsin photoreceptors in the retina. The retinohypothalamic tract (RHT) utilizes two neurotransmitters: glutamate and PACAP, so photic information is transduced to the brain master clock located in the suprachiasmatic nucleus (SCN). From the SCN, neuronal signals reach neuroendocrine cells in the hypothalamus (TRH, CRH, and GnRH), and through the midbrain and brainstem, via neurons in the intermediolateral column in the spinal cord and the noradrenergic neurons of the superior cervical ganglion to the pineal gland. Hormones (TSH, ACTH, FSH, and LH) are released upon stimulation of pituitary cells into the blood, reaching their endocrine target glands (thyroid, adrenal, gonads) causing release of thyroid hormones, cortisol/corticosterone, and sex steroids

HNS consists of neuroendocrine neurons located in the "magnocellular" PVN and in the hypothalamic supraoptic nucleus (SON). Two distinct populations of neurosecretory neurons release oxytocin and AVP via neurosecretory axon terminals in the neural lobe of the pituitary and into the blood. Oxytocin plays several roles during sexual reproduction, and during and after childbirth. AVP, also known as the "antidiuretic hormone (ADH)," is regulated in part by the circadian-timing system, and targets AVP receptors in the kidney distal tubules controlling reabsorption of water. AVP also has vasoconstrictor effects on blood pressure regulation (Engelmann and Landgraf 1997). An important regulator of the neuroendocrine axis is the nocturnal release of melatonin secreted from the pineal gland. The rhythm of melatonin production is tightly controlled by the SCN and provides information on day length for the organization of biological rhythms. It appears to be the best-established humoral factor of signaling time of day and time of year to other physiological systems (Pevet and Challet 2011; Arendt 2009; Hazlerigg and Loudon 2008).

8.3   The Mammalian Circadian Timing System

The mammalian circadian system consists of a central oscillator located in the SCN and a network of endogenous clocks in the brain and in peripheral tissues coupled by internal hormonal signals and the autonomic nervous system. 10,000–20,000 neurons constitute the neuronal network of the SCN, many of which express a molecular clockwork based on positive and negative feedback loops of so-called clock proteins and their respective genes (Mohawk and Takahashi 2011). The molecular clock (described in detail in Chap. 11) generates circadian rhythms of approximately 24 h (*circa dies* = approximately a day). The endogenous period length of the individual ("tau") varies between mammalian species. In mice, it is often shorter than 24 h, while humans often have a tau longer than 24 h (Czeisler et al. 1999; Daan and Pittendrigh 1976a). Due to this deviation from the astronomical day length of 24 h, the clock needs daily adjustment to the solar cycle. This process is known as photo- or light entrainment (Golombek and Rosenstein 2010; Roenneberg and Foster 1997). The light-dark cycle is the most powerful "time giver" (German: zeitgeber or zeitgeber time; ZT), which interacts with other inputs to the circadian system. These other "nonphotic" signals include metabolic cues, physical activity, sleep, temperature, and immune signals (Daan and Aschoff 2001). Of these nonphotic inputs, metabolic cues representing caloric status represent the most important signal, but are beyond the scope of this chapter (Challet 2015). An integrated output from the entrained clock is conveyed by neuronal and humoral signals to the brain and body. Among the target areas innervated directly or indirectly from SCN neurons are cells in the neuroendocrine system of the hypothalamus and the pineal gland (Kalsbeek and Buijs 2002; Larsen et al. 1998) (Fig. 8.1). These signals secure the secretion of several of the releasing hormones of the three major neuroendocrine axes in a time (circadian and circannual)-dependent manner, which causes the temporal changes in peripheral hormone levels in the blood (Kalsbeek et al. 2006).

8.3.1   Light Regulation of Circadian Rhythms: The Photic Phase Response Curve (PRC)

Light has a time-dependent effect on the circadian clock that is a fundamental property of the clock (Golombek and Rosenstein 2010; Daan and Pittendrigh 1976b). In nature, this ability ensures the individual to stay entrained with the solar and annual cycle. The mechanism and physiology of the entrainment process has been studied in detail and both light intensity, wavelength and time are important for entrainment of the circadian pacemaker (Golombek and Rosenstein 2010; Duffy and Czeisler 2009). The SCN is sensitive to light at the end of the subjective day, throughout the night and during the early day, whereas light in the middle of the subjective day has little or no effect on clock phasing (Daan and Pittendrigh 1976a). This time-dependent sensitivity and response to light stimulation is referred to as the phase-response curve (PRC) to light (Fig. 8.2). In individuals with a short tau

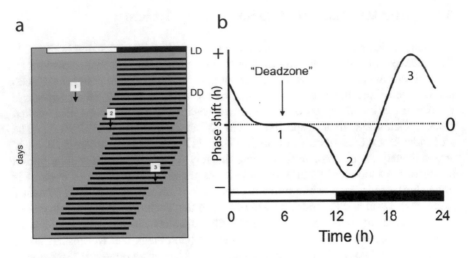

Fig. 8.2 Light regulation of circadian rhythms; the photic-phase response curve (PRC). (**a**) Schematic presentation of the activity rhythms of a nocturnal animal, where each horizontal line represents the activity of the animal in one day. The animal is entrained to a light/dark photoperiod (LD) as represented on the top of the record. The animal is then released into constant darkness (DD) and the activity rhythm is now "free-running". During the free-running period, the animal experiences light pulses during subjective day (Daan and Aschoff 2001), early subjective night (Golombek and Rosenstein 2010), and late subjective night (Klein et al. 1991). The light pulse given during the day has little or no effect on the phase of the endogenous rhythm. Light pulses given in the early subjective night result in a phase delay of the overt rhythm as indicated by (Golombek and Rosenstein 2010) in panels (**a**) and (**b**), and a light pulse given in the late subjective night results in a phase advance of the overt rhythm as indicated by (Klein et al. 1991) in panels (**a**) and (**b**). A complete phase-response curve to light stimulation during a 24-h period is drawn in (**b**). Phase delays are plotted in the negative direction (downward) and phase advances are plotted in the upwards direction. The horizontal axis in (**b**) represents one circadian cycle

(<24 h), the subjective night will occur before the end of the solar day. To adjust this deviation, light at early night results in a phase delay of the circadian phase causing the clock to slow down. Individuals with a long tau (>24 h) will, on the other hand, meet the morning light while the subjective clock still shows nighttime. Light at the end of the subjective night speeds up the clock and causes phase advance of the circadian clock to stay entrained with the solar cycle. During the changing seasons, life in the northern and southern hemispheres adapts circadian rhythms to the daily change in day and night length, due to the time-dependent phase responses to light of the circadian pacemaker (Hughes et al. 2015).

8.4   The Retinohypothalamic Tract

In mammals, photic information to the SCN is solely received in the retina (Nelson and Zucker 1981) and transmitted via a monosynaptic neuronal pathway, originally described by Moore and Lenn (Moore and Lenn 1972), which led to the identification of the SCN as the brain's clock (Klein et al. 1991). The origin of this pathway was shown to be a distinct subpopulation of retinal ganglion cells (RGCs) widely distributed in the entire retina (Moore et al. 1995). RHT projections from each eye reach the ventral bilateral SCN (Morin and Allen 2005) and bifurcating axon terminals also reach the intergeniculate leaflet (IGL) of the lateral geniculate complex, which can be considered as part of the circadian timing system (Pickard 1985). Cells in the IGL integrate photic and nonphotic information and project to the SCN, providing feedback regulation of the pacemaker via the geniculo-hypothalamic tract (GHT) (Moore 1995). Nerve fibers from the RHT target several areas not directly involved in circadian timing, such as the ventral preoptic area (VLPO) and the hypothalamic subparaventricular zone (subPVN). The VLPO is involved in regulation of the homeostatic regulation of sleep (Saper et al. 2005a), and light indirectly affects hormone secretion via effects on sleep homeostasis (Saper et al. 2005b). The subPVN has been suggested to play a role in light-regulated masking behavior (see later).

8.4.1 Photoreceptors of the RHT: Role of Melanopsin

The role of the eyes in photoentrainment has in mammals been documented by showing "free-running" rhythms following enucleation of the eye (Nelson and Zucker 1981; Foster et al. 1991). However, examination of blind people (Kleinman et al. 2002; Czeisler et al. 1995) and mice lacking the outer photoreceptors (the rods and cones) demonstrated in the 1990s that light-induced melatonin suppression and photoentrainment were preserved despite visual blindness (Foster et al. 1991; Freedman et al. 1999). These studies indicated that an unidentified photoreceptor located in the inner retina could be involved in the NIF system. In 1998, Provencio et al. identified a new opsin photoreceptor in frog skin that was named melanopsin (Provencio et al. 1998). Shortly after, Provencio et al. showed that OPN4-encoding melanopsin was expressed in a subset of RGCs in the mammalian retina (Provencio et al. 2000). This observation was followed by studies confirming that the melanopsin locates to their surface membrane (Hannibal et al. 2002; Hattar et al. 2002; Gooley et al. 2001), and in an elegant study, the melanopsin-expressing RGCs were shown to be intrinsically photosensitive independent of signals from the outer retina (Berson et al. 2002). During the following years, melanopsin was established as a new mammalian photoreceptor (Hattar et al. 2003; Panda et al. 2003) located exclusively in RGCs of the RHT being sensitive to blue light of approximately 480 nm (Do and Yau 2010; Lucas et al. 2014). The melanopsin-expressing RGCs (mRGCs) are a heterogeneous group represented by 5–7 subtypes of RGCs (Ecker et al. 2010; Hannibal et al. 2017), which together constitute just 0.6–1.0% of the total number of RGCs in the mammalian retina (Hannibal et al. 2002, 2017; Hattar et al. 2002; Liao et al. 2016; Hughes et al. 2013; Schmidt and Kofuji 2009). In addition to the direct light response, the mRGCs receive light information from rods and cones. The information is integrated in the mRGCs via bipolar and amacrine cells. Differences in dendritic morphology of the mRGCs suggest that afferent connections may differ qualitatively, making the NIF system sensitive to the broad spectrum of light found from sunrise to sunset (Lucas et al. 2014; Dacey et al. 2005). Light perception to the circadian timing system and other NIF functions are dependent on the mRGCs, since all NIF-controlled functions are lost or severely affected after genetic or toxic elimination of melanopsin-expressing RGCs (Lucas et al. 2014; Hatori et al. 2008; Guler et al. 2008).

8.4.2   Neurotransmitters of the RHT

RHT projecting axon terminals are found in retino-recipient areas of the brain, which include the SCN, the IGL, the sleep-regulation neurons in the ventrolateral preoptic nucleus (VLPO), the subparaventicular zone of the PVN, and nuclei in the pretectal area, including the olivary pretectal nucleus (OPN) controlling the pupillary reflex (Hannibal and Fahrenkrug 2004; Hattar et al. 2006; Hannibal et al. 2014). In mammals, these projections costore two neurotransmitters, the classic neurotransmitter glutamate and the neuropeptide pituitary adenylate cyclase–activating polypeptide (PACAP) (Hannibal et al. 2000). The excitatory neurotransmitter glutamate is considered as the primary neurotransmitter due to its "light like"–phase shifting capacity on SCN neurons (Hannibal 2002), while PACAP seems to have a neuromodulatory effect by gating the glutamate-induced resetting of the circadian phase (Hannibal 2006, 2016). The contribution of photoreceptors that initiate light signaling and release of the two neurotransmitters, glutamate and PACAP, has been studied in another NIF-regulated function, the pupillary light reflex (Keenan et al. 2016). This study shows that transient responses utilize input from rod photoreceptors and glutamate signaling, whereas sustained stimulation primarily involves melanopsin and PACAP release (Keenan et al. 2016). Several subtypes of glutamate receptors, including both NMDA and non-NMDA, and metabotropic receptors have been identified in the SCN, whereas PACAP seems to exert its effects via the specific PACAP type 1 receptor (PAC1) expressed in the SCN (Chen et al. 1999; Hannibal et al. 2001, 2008).

8.5   Impact of Light on Clock Function and Neuroendocrine Regulation: Circadian Regulation and Masking

Photoentrainment is the main factor that keeps the circadian clock aligned with the light/dark cycle (see earlier) and makes SCN-controlled physiological processes under indirect retinal control. This ensures the daily variation in the secretion of cortisol/corticosterone, which in nocturnal animals peaks when activity is initiated at sunset, while in humans and other day-active animals the secretion of cortisol peaks in the morning. TSH also demonstrates daily oscillation with a pattern similar to the HPA-axis. Melatonin, on the other hand, is rhythmically released in the beginning of the night in both nocturnal and diurnal animals. During altering photoperiods, the neuroendocrine secretion under SCN control adapts hormone release corresponding to the day length. However, light also directly influences rhythmic physiology, behavior, and hormone secretion. This effect of light is often referred to as masking (Mrosovsky 1999). Masking is independent of the SCN clock (Redlin and Mrosovsky 1999), and is an important factor that controls rhythmic behavior and physiology during clock arrhythmicity caused by clock gene mutation (Husse et al. 2014; Bunger et al. 2000) or disrupted synchronization of individual clock neurons (Hannibal et al. 2011; Bechtold et al. 2008; Vosko et al. 2007).

Lights at night initiates a response affecting the circadian regulation of hormone secretion by altering the circadian phase (see earlier) through neuronal pathways independent of the SCN, which directly or indirectly target areas involved in physiology and behavior. Melatonin secretion is an example of a very light-sensitive system, where the rhythmic control is overridden by light-induced inhibition at night, resulting in low level of nocturnal melatonin even after a short pulse of light at night (Pevet and Challet 2011). A direct effect (masking) of light also seems to explain the continued oscillation in peripheral clocks and hormone secretion in genetic SCN-ablated animals (Husse et al. 2014), as the effects of light stimulation on the adrenal glands are independent of the SCN (Kiessling et al. 2014).

8.6   Effects of Artificial Light at Night (ALAN) on the Neuroendocrine Axis

The circadian timing system in all living species, including mammals, evolved long before the occurrence of our modern society. Although many people on earth live in "rural" areas where light is "natural" coming primarily from daylight, most of the industrial parts of the world are exposed to artificial light at night (ALAN) (Fig. 8.3). The increasing use of electrical light has changed the temporal niche for humans,

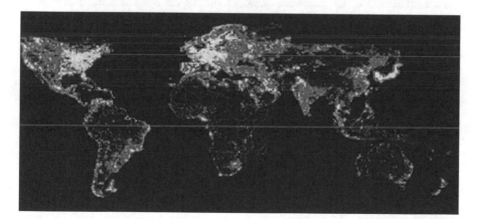

Fig. 8.3 Artificial light at night (ALAN). ALAN levels detected by the US-DMPS satellites' sensors in 2010. Note areas emitting the highest ALAN levels are marked in red, less-lit areas are marked in orange and yellow. Areas with no stable light appear in black (Cinzano and Elvidge 2001). Source: mapped using DMSP (2014) data

allowing them to be active at nighttime. Although this has been an important factor for the growing development in our societies, light at night is a factor with potentially great impact on health and the development of diseases, including metabolic syndrome, sleep disorders, and cancer (Navara and Nelson 2007). Because hormone levels vary in accordance with the light/dark cycle corresponding to metabolic, reproductive, and immunological functions, ALAN is a potential disruptor of the endocrine functions due to its impact on circadian regulation and by direct effects of light independent of the circadian system (see Sect. 8.5). Nocturnal melatonin secretion is probably the most sensitive of the neuroendocrine axes affected by ALAN (Ouyang et al. 2018). Disruption in nocturnal melatonin has been associated with increased risk of developing different forms of cancers (Hansen 2001; Van Dycke et al. 2015; Kloog et al. 2010) and with the higher occurrence of health problems found in people at shift work, such as metabolic syndrome, sleep disturbances, and depression (Navara and Nelson 2007; Fonken et al. 2010; Shivers et al. 1991). ALAN-induced suppression of melatonin signaling also seems to affect seasonal regulation of the reproductive axis primarily observed in seasonal breeders (Ouyang et al. 2018). ALAN may also cause a change in HPT-axis, metabolism, and seasonal adaptation targeting not only thyroid hormone release, but also via hormone action in the pars tuberalis of the pituitary gland (Hut 2011). Melatonin, a critical hormone for seasonal regulation of the reproductive axis in mammals, interacts with thyroid hormones in the pars tuberalis (Reiter et al. 2014). ALAN may affect this regulation by a direct suppression of melatonin expression and by a phase disruption of the circadian system (Pevet and Challet 2011; Hut 2011).

8.7   Perspectives

Photoentrainment of the circadian clock located in the SCN is fundamental for a stable regulation of neuroendocrine secretion into temporal niche controlling physiological functions such as metabolism, sleep, immune systems, and reproduction. Masking by light directly suppresses melatonin secretion independent of the circadian system, with impact on several neuroendocrine axes. In modern societies, ALAN seems to affect circadian and neuroendocrine systems and should be considered in the understanding of health problems in the industrialized human population.

Acknowledgments This work was supported by the Danish Biotechnology Center for Cellular Communication.

References

Arendt J (2009) Melatonin. In: Binder MD, Hirokawa N, Windhorst U (eds) Encyclopedia of neuroscience. Springer, Berlin, pp 2297–2302
Bechtold DA, Brown TM, Luckman SM, Piggins HD (2008) Metabolic rhythm abnormalities in mice lacking VIP-VPAC2 signaling. Am J Physiol Regul Integr Comp Physiol 294(2):R344–RR51

Berson DM, Dunn FA, Takao M (2002) Phototransduction by retinal ganglion cells that set the circadian clock. Science 295(5557):1070–1073

Binder MD, Hirokawa N, Windhorst U (2009) Neuroendocrine axis. In: Binder MD, Hirokawa N, Windhorst U (eds) Encyclopedia of neuroscience. Springer, Berlin

Bunger MK, Wilsbacher LD, Moran SM, Clendenin C, Radcliffe LA, Hogenesch JB et al (2000) Mop3 is an essential component of the master circadian pacemaker in mammals. Cell 103 (7):1009–1017

Challet E (2015) Keeping circadian time with hormones. Diabetes Obes Metab 17(Suppl 1):76–83. https://doi.org/10.1111/dom.12516

Chen D, Buchanan GF, Ding JM, Hannibal J, Gillette MU (1999) PACAP: a pivotal modulator of glutamatergic regulation of the suprachiasmatic circadian clock. Proc Natl Acad Sci U S A 96 (23):13409–13414

Cinzano PFF, Elvidge CD (2001) The first world atlas of the artificial night sky brightness. Mon Not R Astron Soc 328:689–707

Czeisler CA, Shanahan TL, Klerman EB, Martens H, Brotman DJ, Emens JS et al (1995) Suppression of melatonin secretion in some blind patients by exposure to bright light. N Engl J Med 332(1):6–11

Czeisler CA, Duffy JF, Shanahan TL, Brown EN, Mitchell JF, Rimmer DW et al (1999) Stability, precision, and near-24-hour period of the human circadian pacemaker. Science 284 (5423):2177–2181

Daan S, Aschoff J (2001) The entrainment of circadian systems. In: Takahashi JS, Turek FW, Moore RY (eds) Circadian clocks. Handbook of behavioral neurobiology. Kluwer Academic/Plenum Publisher, New York, pp 7–43

Daan S, Pittendrigh CS (1976a) A functional analysis of circadian pacemakers in nocturnal rodents. II. The variability of phase response curves. J Comp Physiol 106:253–266

Daan S, Pittendrigh CS (1976b) A functional analysis of the circadian pacemakers in nocturnal rodents. IV. Entrainment: pacemaker and clock. J Comp Physiol 106:253–266

Dacey DM, Liao HW, Peterson BB, Robinson FR, Smith VC, Pokorny J et al (2005) Melanopsin-expressing ganglion cells in primate retina signal color and irradiance and project to the LGN. Nature 433(7027):749–754

Do MT, Yau KW (2010) Intrinsically photosensitive retinal ganglion cells. Physiol Rev 90 (4):1547–1581

Duffy JF, Czeisler CA (2009) Effect of light on human circadian physiology. Sleep Med Clin 4 (2):165–177

Ecker JL, Dumitrescu ON, Wong KY, Alam NM, Chen SK, LeGates T et al (2010) Melanopsin-expressing retinal ganglion-cell photoreceptors: cellular diversity and role in pattern vision. Neuron 67(1):49–60

Engelmann M, Landgraf R (1997) Intracerebral release of vasopressin and oxytocin: new aspects of the old concept of neurosecretion. In: Korf H-W, Usadel K-H (eds) Neuroendocrinology Retrospect and perspectives. Springer, Berlin, pp 87–97

Fonken LK, Workman JL, Walton JC, Weil ZM, Morris JS, Haim A et al (2010) Light at night increases body mass by shifting the time of food intake. Proc Natl Acad Sci U S A 107 (43):18664–18669

Foster RG, Provencio I, Hudson D, Fiske S, De Grip W, Menaker M (1991) Circadian photoreception in the retinally degenerate mouse (rd/rd). J Comp Physiol A 169(1):39–50

Freedman MS, Lucas RJ, Soni B, von Schantz M, Muñoz M, David-Gray Z et al (1999) Regulation of mammalian circadian behavior by non-rod, non-cone, ocular photoreceptors. Science 284:502–504

Golombek DA, Rosenstein RE (2010) Physiology of circadian entrainment. Physiol Rev 90 (3):1063–1102

Gooley JJ, Lu J, Chou TC, Scammell TE, Saper CB (2001) Melanopsin in cells of origin of the retinohypothalamic tract. Nat Neurosci 12:1165

Grattan DR (2015) 60 years of neuroendocrinology: the hypothalamo-prolactin axis. J Endocrinol 226(2):T101–T122

Guler AD, Ecker JL, Lall GS, Haq S, Altimus CM, Liao HW et al (2008) Melanopsin cells are the principal conduits for rod-cone input to non-image-forming vision. Nature 453(7191):102–105

Hannibal J (2002) Neurotransmitters of the retino-hypothalamic tract. Cell Tissue Res 309 (1):73–88

Hannibal J (2006) Roles of PACAP-containing retinal ganglion cells in circadian timing. Int Rev Cytol 251:1–39

Hannibal J (2016) PACAP in the circadian timing system: learning from knockout models. Pituitary adenylate activating polypeptide—PACAP. Current topics in neurotoxicity. Springer, Switzerland, pp 227–237

Hannibal J, Fahrenkrug J (2004) Target areas innervated by PACAP immunoreactive retinal ganglion cells. Cell Tissue Res 316(1):99–113

Hannibal J, Moller M, Ottersen OP, Fahrenkrug J (2000) PACAP and glutamate are co-stored in the retinohypothalamic tract. J Comp Neurol 418:147–155

Hannibal J, Brabet P, Jamen F, Nielsen HS, Journot L, Fahrenkrug J (2001) Dissociation between light induced phase shift of the circadian rhythm and clock gene expression in mice lacking the PACAP type 1 receptor (PAC1). J Neurosci 21(13):4883–4890

Hannibal J, Hindersson P, Knudsen SM, Georg B, Fahrenkrug J (2002) The photopigment melanopsin is exclusively present in PACAP containing retinal ganglion cells of the retinohypothalamic tract. J Neurosci 22:RC191:1–7

Hannibal J, Brabet P, Fahrenkrug J (2008) Mice lacking the PACAP type I receptor have impaired photic entrainment and negative masking. Am J Physiol Regul Integr Comp Physiol 295(6): R2050–R20R8

Hannibal J, Hsiung HM, Fahrenkrug J (2011) Temporal phasing of locomotor activity, heart rate rhythmicity, and core body temperature is disrupted in VIP receptor 2-deficient mice. Am J Physiol Regul Integr Comp Physiol 300(3):R519–R530. https://doi.org/10.1152/ajpregu.00599. 2010

Hannibal J, Kankipati L, Strang CE, Peterson BB, Dacey D, Gamlin PD (2014) Central projections of intrinsically photosensitive retinal ganglion cells in the macaque monkey. J Comp Neurol 522 (10):2231–2248

Hannibal J, Christiansen AT, Heegaard S, Fahrenkrug J, Kiilgaard JF (2017) Melanopsin expressing human retinal ganglion cells: subtypes, distribution, and intraretinal connectivity. J Comp Neurol 525(8):1934–1961. https://doi.org/10.1002/cne.24181

Hansen J (2001) Light at night, shiftwork, and breast cancer risk. J Natl Cancer Inst 93 (20):1513–1515

Hatori M, Le H, Vollmers C, Keding SR, Tanaka N, Schmedt C et al (2008) Inducible ablation of melanopsin-expressing retinal ganglion cells reveals their central role in non-image forming visual responses. PLoS One 3(6):e2451

Hattar S, Liao HW, Takao M, Berson DM, Yau KW (2002) Melanopsin-containing retinal ganglion cells: architecture, projections, and intrinsic photosensitivity. Science 295(5557):1065–1070

Hattar S, Lucas RJ, Mrosovsky N, Thompson S, Douglas RH, Hankins MW et al (2003) Melanopsin and rod-cone photoreceptive systems account for all major accessory visual functions in mice. Nature 424(6944):76–81

Hattar S, Kumar M, Park A, Tong P, Tung J, Yau KW et al (2006) Central projections of melanopsin-expressing retinal ganglion cells in the mouse. J Comp Neurol 497(3):326–349

Hazlerigg D, Loudon A (2008) New insights into ancient seasonal life timers. Curr Biol 18(17): R795–R804. https://doi.org/10.1016/j.cub.2008.07.040

Hughes S, Watson TS, Foster RG, Peirson SN, Hankins MW (2013) Nonuniform distribution and spectral tuning of photosensitive retinal ganglion cells of the mouse retina. Curr Biol 23 (17):1696–1701

Hughes S, Jagannath A, Hankins MW, Foster RG, Peirson SN (2015) Photic regulation of clock systems. Methods Enzymol 552:125–143. https://doi.org/10.1016/bs.mie.2014.10.018

Husse J, Leliavski A, Tsang AH, Oster H, Eichele G (2014) The light-dark cycle controls peripheral rhythmicity in mice with a genetically ablated suprachiasmatic nucleus clock. FASEB J 28 (11):4950–4960. https://doi.org/10.1096/fj.14-256594

Hut RA (2011) Photoperiodism: shall EYA compare thee to a summer's day? Curr Biol 21(1):R22–R25. https://doi.org/10.1016/j.cub.2010.11.060

Kalsbeek A, Buijs RM (2002) Output pathways of the mammalian suprachiasmatic nucleus: coding circadian time by transmitter selection and specific targeting. Cell Tissue Res 309(1):109–118. https://doi.org/10.1007/s00441-002-0577-0

Kalsbeek A, Palm IF, La Fleur SE, Scheer FA, Perreau-Lenz S, Ruiter M et al (2006) SCN outputs and the hypothalamic balance of life. J Biol Rhythms 21(6):458–469. https://doi.org/10.1177/0748730406293854

Keenan WT, Rupp AC, Ross RA, Somasundaram P, Hiriyanna S, Wu Z et al (2016) A visual circuit uses complementary mechanisms to support transient and sustained pupil constriction. Elife 5: e15392

Kennett JE, Poletini MO, Freeman ME (2008) Vasoactive intestinal polypeptide modulates the estradiol-induced prolactin surge by entraining oxytocin neuronal activity. Brain Res 1196:65–73

Kiessling S, Sollars PJ, Pickard GE (2014) Light stimulates the mouse adrenal through a retinohypothalamic pathway independent of an effect on the clock in the suprachiasmatic nucleus. PLoS One 9(3):e92959

Klein DC, Moore RY, Reppert SM (1991) Suprachiasmatic nucleus. The mind's clock. Oxford University Press, New York

Klerman EB, Shanahan TL, Brotman DJ, Rimmer DW, Emens JS, Rizzo JF III et al (2002) Photic resetting of the human circadian pacemaker in the absence of conscious vision. J Biol Rhythms 17(6):548–555

Kloog I, Stevens RG, Haim A, Portnov BA (2010) Nighttime light level co distributes with breast cancer incidence worldwide. Cancer Causes Control 21(12):2059–2068. https://doi.org/10.1007/s10552-010-9624-4

Larsen PJ, Enquist LW, Card JP (1998) Characterization of the multisynaptic neuronal control of the rat pineal gland using viral transneuronal tracing. Eur J Neurosci 10(1):128–145

Liao HW, Ren X, Peterson BB, Marshak DW, Yau KW, Gamlin PD et al (2016) Melanopsin-expressing ganglion cells in macaque and human retinas form two morphologically distinct populations. J Comp Neurol 524(14):2845–2872. https://doi.org/10.1002/cne.23995

Lincoln GA, Clarke IJ, Hut RA, Hazlerigg DG (2006) Characterizing a mammalian circannual pacemaker. Science 314(5807):1941–1944. https://doi.org/10.1126/science.1132009

Lucas RJ, Peirson SN, Berson DM, Brown TM, Cooper HM, Czeisler CA et al (2014) Measuring and using light in the melanopsin age. Trends Neurosci 37(1):1–9

Mohawk JA, Takahashi JS (2011) Cell autonomy and synchrony of suprachiasmatic nucleus circadian oscillators. Trends Neurosci 34(7):349–358

Moore RY (1995) Organization of the mammalian circadian system. Ciba Found Symp 183:88 99

Moore RY, Lenn NJ (1972) A retinohypothalamic projection in the rat. J Comp Neurol 146:1–14

Moore RY, Speh JC, Card JP (1995) The retinohypothalamic tract originates from a distinct subset of retinal ganglion cells. J Comp Neurol 352:351–366

Morin LP, Allen CN (2005) The circadian visual system, 2005. Brain Res Rev 51(1):1–60

Mrosovsky N (1999) Masking: history, definitions, and measurement. Chronobiol Int 16 (4):415–429

Navara KJ, Nelson RJ (2007) The dark side of light at night: physiological, epidemiological, and ecological consequences. J Pineal Res 43(3):215–224. https://doi.org/10.1111/j.1600-079X.2007.00473.x

Nelson RJ, Zucker I (1981) Absence of extraocular photoreception in diurnal and nocturnal rodents exposed to direct sunlight. Comp Biochem Physiol 69A:145–148

Ouyang JQ, Davies S, Dominoni D (2018) Hormonally mediated effects of artificial light at night on behavior and fitness: linking endocrine mechanisms with function. J Exp Biol 221(Pt 6): jeb156893

Panda S, Provencio I, Tu DC, Pires SS, Rollag MD, Castrucci AM et al (2003) Melanopsin is required for non-image-forming photic responses in blind mice. Science 301(5632):525–527

Pevet P, Challet E (2011) Melatonin: both master clock output and internal time-giver in the circadian clocks network. J Physiol Paris 105(4–6):170–182. https://doi.org/10.1016/j.jphysparis.2011.07.001

Pickard GE (1985) Bifurcating axons of retinal ganglion cells terminate in the hypothalamic suprachiasmatic nucleus and the intergeniculate leaflet of the thalamus. Neurosci Lett 55:211–217

Provencio I, Jiang G, De Grip WJ, Hayes WP, Rollag MD (1998) Melanopsin: an opsin in melanophores, brain, and eye. Proc Natl Acad Sci U S A 95(1):340–345

Provencio I, Rodriguez IR, Jiang G, Hayes WP, Moreira EF, Rollag MD (2000) A novel human opsin in the inner retina. J Neurosci 20(0270-6474):600–605

Redlin U, Mrosovsky N (1999) Masking by light in hamsters with SCN lesions. J Comp Physiol A 184(4):439–448

Reiter RJ, Tan DX, Galano A (2014) Melatonin: exceeding expectations. Physiology (Bethesda) 29 (5):325–333. https://doi.org/10.1152/physiol.00011.2014

Roenneberg T, Foster RG (1997) Twilight times: light and the circadian system. Photochem Photobiol 66(5):549–561

Saper CB, Cano G, Scammell TE (2005a) Homeostatic, circadian, and emotional regulation of sleep. J Comp Neurol 493(1):92–98

Saper CB, Scammell TE, Lu J (2005b) Hypothalamic regulation of sleep and circadian rhythms. Nature 437(7063):1257–1263

Schmidt TM, Kofuji P (2009) Functional and morphological differences among intrinsically photosensitive retinal ganglion cells. J Neurosci 29(2):476–482

Shivers BD, Gorcs TJ, Gottschall PE, Arimura A (1991) Two high affinity binding sites for pituitary adenylate cyclase- activating polypeptide have different tissue distributions. Endocrinology 128:3055–3065

Van Dycke KC, Rodenburg W, van Oostrom CT, van Kerkhof LW, Pennings JL, Roenneberg T et al (2015) Chronically alternating light cycles increase breast cancer risk in mice. Curr Biol 25 (14):1932–1937. https://doi.org/10.1016/j.cub.2015.06.012

Vosko AM, Schroeder A, Loh DH, Colwell CS (2007) Vasoactive intestinal peptide and the mammalian circadian system. Gen Comp Endocrinol 152(2–3):165–175

Recommended Further Reading

Do MT, Yau KW (2010) Intrinsically photosensitive retinal ganglion cells. Physiol Rev 90 (4):1547–1581. A small population of retinal ganglion cells in the mammalian eye that express a unique visual pigment called melanopsin. This review describes the anatomy and physiology of this remarkable system.

Golombek DA, Rosenstein RE (2010) Physiology of circadian entrainment. Physiol Rev 90 (3):1063–1102. This paper reviews the anatomy and physiology of the circadian timing system in mammals.

Kalsbeek A, Palm IF, La Fleur SE, Scheer FA, Perreau-Lenz S, Ruiter M et al (2006) SCN outputs and the hypothalamic balance of life. J Biol Rhythms 21(6):458–469. This review considers the anatomical connections and neurotransmitters used by the SCN to control the daily rhythms in hormone release.

Seasons, Clocks and Mood

9

Timo Partonen

Abstract

Tendency to experience the seasonal changes in mood and behaviour is manifested to a different degree in individuals, ranging from the patients with mood disorder through milder forms to the normal. In addition, clinical data have demonstrated abnormalities in the circadian rhythms in patients with mood disorders. Inside a cell, the key molecular events and mechanisms controlling the circadian rhythms have been elucidated. Thus, circadian clock gene variants are a fruitful target for elucidation of the pathogenesis of mood disorders. In humans, there are about 20 key genes of the circadian transcription-to-translation feedback loops which generate and maintain the circadian rhythms. The findings which have gained support thus far indicate that genetic variants of certain, but not all, circadian clock genes contribute to the pathogenesis of depressive episodes emerging from seasonal affective disorder, major depressive disorder or bipolar disorder. The circadian genes encoding proteins for repression of transcription, as "the breaks" of the circadian transcription-to-translation feedback loops, are essential to the functions of circadian clocks. Here, the cryptochrome circadian regulator proteins CRY1 and CRY2 are keys, as they are strategically positioned to modulate not only circadian rhythms of a cell, but also to influence emotional reactions and mood of the individual.

Keywords

Circadian clock · Genetic variant · Seasonal affective disorder

T. Partonen (✉)
Department of Public Health Solutions, National Institute for Health and Welfare (THL), Helsinki, Finland
e-mail: timo.partonen@thl.fi

F. J. P. Ebling, H. D. Piggins (eds.), *Neuroendocrine Clocks and Calendars*, Masterclass in Neuroendocrinology 10, https://doi.org/10.1007/978-3-030-55643-3_9

9.1   Introduction

In the beginning of life, 3.5 to 3.9 billion years ago, the length of day was about 14 h and ultraviolet radiation was not filtered by Earth's atmosphere. Thus, the intrinsic clock of an organism (Schmelling et al. 2017) met the night–day transitions with the approximate period of 14 h, and was primarily involved in protection from ultraviolet radiation. During evolution, two cryptochrome genes, i.e., the *Cryptochrome circadian regulator 1* (*Cry1*) and *Cryptochrome circadian regulator 2* (*Cry2*) which encode the proteins CRY1 and CRY2, evolved from the family of DNA photolyase proteins (Heijde et al. 2010), and potentially played a role in control of the light-induced effects. Thereafter, the period for the night–day transitions has lengthened, so the intrinsic clock has evolved a slowing-down mechanism (Abe et al. 2015) and adopted periods of longer than 14 h up to the current one of about 24 h as the reference.

Exposures to environmental light and ambient temperature following the terrestrial 24-h cycle together synchronize the phase of the intrinsic clock (Boothroyd et al. 2007). To keep precise timing, the principal circadian clock must generate temperature-compensated signals throughout the organism. Evolution of the mechanisms for anticipation of the effects of day-to-day and season-to-season changes in ambient temperature has been seen as beneficial to a population as well as to the individual, and to favour adaptation to the habitat (François et al. 2012).

Physiological functions and behaviours demonstrate routine daily as well as seasonal fluctuations that are intrinsically generated and maintained by a network of intrinsic clocks in multicellular species (Meijer et al. 2007). These clocks are known as circadian clocks. In addition, there are still intrinsic rhythms with periods of shorter than 24 h. These rhythms are generated by intrinsic clocks known as ultradian oscillators and integrated into the circadian and seasonal rhythms (Kleitman 1949).

9.1.1   Intrinsic Clocks

Circadian clocks are endogenous pacemakers that evolve their properties, when subjected to selection, but have been conserved during evolution (Rosbash 2009). Inside a cell, the key molecular events and mechanisms of these clocks have been elucidated (Ibáñez 2017), and see Chap. 11. However, it is not yet known how the coupling of ultradian oscillators to produce the circadian rhythm at the organism level is achieved (Dowse et al. 1987).

In humans, there are about 20 key genes of the circadian transcription-to-translation feedback loops (Zhang et al. 2009). In addition, there are about 140 key genes cycling with a 12-h period at the mRNA as well as the protein levels, which are functionally distinct from the circadian genes (Zhu et al. 2017), and about 60 key genes cycling with an 8-h period (Hughes et al. 2009). A recent estimate is that of all the genes, for example in the liver, 35% are 8-h ultradian genes, 28% are 24-h circadian genes and 20% are 12-h ultradian genes (Zhu et al. 2017). It is of note that

Cry2 belongs to each of the aforementioned groups of genes, the *Circadian-associated repressor of transcription* (*Ciart*) to those with 8-h and 12-h cycles, and *Cry1* to that with 24-h cycles (Zhu et al. 2017).

The relative abundance and robustness of rhythms in transcription tend to vary from tissue to tissue. In olive baboons that are day-active primate relatives of humans, at the organism level, transcription is organized into major bursts during early morning, such as that of CRY2, and late afternoon (Mure et al. 2018). Only 700 rhythmic gene transcripts, such as those of CRY1, reach their peak during early evening. Across tissues, the most frequent cycling clock component is CIART (Mure et al. 2018).

Genes encoding proteins for repression of transcription, as "the breaks" of a system, are essential to the functions of circadian clocks (Dardente et al. 2007). CRY1 and CRY2 (Hsu et al. 1996) are the key repressors which act in the core of the circadian clocks (Griffin Jr et al. 1999; Kume et al. 1999; Miyamoto and Sancar 1999; van der Horst et al. 1999). Similar to CRY1, CIART is a repressor in the feedback loop that involves transcriptional activators of the circadian clock genes (Annayev et al. 2014). CRY1 and CRY2 are sensitive to signals of a wide range of the electromagnetic spectrum, as they react not only to ultraviolet radiation but also to light exposure (Partch et al. 2005; Foley et al. 2011), which fluctuate in their activity across seasons.

CRY1 is needed for a slowing-down mechanism and as a strong repressor in the evening for a robust signal of morning phase (Ukai-Tadenuma et al. 2011). However, CRY2 plays a leading role, as it not only acts as a repressor in general, but also balances and opposes the actions of CRY1. CRY2 inhibits CRY1 from accessing to its DNA targets too early, and it is facilitated by the proteins (PER1 and PER2) encoded by the *Period circadian regulator 1* gene and the *Period circadian regulator 2* gene (Anand et al. 2013). On the other hand, due to its stronger physical interaction with the complex of ARNTL, being encoded by the *Aryl hydrocarbon receptor nuclear translocator like* gene, and CLOCK, being encoded by the *Clock circadian regulator* gene, on DNA, CRY1 is capable of forming a stable complex without PER1 or PER2. It is only CRY2 which can inhibit the activated forms of ARNTL, while CRY1 and PER proteins have no effect (Dardente et al. 2007).

9.2 Seasons and Mood

Changes in mood are part of a broader range of changes in behaviour, welfare and health that follows the change of seasons. This concept, or seasonality, refers to season-to-season changes in sleep duration, social activity, mood, appetite, weight or energy level that are common in a population (Grimaldi et al. 2009). The seasonal course is usually characterized by recurrent emergence which coincides with the reduced hours of daylight during the winter season and disappearance in summer. Tendency to experience these seasonal changes is manifested to a different degree in individuals, ranging from the patients with seasonal affective disorder (SAD) through milder or subsyndromal forms of SAD to the normal.

SAD was originally defined as a syndrome in which depression occurred during the autumn or winter and remitted the following spring or summer for at least two successive years. In addition, the SAD patient had to show a history of major depressive or bipolar disorder. Since then, two subtypes of SAD have been described in the literature: winter SAD and summer SAD, of which the former is far more frequent (Partonen and Lönnqvist 1998). Approximately 10% of recurrent depressive episodes follow the seasonal pattern, yielding the prevalence rates of 0.4% for major to 1.0% for minor depressive disorder with a seasonal pattern (Blazer et al. 1998).

9.3   Seasons and Clocks

The intrinsic clocks align their pace with the seasons on the globe. As the levels of PER2 in the correct phase is far more critical than PER2 levels as such for synchronization of the circadian clocks (Chen et al. 2009), the dimerization of PER2 with CRY1, CRY2 or CIART might play a major role in alignment of physiology of the individual with seasons.

In sheep, CRY1 and CRY2 proteins in the pars tuberalis of the pituitary gland give a signal of dusk, whereas PER1 and PER2 proteins give a signal of dawn (Lincoln et al. 2002). They create an interval of time between the peaks of transcription of the *Period circadian regulator* genes and those of the *Cryptochrome circadian regulator* genes, and thus with the dimers also a mechanism to track the timing of dawn and dusk over the year. When the pineal gland is activated by the sympathetic nervous system, melatonin is excreted in large quantities into the circulation only at night and induces the transcription of *Cry1* (Hazlerigg et al. 2004). This cascade of events influences the timing of the peaks in transcription and the control of a summer or winter physiology of the individual.

Currently, it is not known whether the dynamics between PER and CRY proteins holds for humans. Data from baboons suggest that it does not (Mure et al. 2018). PER1, PER2, CRY1 and CRY2 are cycling and generating peaks of transcription in only 10 of the 64 tissues, none in the brain. These data support another hypothesis as follows. Although CRY2 is not cycling robustly in the suprachiasmatic nucleus, its maximum levels occur precisely at the lights-on, while those of PER1 and PER2 occur 2 to 3 h later and those of CRY1 about 8 h later (Mure et al. 2018). So, CRY2, PER1 and PER2 track the timing of dawn, and CRY1 tracks dusk. A tissue where tracking of the night–day transitions might begin is the retinal pigment epithelium. There, the peak of transcription occurs at 4 h before the lights-on for CRY2, but after the lights-on by 53 min, 1 h 37 min and 11 h for PER1, PER2 and CRY1, respectively. These phases of transcription might tag the intervals of time along the seasons.

In baboons, first-hand information on the photoperiod might not be processed in the pituitary gland nor mediated by melatonin as extensively studied in sheep, but directly in the retina. Cryptochromes within the cytoplasm may play a photoreceptive role in the retina separate from but coupled with their nuclear role in the transcription-translation feedback loop of the circadian clock (Nießner et al. 2016). Dysfunction of cryptochromes in the retina compromises the spontaneous firing rates in the optic nerve fibres and their response to light exposure, and this disturbance affects the retinorecipient neurons of the suprachiasmatic nucleus (Nakamura et al. 2011). Patients with SAD display retinal abnormalities at the level of the photoreceptors or retinal pigment epithelium and are therefore less sensitive to light exposure (Lam et al. 1991). Such abnormalities might enhance ultradian rhythm activity (Glod et al. 1997) and cause a reset error of circadian rest-activity cycles (Teicher et al. 1997).

In a longitudinal analysis over 11 years, *Cry2* rs61884508 G allele had a protective effect against the worsening of problems with seasonal changes in mood and behaviour (Kovanen et al. 2016). Whether it tracks the timing of dawn, it is currently not known. In addition, *Npas2* (*Neuronal PAS domain protein 2*) rs2305160 A allele carriers have lower levels of global seasonality, i.e., their scores on the seasonal variations in sleep length, social activity, mood, weight, appetite and energy level, and *Npas2* rs6725296 A allele carriers have greater changes in weight and appetite in particular (Kovanen et al. 2010). These findings extend the role of NPAS2 in seasonality from the clinical SAD (Johansson et al. 2003) to a population at large.

An additional tag might be provided by transcription of the *Period circadian regulator 3* (*Per3*) gene that, in baboons, tracks dawn with its peak of transcription at 2 h 10 min before the lights-on (Mure et al. 2018). In humans, two rare mutations in *Per3* reduce the ability of PER3 to stabilize PER2 (Zhang et al. 2016). It might change the alignment of PER2 with CRY2 at dawn and with CRY1 for dusk. Mutation carriers tend to have greater seasonal changes in mood and behaviour as well as more severe depressive symptoms (Zhang et al. 2016).

The change of seasons challenges the functions of the circadian clocks. Especially, the change of winter to spring, when the lengthening days are already warm but nights are still cold, sends a conflicting signal for timing to the intrinsic clocks, and is a stressful period to the organism. Brown adipose tissue is a unique characteristic of mammals that generates heat by uncoupling mitochondrial respiration from adenosine triphosphate production independently of shivering and locomotor activity, and when activated by the sympathetic nervous system it warms up the mammalian body (Enerbäck 2010). In adult humans, the activity of brown adipose tissue not only fluctuates with changes in the photoperiod and ambient temperature across seasons (Bahler et al. 2016), but also follows a circadian rhythm with its greatest thermogenic effect occurring at night (Lee et al. 2016). Thus, it is capable of acting as a pacemaker of the organism, if the view of body temperature as a universal time cue holds (Buhr et al. 2010). Indeed, at least in rats, the activity of brown adipose tissue seems to guide the circadian rhythm of core body temperature that is the anchorage for other circadian rhythms (Yang et al. 2011).

There are two neural feedback circuits involving brown adipose tissue. First, the efferent sympathetic brain-to-brown-adipose-tissue and the afferent sensory brown-adipose-tissue-to-brain pathways are in control of the activity of brown adipose tissue (Ryu et al. 2015). Second, the spinoparabrachial pathway, which senses warm cutaneous temperatures, projects to the dorsal raphe nucleus and a pathway from there back to the skin are involved as well (Hale et al. 2013). CRY1 and CRY2 take part in regulation of energy balance to which they couple the activity of brown adipose tissue (López et al. 2010).

When the cues from the daily changes in exposures to light and temperature conflict with one another, dysfunction of CRY2, CRY1 or CIART is likely to compromise the synchronization of peripheral clocks to the photoperiod, for example in the skin, leaving it exposed to ambient temperatures, as demonstrated in a model organism of biology (Harper et al. 2017). Such dysfunction in the skin or brown adipose tissue may let cold ambient temperatures and the subsequent deactivation of serotonergic neurotransmission and activation of brown adipose tissue affect the brain more easily. If so, the shortage of serotonergic in contrast to overwhelming signalling from brown adipose tissue to the brain might disturb the slowing-down mechanism of the circadian clocks. This disturbance might induce desynchronization of the circadian rhythms, their misalignment and seasonal mismatch (Partonen 2012), and cause changes in mood and behaviour, and a contribution to the pathogenesis of mood disorders.

9.4   Clocks and Mood

Clinical data have demonstrated abnormalities in the circadian rhythms in patients with mood disorders. Thus, circadian clock gene variants are a fruitful target for elucidation of the pathogenesis. The findings which have gained support thus far indicate that genetic variants of *Rora* (*RAR related orphan receptor A*) (rs2028122) and *Cry1* (rs2287161) are associated with depressive disorder, *Rorb* (*RAR related orphan receptor B*) (rs7022435, rs3750420, rs1157358, rs3903529) and *Nr1d1* (*Nuclear receptor subfamily 1 group D member 1*) (rs2314339) with bipolar disorder, and *Npas2* (rs11541353, rs6738097) and *Cry2* (rs10838524, rs1554338) with SAD.

Cry2 rs10838524 G allele, rs7121611 A allele, rs7945565 G allele, rs1401419 G allele and rs3824872 G allele are associated with dysthymia, which was supported by haplotype analysis, whereas *Cry2* rs7123390 G allele and rs2292910 C allele are associated with major depressive disorder (Kovanen et al. 2013; Kovanen et al. 2017). Of these, rs10838524 allele G and rs7123390 allele G in a Finnish sample, and rs10838524 allele A, rs10838527 allele G and rs3824872 allele A in a Swedish sample were associated with SAD (Lavebratt et al. 2010b), rs10838524 A allele with greater chronicity of depressive symptoms (Fiedorowicz et al. 2012), and rs10838524 G allele as well as the haplotype GG of rs10838524 and rs7123390 with depressed female patients with early morning awakening (Utge et al. 2010). To balance this view, there are also reports of no association of rs10838524 with major depressive disorder nor rs7121611 or rs2292910 with major depressive disorder or bipolar disorder. The first genome-wide association study of SAD found no susceptibility loci at a genome-wide significant level, and its strongest association was at *Zbtb20* (*Zinc finger and BTB domain containing 20*) rs139459337 (Ho et al. 2018).

This gene encodes a repressor of transcription, and the expression quantitative trait loci analysis shows that the risk allele T is linked to reduced mRNA expression in human temporal cortex.

The mechanism by which *Cry2* rs10838524 might be linked to SAD was modelled using mathematical simulation to yield the observed phenotype as measured in *Per2* mRNA (Liberman et al. 2018). It demonstrated a decrease in winter amplitude by at least 30% from summer amplitude, indicative of SAD, while the amplitude in the summer condition remained within 15% of the wild type. On the other hand, *Cry1* rs2287161 (Soria et al. 2010) may increase transcription, while *Per2* rs10462023 (Lavebratt et al. 2010a) may increase nuclear export of mRNA, and both these variants as representative of major depressive disorder eventually cause a decrease in amplitude by at least 30% from the wild type (Liberman et al. 2018).

In the first study with a set of key circadian clock gene variants (Johansson et al. 2003), *Npas2* rs11541353 was discovered to associate with SAD. The focus was enlarged on *Npas2*, *Arntl* and *Per2*, since a genetic risk profile for SAD was identified, with carriers of the risk genotype combination having the odds ratio of 4.43 of SAD as compared with the remaining, and that of 10.67 as compared with the most protective genotype combination (Partonen et al. 2007). Here, *Per2* rs56013859 G allele is the rare risk allele and increases the transcription of *Per2*. Depressive-like behaviour is linked to the increased transcription of *Per2* in the mesolimbic dopaminergic cells, which intensifies the activity of the enzyme monoamine oxidase A and reduces the availability of dopamine for neurotransmission (Hampp et al. 2008).

Beyond, the *Caveolae-associated protein 3* (*Cavin3*) regulates the PER-to-CRY protein abundance and interactions (Schneider et al. 2012), and thus this may influence the intervals of time for transcription tracking the dawn and dusk. The *Cavin3* loss-of-function shortens the circadian period, similar to knockout animal models of each key circadian clock gene except that of *Cry2* (Ko and Takahashi 2006). *Cry2* knockout mice have a prolonged circadian period, and it resembles the gain-of-function for *Cavin3* which lengthens the circadian period. *Cavin3* rs1488864 A allele is associated with major depressive disorder, which was supported by haplotype analysis (Kovanen et al. 2017).

9.5 Conclusion

Elucidation of the effects of seasons and intrinsic clocks on mood has yielded the first insight into the targets of interest. CRY1 and CRY2 are keys, as they are strategically positioned to modulate not only circadian rhythms of a cell, but also to influence emotional reactions and mood of the individual. Currently, there is evidence to conclude that *Cry2* may be "a mood gene", as its genetic variants are associated with a range of depressive states in particular, and deserves further study.

References

Abe J, Hiyama TB, Mukaiyama A, Son S, Mori T, Saito S, Osako M, Wolanin J, Yamashita E, Kondo T, Akiyama S (2015) Atomic-scale origins of slowness in the cyanobacterial circadian clock. Science 349:312–316

Anand SN, Maywood ES, Chesham JE, Joynson G, Banks GT, Hastings MH, Nolan PM (2013) Distinct and separable roles for endogenous CRY1 and CRY2 within the circadian molecular clockwork of the suprachiasmatic nucleus, as revealed by the Fbxl3^{Afh} mutation. J Neurosci 33:7145–7153

Annayev Y, Adar S, Chiou YY, Lieb JD, Sancar A, Ye R (2014) Gene model 129 (*Gm129*) encodes a novel transcriptional repressor that modulates circadian gene expression. J Biol Chem 289:5013–5024

Bahler L, Deelen JW, Hoekstra JB, Holleman F, Verberne HJ (2016) Seasonal influence on stimulated BAT activity in prospective trials: a retrospective analysis of BAT visualized on ^{18}F-FDG PET-CTs and ^{123}I-*m*IBG SPECT-CTs. J Appl Physiol 120:1418–1423

Blazer DG, Kessler RC, Swartz MS (1998) Epidemiology of recurrent major and minor depression with a seasonal pattern: the National Comorbidity Survey. Br J Psychiatry 172:164–167

Boothroyd CE, Wijnen H, Naef F, Saez L, Young MW (2007) Integration of light and temperature in the regulation of circadian gene expression in *Drosophila*. PLoS Genet 3:e54

Buhr ED, Yoo SH, Takahashi JS (2010) Temperature as a universal resetting cue for mammalian circadian oscillators. Science 330:379–385

Chen R, Schirmer A, Lee Y, Lee H, Kumar V, Yoo SH, Takahashi JS, Lee C (2009) Rhythmic PER abundance defines a critical nodal point for negative feedback within the circadian clock mechanism. Mol Cell 36:417–430

Dardente H, Fortier EE, Martineau V, Cermakian N (2007) Cryptochromes impair phosphorylation of transcriptional activators in the clock: a general mechanism for circadian repression. Biochem J 402:525–536

Dowse HB, Hall JC, Ringo JM (1987) Circadian and ultradian rhythms in *period* mutants of *Drosophila melanogaster*. Behav Genet 17:19–35

Enerbäck S (2010) Human brown adipose tissue. Cell Metab 11:248–252

Fiedorowicz JG, Coryell WH, Akhter A, Ellingrod VL (2012) Chryptochrome 2 variants, chronicity, and seasonality of mood disorders. Psychiatr Genet 22:305–306

Foley LE, Gegear RJ, Reppert SM (2011) Human cryptochrome exhibits light dependent magnetosensitivity. Nat Commun 2:356

François P, Despierre N, Siggia ED (2012) Adaptive temperature compensation in circadian oscillations. PLoS Comput Biol 8:e1002585

Glod CA, Teicher MH, Polcari A, McGreenery CE, Ito Y (1997) Circadian rest-activity disturbances in children with seasonal affective disorder. J Am Acad Child Adolesc Psychiatry 36:188–195

Griffin EA Jr, Staknis D, Weitz CJ (1999) Light-independent role of CRY1 and CRY2 in the mammalian circadian clock. Science 286:768–771

Grimaldi S, Partonen T, Haukka J, Aromaa A, Lönnqvist J (2009) Seasonal vegetative and affective symptoms in the Finnish general population: testing the dual vulnerability and latitude effect hypotheses. Nord J Psychiatry 63:397–404

Hale MW, Raison CL, Lowry CA (2013) Integrative physiology of depression and antidepressant drug action: implications for serotonergic mechanisms of action and novel therapeutic strategies for treatment of depression. Pharmacol Ther 137:108–118

Hampp G, Ripperger JA, Houben T, Schmutz I, Blex C, Perreau-Lenz S, Brunk I, Spanagel R, Ahnert-Hilger G, Meijer JH, Albrecht U (2008) Regulation of monoamine oxidase a by circadian-clock components implies clock influence on mood. Curr Biol 18:678–683

Harper REF, Ogueta M, Dayan P, Stanewsky R, Albert JT (2017) Light dominates peripheral circadian oscillations in *Drosophila melanogaster* during sensory conflict. J Biol Rhythm 32:423–432

Hazlerigg DG, Andersson H, Johnston JD, Lincoln G (2004) Molecular characterization of the long-day response in the Soay sheep, a seasonal mammal. Curr Biol 14:334–339

Heijde M, Zabulon G, Corellou F, Ishikawa T, Brazard J, Usman A, Sanchez F, Plaza P, Martin M, Falciatore A, Todo T, Bouget FY, Bowler C (2010) Characterization of two members of the cryptochrome/photolyase family from *Ostreococcus tauri* provides insights into the origin and evolution of cryptochromes. Plant Cell Environ 33:1614–1626

Ho KWD, Han S, Nielsen JV, Jancic D, Hing B, Fiedorowicz J, Weissman MM, Levinson DF, Potash JB (2018) Genome-wide association study of seasonal affective disorder. Transl Psychiatry 8:190

Hsu DS, Zhao X, Zhao S, Kazantsev A, Wang RP, Todo T, Wei YF, Sancar A (1996) Putative human blue-light photoreceptors hCRY1 and hCRY2 are flavoproteins. Biochemistry 35:13871–13877

Hughes ME, DiTacchio L, Hayes KR, Vollmers C, Pulivarthy S, Baggs JE, Panda S, Hogenesch JB (2009) Harmonics of circadian gene transcription in mammals. PLoS Genet 5:e1000442

Ibáñez C (2017). Scientific background discoveries of molecular mechanisms controlling the circadian rhythm retention. www.nobelprize.org/nobel_prizes/medicine/laureates/2017/advanced-medicineprize2017.pdf (accessed 3 October 2017)

Johansson C, Willeit M, Smedh C, Ekholm J, Paunio T, Kieseppä T, Lichtermann D, Praschak-Rieder N, Neumeister A, Nilsson LG, Kasper S, Peltonen L, Adolfsson R, Schalling M, Partonen T (2003) Circadian clock-related polymorphisms in seasonal affective disorder and their relevance to diurnal preference. Neuropsychopharmacology 28:734–739

Kleitman N (1949) Biological rhythms and cycles. Physiol Rev 29:1–30

Ko CH, Takahashi JS (2006) Molecular components of the mammalian circadian clock. Hum Mol Genet 15:R271–R277

Kovanen L, Donner K, Kaunisto M, Partonen T (2016) CRY1 and CRY2 genetic variants in seasonality: a longitudinal and cross-sectional study. Psychiatry Res 242:101–110

Kovanen L, Donner K, Kaunisto M, Partonen T (2017) PRKCDBP (CAVIN3) and CRY2 associate with major depressive disorder. J Affect Disord 207:136–140

Kovanen L, Kaunisto M, Donner K, Saarikoski ST, Partonen T (2013) CRY2 genetic variants associate with dysthymia. PLoS One 8:e71450

Kovanen L, Saarikoski ST, Aromaa A, Lönnqvist J, Partonen T (2010) ARNTL (BMAL1) and NPAS2 gene variants contribute to fertility and seasonality. PLoS One 5:e10007

Kume K, Zylka MJ, Sriram S, Shearman LP, Weaver DR, Jin X, Maywood ES, Hastings MH, Reppert SM (1999) mCRY1 and mCRY2 are essential components of the negative limb of the circadian clock feedback loop. Cell 98:193–205

Lam RW, Beattie CW, Buchanan A, Remick RA, Zis AP (1991) Low electrooculographic ratios in patients with seasonal affective disorder. Am J Psychiatry 148:1526–1529

Lavebratt C, Sjöholm LK, Partonen T, Schalling M, Forsell Y (2010a) PER2 variation is associated with depression vulnerability. Am J Med Genet B Neuropsychiatr Genet 153B:570–581

Lavebratt C, Sjöholm LK, Soronen P, Paunio T, Vawter MP, Bunney WE, Adolfsson R, Forsell Y, Wu JC, Kelsoe JR, Partonen T, Schalling M (2010b) CRY2 is associated with depression. PLoS One 5:e9407

Lee P, Bova R, Schofield L, Bryant W, Dieckmann W, Slattery A, Govendir MA, Emmett L, Greenfield JR (2016) Brown adipose tissue exhibits a glucose-responsive thermogenic biorhythm in humans. Cell Metab 23:602–609

Liberman AR, Halitjaha L, Ay A, Ingram KK (2018) Modeling strengthens molecular link between circadian polymorphisms and major mood disorders. J Biol Rhythm 33:318–336

Lincoln G, Messager S, Andersson H, Hazlerigg D (2002) Temporal expression of seven clock genes in the suprachiasmatic nucleus and the pars tuberalis of the sheep: evidence for an internal coincidence timer. Proc Natl Acad Sci U S A 99:13890–13895

López M, Varela L, Vázquez MJ, Rodríguez-Cuenca S, González CR, Velagapudi VR, Morgan DA, Schoenmakers E, Agassandian K, Lage R, Martínez de Morentin PB, Tovar S,

Nogueiras R, Carling D, Lelliott C, Gallego R, Oresic M, Chatterjee K, Saha AK, Rahmouni K, Diéguez C, Vidal-Puig A (2010) Hypothalamic AMPK and fatty acid metabolism mediate thyroid regulation of energy balance. Nat Med 16:1001–1008

Meijer JH, Michel S, Vansteensel MJ (2007) Processing of daily and seasonal light information in the mammalian circadian clock. Gen Comp Endocrinol 152:159–164

Miyamoto Y, Sancar A (1999) Circadian regulation of cryptochrome genes in the mouse. Brain Res Mol Brain Res 71:238–243

Mure LS, Le HD, Benegiamo G, Chang MW, Rios L, Jillani N, Ngotho M, Kariuki T, Dkhissi-Benyahya O, Cooper HM, Panda S (2018) Diurnal transcriptome atlas of a primate across major neural and peripheral tissues. Science 359:eaao0318

Nakamura TJ, Ebihara S, Shinohara K (2011) Reduced light response of neuronal firing activity in the suprachiasmatic nucleus and optic nerve of cryptochrome-deficient mice. PLoS One 6: e28726

Nießner C, Denzau S, Malkemper EP, Gross JC, Burda H, Winklhofer M, Peichl L (2016) Cryptochrome 1 in retinal cone photoreceptors suggests a novel functional role in mammals. Sci Rep 6:21848

Partch CL, Clarkson MW, Ozgür S, Lee AL, Sancar A (2005) Role of structural plasticity in signal transduction by the cryptochrome blue-light photoreceptor. Biochemistry 44:3795–3805

Partonen T (2012) Hypothesis: cryptochromes and brown fat are essential for adaptation and affect mood and mood-related behaviors. Front Neurol 3:157

Partonen T, Lönnqvist J (1998) Seasonal affective disorder. Lancet 352:1369–1374

Partonen T, Treutlein J, Alpman A, Frank J, Johansson C, Depner M, Aron L, Rietschel M, Wellek S, Soronen P, Paunio T, Koch A, Chen P, Lathrop M, Adolfsson R, Persson ML, Kasper S, Schalling M, Peltonen L, Schumann G (2007) Three circadian clock genes Per2, Arntl, and Npas2 contribute to winter depression. Ann Med 39:229–238

Rosbash M (2009) The implications of multiple circadian clock origins. PLoS Biol 7:e62

Ryu V, Garretson JT, Liu Y, Vaughan CH, Bartness TJ (2015) Brown adipose tissue has sympathetic-sensory feedback circuits. J Neurosci 35:2181–2190

Schmelling NM, Lehmann R, Chaudhury P, Beck C, Albers SV, Axmann IM, Wiegard A (2017) Minimal tool set for a prokaryotic circadian clock. BMC Evol Biol 17:169

Schneider K, Köcher T, Andersin T, Kurzchalia T, Schibler U, Gatfield D (2012) CAVIN-3 regulates circadian period length and PER:CRY protein abundance and interactions. EMBO Rep 13:1138–1144

Soria V, Martínez-Amorós E, Escaramís G, Valero J, Pérez-Egea R, García C, Gutiérrez-Zotes A, Puigdemont D, Bayés M, Crespo JM, Martorell L, Vilella E, Labad A, Vallejo J, Pérez V, Menchón JM, Estivill X, Gratacòs M, Urretavizcaya M (2010) Differential association of circadian genes with mood disorders: CRY1 and NPAS2 are associated with unipolar major depression and CLOCK and VIP with bipolar disorder. Neuropsychopharmacology 35:1279–1289

Teicher MH, Glod CA, Magnus E, Harper D, Benson G, Krueger K, McGreenery CE (1997) Circadian rest-activity disturbances in seasonal affective disorder. Arch Gen Psychiatry 54:124–130

Ukai-Tadenuma M, Yamada RG, Xu H, Ripperger JA, Liu AC, Ueda HR (2011) Delay in feedback repression by cryptochrome 1 is required for circadian clock function. Cell 144:268–281

Utge SJ, Soronen P, Loukola A, Kronholm E, Ollila HM, Pirkola S, Porkka-Heiskanen T, Partonen T, Paunio T (2010) Systematic analysis of circadian genes in a population-based sample reveals association of TIMELESS with depression and sleep disturbance. PLoS One 5: e9259

van der Horst GT, Muijtjens M, Kobayashi K, Takano R, Kanno S, Takao M, de Wit J, Verkerk A, Eker AP, van Leenen D, Buijs R, Bootsma D, Hoeijmakers JH, Yasui A (1999) Mammalian Cry1 and Cry2 are essential for maintenance of circadian rhythms. Nature 398:627–630

Yang YL, Shen ZL, Tang Y, Wang N, Sun B (2011) Simultaneous telemetric analyzing of the temporal relationship for the changes of the circadian rhythms of brown adipose tissue thermogenesis and core temperature in the rat [in Chinese]. Zhongguo Ying Yong Sheng Li Xue Za Zhi 27:348–352

Zhang L, Hirano A, Hsu PK, Jones CR, Sakai N, Okuro M, McMahon T, Yamazaki M, Xu Y, Saigoh N, Saigoh K, Lin ST, Kaasik K, Nishino S, Ptáček LJ, Fu YH (2016) A PERIOD3 variant causes a circadian phenotype and is associated with a seasonal mood trait. Proc Natl Acad Sci U S A 113:E1536–E1544

Zhang EE, Liu AC, Hirota T, Miraglia LJ, Welch G, Pongsawakul PY, Liu X, Atwood A, Huss JW 3rd, Janes J, Su AI, Hogenesch JB, Kay SA (2009) A genome-wide RNAi screen for modifiers of the circadian clock in human cells. Cell 139:199–210

Zhu B, Zhang Q, Pan Y, Mace EM, York B, Antoulas AC, Dacso CC, O'Malley BW (2017) A cell-autonomous mammalian 12 hr clock coordinates metabolic and stress rhythms. Cell Metab 25:1305–1319

Further Recommended Reading

Hühne A, Welsh DK, Landgraf D (2018) Prospects for circadian treatment of mood disorders. *Ann Med.* 50:637–654

This review provides a view on specific potential mechanisms by which disrupted intrinsic clocks may contribute to the development of mood disorders.

Ketchesin KD, Becker-Krail D, McClung CA (2020) Mood-related central and peripheral clocks. *Eur J Neurosci.* 51:326–345

This review delivers a summary of studies in animal models attempting to elucidate the molecular and cellular mechanisms in which circadian genes regulate mood.

McCarthy MJ (2019) Missing a beat: assessment of circadian rhythm abnormalities in bipolar disorder in the genomic era. *Psychiatr Genet.* 29:29–36

This review summarizes the findings from genome-wide association studies of bipolar disorder and elucidates a potentially novel circadian mechanism which may be partly distinct from those identified in animal models.

Photoperiodic Modulation of Clock Gene Expression in the SCN

10

Alena Sumova and Helena Illnerova

Abstract

In temperate zones, photoperiod changes dramatically over the course of the year, so organisms have evolved mechanisms allowing anticipation of these environmental changes. The information about changes in duration of daylight is conveyed to the organism via neuroendocrine pathways. These pathways involve photoperiodic modulation of rhythmic production of the pineal hormone melatonin which is under control of the circadian system. This chapter will consider the role of the central circadian clock located in the suprachiasmatic nuclei in the adaptation to the photoperiodic changes, focusing on how photoperiod modulates circadian clock mechanisms at the molecular level.

Keywords

Suprachiasmatic nucleus · Photoperiod · Entrainment · Circadian clock

10.1 Introduction

10.1.1 Photoperiodic Modulation of Physiological Functions

Functions of many organisms living in temperate zones are significantly modulated during the year. These modulations are to adopt appropriate strategies for surviving severe conditions in winter and to ensure birth of offspring during optimal conditions in spring and summer.

A. Sumova (✉) · H. Illnerova
Institute of Physiology, Czech Academy of Sciences, Prague, Czechia
e-mail: alena.sumova@fgu.cas.cz; illnerova@kav.cas.cz

© The Editor(s) (if applicable) and The Author(s), under exclusive license to
Springer Nature Switzerland AG 2020
F. J. P. Ebling, H. D. Piggins (eds.), *Neuroendocrine Clocks and Calendars*,
Masterclass in Neuroendocrinology 10, https://doi.org/10.1007/978-3-030-55643-3_10

Organisms need to be prepared for upcoming seasonal changes to start these physiological, morphological, and behavioral adaptations before the seasonal changes actually occur. To do so, they need to be equipped with a mechanism allowing them to anticipate seasonal changes and modulate their biology accordingly, for example to change their gonadal activity, pelage color and quality, body fat composition, and related body weight. In temperate zones, the major factor used for the prediction of seasonal changes is the changing duration of day length (photoperiod) across the year. The photoperiod shortening indicates upcoming winter, and photoperiod lengthening indicates upcoming summer. It has been known for a long time that photoperiod modulates physiological functions via its effect on the pineal gland in mammals. For example, in Djungarian hamsters, removal of the pineal gland (pinealectomy) prevents the normal inhibition of reproductive activity following the transfer of animals from long summer days to short winter days. This and other observations provided compelling evidence that the pineal gland is involved in the transmission of information about photoperiod to the reproductive system and to the organism as a whole, and is thus involved in photoperiodic time measurement (Reiter 1974).

10.1.2 Photoperiodic Regulation of Pineal Function

In 1958, the pineal gland was recognized as an endocrine organ producing the hormone melatonin, whose chemical structure was discovered by Lerner and colleagues (Lerner et al. 1959). The pineal gland produces melatonin rhythmically via signals delivered from a circadian clock in the suprachiasmatic nucleus of the hypothalamus (SCN). Upon these signals, melatonin levels are elevated during the subjective night and almost undetectable during the subjective day. As a result of this regulation from the SCN, melatonin production in the pineal gland remains rhythmic even in the absence of external light/dark cycles, that is, in prolonged constant darkness (Klein and Moore 1979). The duration of melatonin secretion changes according to the duration of the subjective night. In all mammalian animal models studied so far, the duration is shorter on short summer nights whereas it is longer on long winter nights (Illnerová and Vaněček 1980; Arendt et al. 1985; Illnerová and Vaněček 1988). Importantly, with the change in photoperiod, the melatonin production is modulated via independent shifts of its evening rise and morning decline (Illnerová 1988), so the changed phase-relationship between these two parameters determines the duration of high melatonin production. The fact that the evening rise and morning decline in melatonin levels may change independently indicates that the mechanism controlling the melatonin production in the pineal gland is driven by a complex mechanism. The duration of elevated melatonin levels is decoded as a major signal informing the body about seasonal changes in the environment (Carter and Goldman 1983; Carter et al. 2016; Bittman et al. 1983). The code driving the photoperiodic responses is not the absolute value of the melatonin signal duration, but rather change of the duration and the direction of this change (Hoffmann and Illnerova 1986; Illnerová et al. 1986).

In contrast to most mammalian species, humans, at least urbanized subjects, do not seem to respond to short days in winter by extension of the duration of elevated melatonin concentrations (Illnerová et al. 1985). This is likely due to the fact that nowadays humans experience photoperiod longer than 12 h even in winter, when the shortened natural light interval is extended by the artificial light. Nevertheless, human subjects have retained the ability to respond to photoperiodic changes, because in situations when they experience a real natural photoperiod without artificial light, the interval of high nocturnal melatonin is reduced in the summer photoperiod, as compared with the winter photoperiod (Vondrašová et al. 1997).

10.2   Suprachiasmatic Nuclei Are the Central Circadian Clock Directly Entrained by External Light/Dark Cycles

The SCN are a paired structure composed of individual oscillating cells (Welsh et al. 1995; Welsh et al. 2010). These individual SCN cells differ in their morphological parameters, peptidergic phenotypes, and function. Whereas cells located predominantly in the ventrolateral part (core) receive photic information from the retina and express mostly light-dependent rhythmicity, cells located prevalently in the dorsomedial part (shell) do not receive any direct retinal input and are spontaneously rhythmic (van den Pol 1991; Sumová et al. 1998; Schwartz et al. 2000). The neurons in the core send the information about actual light/dark cycle to the cells in the shell to entrain their rhythmicity accordingly. Therefore, communication not only among the individual cells but also between the two cellular subpopulations is important for the integration of the rhythms into the resulting SCN output.

In the absence of environmental cycles, the SCN clock determines intervals of subjective day and subjective night during which various processes change specifically. For example, at the systemic level, the subjective day represents intervals of inactivity and subjective night interval of activity for nocturnal species; for diurnal species the opposite holds true. At the SCN level, irrespective of diurnality or nocturnality, the subjective day is represented by elevated neuronal firing in the shell part of the SCN, whereas the subjective night is clearly defined by an interval of higher neuronal responsiveness to light in its core part. These light-induced responses in the core are controlled by the clock and were first detected as photic induction of immediate early gene expression, for example, c-fos (Kornhauser et al. 1993; Sumová and Illnerová 1998). Expression of c-fos is an indirect marker of neuronal activity because its expression is often increased when neurons fire action potentials. Therefore, its upregulation in a neuron indicates its recent activity.

The circadian clock in the SCN can be reset by light only during the subjective night but not during the subjective day (Pittendrigh and Daan 1976). Photic stimuli reset the SCN clock and its output rhythmicity (e.g., melatonin production) by phase-delaying when they are intruding into the early subjective night, and by phase-advancing when they are present during the late subjective night (Illnerová et al. 1989; Illnerová 1991). In consequence of this basic mechanism, a clock which is advanced so that its subjective night occurs too early relative to the external light/

dark cycle receives a light stimulus in its early subjective night which delays the clock's phase. Conversely, for a delayed clock, light in the morning intrudes into the delayed subjective night and shifts the clock forward. Thus, on the daily basis both complementary mechanisms "repair" the deviation of the clock's phase according to external light/dark cycle and keep it entrained with the 24 h solar day.

10.3 Photoperiodic Modulation of Output Rhythmicity within the SCN

10.3.1 Photoperiod Controls the SCN Output Rhythms at the Systemic Level

The SCN drive output rhythms, that can be recognized at various levels in the organism, include both behavioral (including locomotion, sleep, feeding) and humoral (including melatonin) functions. These output rhythms are modulated by changes in photoperiod. Compared to photoperiodic modulation of behavioral rhythms, the mechanisms underlying modulation of melatonin production have been better described. The SCN controls rhythmic melatonin production via its multisynaptic connection with the pineal gland (Hastings 1991). The mechanism responsible for photic entrainment of the melatonin signal with external environment is dual: light can acutely suppress melatonin production anytime during the day or night. Secondly, under a light/dark cycle, light first entrains the SCN clock and the information is conveyed to the pineal. Therefore, under the changing photoperiods, this latter mechanism requires photoperiodic modulation of the functional state of the central circadian clock at neuronal and molecular levels. Based on this understanding, the SCN has been recognized to serve in the body not only as a daily clock but also as a calendar (Sumová et al. 1995b).

10.3.2 Photoperiod Modulates Specific SCN Regions

Within the SCN, photoperiod modulates mutual phasing among cellular subpopulations located in the photosensitive core region as well as the spontaneously rhythmic shell region. Additionally, it modulates mutual phasing among oscillators in subpopulations located in the rostral and caudal part of the SCN (Fig. 10.1).

10.3.3 Photoperiodic Modulation of the Photic Sensitivity in the SCN Core Region

The effect of photoperiod on the SCN clock was first demonstrated using the clock-controlled interval of photosensitivity of the SCN core region as a marker of duration of subjective night (see above). To test the photoperiodic changes in this interval, the

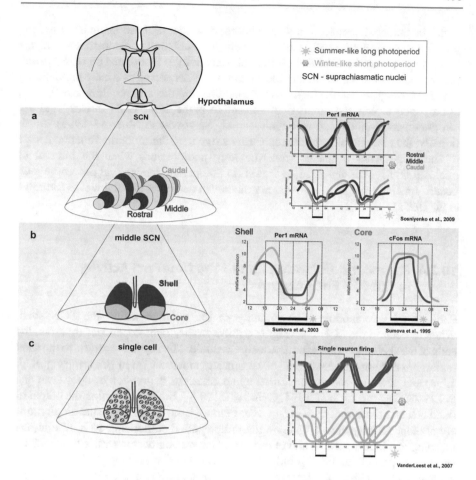

Fig. 10.1 Schematic overview of the effect of photoperiod on the suprachiasmatic nuclei (SCN). Three levels of photoperiodic modification are shown: (**a**) In the nuclei, photoperiod changes mutual phasing among clocks in their rostral, middle, and caudal parts. (**b**) In the middle SCN, photoperiod changes duration on endogenously elevated clock gene Per1 expression in the shell, and interval of light-induced expression of *cFos* in the core. (**c**) Photoperiod changes mutual phasing among clocks in individual SCN cells. The profiles are schematic representation of data from publications referred to in the figure or summarized in the text

response of the immediate early gene *c-fos* within the SCN core region to light pulses delivered at specific times of a day were examined in animals maintained under various photoperiods (Sumová et al. 1995b; Vuillez et al. 1996). The subjective night was determined as the interval between the evening rise and morning decline in the *c-fos* photoinduction. These two markers were affected by light pulses similarly, as was the case with the evening and morning markers of pineal melatonin production (Sumová and Illnerová 1998). Also, similarly to the rhythm in melatonin production, the interval enabling high nocturnal *c-fos* photoinduction is much wider in animals maintained in short photoperiod than in those maintained in long photoperiod (Sumová et al. 1995b). These data not only demonstrated that the mechanism gating the circadian clock photosensitivity is modulated by photoperiod, but they also provided the first evidence that the SCN serves as a calendar defining the daily program of the organism depending on the season. Importantly, the photoperiod affects the duration of subjective night in the SCN directly and not via photoperiod-modulated melatonin signal (Sumová and Illnerová 1996). Additionally, the photoperiodic effect represents a true modulation of the functional state of the SCN. After a change from the long photoperiod, when the interval of photosensitivity is compressed, to the short photoperiod, the interval decompression occurs gradually and its full extension is achieved only after about 2 weeks (Sumová et al. 1995a).

10.3.4 Photoperiodic Modulation of the Neuronal Activity in the SCN Shell Region

Photoperiod also modulates rhythmicity of the neurons within the SCN shell. Whereas cells in the SCN core region exhibit mostly light-dependent rhythms, the cells of the shell region are spontaneously rhythmic. The rhythms specific to the shell region are rhythms in expression of arginine vasopressin (*Avp*) (Cagampang et al. 1994) and in neural activity measured by spontaneous expression of *c-fos* (van den Pol 1991; Cagampang et al. 1994; Guido et al. 1999), both representing the output of the molecular clock mechanism (see 10.4 below). Both of the shell-specific rhythms are photoperiod-dependent. Under a long photoperiod comprising 16 h of light, the morning rise in *Avp* mRNA and cFos protein expression occurs earlier than under a short photoperiod comprising only 8 h of light, but the evening decline does not change, and therefore, the interval of high *Avp* and cFos expression is longer by several hours under a long than under a short photoperiod (Ják et al. 2000; Sumová et al. 2000). Because cFos is not directly inducible by light in the shell region, photoperiodic change of the interval represents the change of state of the circadian clock. Similarly to the photoperiodic modulation of the SCN core, the adjustment of the interval of spontaneous cFos expression to a change from a long to a short photoperiod in the SCN shell also proceeds gradually, and is fully completed after 2 weeks (Sumová et al. 2000).

The similar adaptation of rhythmicity in both SCN regions to previous photoperiod suggests the existence of internal processing of the photoperiodic signal between both regions. Indeed, photoperiod modulates mutual phasing of the core and shell subpopulations; the longer photoperiod causes larger phase advances of the clock in the core as compared to the shell, leading to desynchrony between the core and shell regions (Evans et al. 2013).

10.3.5 Photoperiod Modulates the Cellular Network Properties

Photoperiod modulates the network organization even at the level of individual cellular activity in the SCN. The electrophysiological recordings of SCN single-unit firing activity demonstrate that under long photoperiod these firing peaks are more dispersed compared to under short photoperiod (VanderLeest et al. 2007). Thus, the peaks of electrical activity of individual SCN neurons are decompressed in long days and compressed in short days. The communication of photoperiodic messages between both subregions as well as individual neurons seems to be provided by the predominant SCN neurotransmitter GABA. Blockade of the neurotransmitter via application of the $GABA_A$ receptor antagonist bicuculline to the SCN slice uncouples the two regions similar to a knife cut (Albus et al. 2005). GABA contributes to the photoperiodic modulation of the SCN via its dual effect in the SCN, acting both as an excitatory and an inhibitory neurotransmitter. Under the long days, GABA excitatory activity is higher during the day than at night but under the short days, GABA inhibitory activity is higher during the day than at night (Farajnia et al. 2014). These data suggest that GABAergic activity is modulated by photoperiod, and this may contribute to changes in the phase distributions among the cellular populations in the SCN.

10.4   Photoperiodic Modulation of the SCN Molecular Clock

10.4.1 Molecular Mechanism of the Mammalian Clock

Starting from the 1990s, the mammalian molecular clockwork underlying rhythmicity in the SCN and other tissues in the body has been gradually elucidated. A set of mammalian clock genes, namely Period (*Per1*, *Per2*, *Per3*), Cryptochrome (*Cry1*, *Cry2*), *Clock*, *Bmal1*, *Bmal2*, *Nr1d1* (also called *Rev-erbα*), *Nr1d2* (also called *Rev-erbβ*), *Rora*, *Rorb*, *Ck1ε*, *CK1δ*, *GSK3β*, are part of the circadian clock. Most of these genes are expressed rhythmically. The list of the clock genes is not complete as recent studies have identified more genes that seem to be significant for the clock mechanism, for example, *Dec1*, *Dec2*. Additionally, other molecules, including miRNA, histone modulators, enzymes, and nuclear receptors are also important modulators of the core clock mechanism. Although the major players of the mechanism have been recognized, research on the fine-tuning of the molecular machinery of the mammalian clock is still very active in order to understand the mutual interlinking of the molecular clock with the cellular processes.

The circadian clock operates at a single cell level, but intercellular communication adds robustness of the molecular oscillation in the SCN. The cellular mechanism generating the circadian signal is based on feedback loop interactions that are a common regulatory mechanism in biology and physiology. The feedback loops operate autonomously to regulate transcription of the clock genes. It means that protein products of clock genes activate or inhibit transcription of their own gene, as well as other genes. The circadian clock uses multiple feedback loops, at least one basic and one accessory loop, which are mutually interlocked. In the basic loop, transcription of a set of genes (e.g., *Per*, *Cry*, *Nr1d1*) is activated via heterodimer composed of CLOCK and BMAL1 (Brain and Muscle ARNT-Like 1) proteins binding to the specific DNA sequences, called E-boxes, on their promoters. Then, PER and CRY proteins form heterodimers which enter the nucleus to inhibit the CLOCK:BMAL1 activity on their promoters. The promoter of *Bmal1* gene is regulated by an accessory feedback loop via its RORE sequence which binds either NR1D1 or RORa to inhibit or activate the transcription, respectively. As a result of this loop, the transcription of *Bmal1* gene is roughly in opposite phase to transcription of all other clock genes. This complexity has evolved to increase stability and robustness of the oscillation and to provide input pathways for adjusting the clock to changes in cellular environment. The feedback loop regulation, together with controlled protein stability, generates autonomous rhythmic signal encoded in rhythmic changes in the clock protein levels. These proteins function as transcriptional factors rhythmically driving expression of a wide array of other genes downstream of the core clock mechanism.

For more details on the molecular clock mechanism, the readers are recommended to go to Chap. 11 and more comprehensive review papers (Takahashi et al. 2008; Reppert 2000; Takahashi 2017).

10.4.2 Photic Entrainment of the Molecular Clock

The molecular clock mechanism described above operates autonomously to run with a period close to, but not exactly equal to, the period of solar day. Thus, the clock can approximately measure time in the absence of external light, but to be accurate, it needs to entrain with external light/dark cycles. Under natural conditions, light regulates the pace of the clockwork via light-sensitive clock genes *Per1,2*. Promoters of these clock genes contain specific DNA binding sites for the signal molecule phosphorylated CREB (Ca2 + -cAMP response element-binding protein), which activates their transcription. The CREB phosphorylation results from a pathway which is initiated by photic stimulation of intrinsically photosensitive cells in the retinal ganglion cell layer. These cells convey the signal to the neurons within the SCN core via release of neurotransmitter glutamate from their terminals. After binding NMDA receptors, intracellular Ca2+ levels are elevated and activate downstream signaling pathways, including CREB phosphorylation, leading to transcriptional activation of *Per1* and *Per2* clock genes. The activation can occur only during the subjective night when the endogenous levels of the clock gene transcripts are low due to the feedback loop mechanism. For more details on the mechanism of photic entrainments, see Meijer and Schwartz 2003.

10.4.3 Photoperiodic Modulation of the Molecular Clock

Data summarized in part 10.3 above demonstrating the modulation of the SCN rhythmicity by the photoperiod suggest that the molecular clock mechanisms underlying the rhythmicity must also be modulated by photoperiod. Extensive data have been accumulated that strongly support this suggestion. The initial evidence came from studies in various rodent species that have indicated that photoperiod modulates expression and protein levels of the light-sensitive *Per* genes in the population of cells in the coronal hypothalamic sections containing the SCN (Messager et al. 2000; Nuesslein-Hildesheim et al. 2000; Steinlechner et al. 2002; Tournier et al. 2003; Sumová et al. 2002; Sumová et al. 2003). Importantly, the photoperiodic SCN modulation was confirmed under conditions of unmasked effect of light, excluding the possibility that the photoperiodic modulation of the light-sensitive clock gene expression was a consequence of direct response to light rather than a reflection of the change in its functional state (Sumová et al. 2002; Sumová et al. 1995b). The spontaneous rise in *Per1* mRNA and PER protein occurs earlier under a long than under a short photoperiod, and consequently the interval of elevated gene and protein expression is significantly extended in long days. The *Per1* mRNA rise seems entrained with the morning light onset. The spontaneous rhythm in *Per1* expression adjusts to changes in photoperiod as previously shown for the rhythm in *c-fos* expression (sections 3.2.1. and 3.2.2 above). After photoperiod shortening via asymmetrical extension of the dark period into the morning hours, the rhythm adjusts gradually to the change, with larger phase delays of the *Per1* expression rise and only small phase delays of its decline, consequently leading to shortening of the interval of high *Per1* expression (Sumová et al. 2007). The data indicate that in rats the morning light onset dominantly entrains the rise in *Per1* expression. Later studies demonstrated that also other clock genes (that is, also clock genes that are not directly light-sensitive) are modulated by photoperiod. Notably, the interval of elevated *Bmal1* expression remains in anti-phase to other clock genes and is, in opposite to *Per1*, longer under a short than under a long photoperiod (Sumová et al. 2003).

Further examination of the photoperiodic modulation of the SCN molecular clock pointed at another level of SCN organization, that is, at its rostro-caudal dimension (Hazlerigg et al. 2005). The photoperiod modulates the mutual phasing of clocks in the rostral, middle, and caudal parts of the SCN that persists also in conditions when animals are exposed to photoperiods with simulated twilight conversion between the light and darkness (Sosniyenko et al. 2009). These studies clearly showed that with gradual extension of the photoperiod, the previously in-phase peaks of the clocks in the rostral, medial, and caudal parts of the SCN become gradually more dispersed so that the interval of elevated expression of *Per1,2* genes and their proteins spreads over the extended light interval. Interestingly, this extension is achieved by attaining a specific phase-relationship between the SCN subpopulations via advancing the phase of clocks in the caudal part relative to those in the rostral part. Consequently, the dynamic of lengthening and shortening of the photoperiod, as occurs with seasonal changes over a year, causes corresponding gradual expansion and compression among the phases of the clocks in the rostro-caudal axis of the SCN (Fig. 10.1). The same pattern persists in vitro when *Per1*- and PER2-driven biolu- minescence is recorded in horizontal SCN sections which preserve the communica- tion between the rostral and caudal SCN regions (Yoshikawa et al. 2017).

10.4.4 Photoperiod Reprograms the Phases of Cellular Oscillators

The important advancement in understanding the molecular mechanism of the photoperiodic modulation of the circadian clock has been achieved with availability to assess the molecular clock in vitro, using transgenic animal models in which activity of the clock components can be recorded in real time. These techniques allow monitoring of the SCN clock not only at the cell-population level but also at the cellular level. It appeared that the waveforms of the rhythms in individual cells do not change with the changing photoperiods whereas the phase-relationships among these cellular clocks are modulated. In accordance with the cellular firing rate rhythms described above, the phasing of cellular molecular oscillations becomes looser with extending photoperiods (Inagaki et al. 2007). When the photoperiod extends to an extreme, that is in constant light, the dispersal of the cellular clock phases exceeds the limit for maintaining a coherent output rhythm at the cell population level, and the animal becomes behaviorally arrhythmic (Ohta et al. 2005).

10.5   Summary and Perspectives

Altogether, the photoperiodic modulation of the SCN requires a plastic rearrange- ment of the cellular oscillators rather than changes in processes governing the generation of the circadian signal within a cell. The circadian clock in the SCN is modulated by photoperiod via a complex multilevel reorganization, changing the mutual phasing of the cellular clocks and clocks in the multidimensional cell populations. Because the individual regions of the SCN deliver signals to specific areas in the brain and elsewhere in the body (Evans et al. 2015), this complexity of SCN photoperiodic modulation affects multiple output regions, though the pineal gland is the principal target in mammals. The correct entrainment of the circadian clocks with changing photoperiods is primarily important for survival of wild animal species, but it may potentially be significant also for human health. Although humans living in modern society are not exposed to full photoperiodic cycles, occurrence of various diseases exhibits seasonal variation. Although artificial light can ameliorate the photoperiodic changes in duration of light and melatonin produc- tion, it seems that in some individuals during the winter, the substitution of intensive natural daylight by artificial light is not sufficient to achieve the same modulation of the human SCN in its complexity herein described. It has been shown that the SCN relays the photic, and thus likely photoperiodic, information to brains regions regulating sleep, cognition, and mood (Deurveilher and Semba 2005), and changes in photoperiod are associated with impairment of mental health in humans (Zelinski et al. 2013). Therefore, it is challenging to understand whether and to what extent variations in the occurrence of these diseases may arise from disordered endogenous photoperiodic programming in humans.

Acknowledgements The preparation of this chapter was supported by the Research Project RV0: 67985823.

References

Albus H et al (2005) A GABAergic mechanism is necessary for coupling dissociable ventral and dorsal regional oscillators within the circadian clock. Curr Biol 15(10):886–893

Arendt J et al (1985) Some effects of melatonin and the control of its secretion in humans. Ciba Found Symp 117:266–283

Bittman EL, Karsch FJ, Hopkins JW (1983) Role of the pineal gland in ovine photoperiodism: regulation of seasonal breeding and negative feedback effects of estradiol upon luteinizing hormone secretion. Endocrinology 113(1):329–336

Cagampang FR et al (1994) Circadian variation of arginine-vasopressin messenger RNA in the rat suprachiasmatic nucleus. Brain Res Mol Brain Res 24(1–4):179–184

Carter DS, Goldman BD (1983) Progonadal role of the pineal in the Djungarian hamster (Phodopus sungorus sungorus): mediation by melatonin. Endocrinology 113(4):1268–1273

Carter SJ et al (2016) A matter of time: study of circadian clocks and their role in inflammation. J Leukoc Biol 99(4):549–560

Deurveilher S, Semba K (2005) Indirect projections from the suprachiasmatic nucleus to major arousal-promoting cell groups in rat: implications for the circadian control of behavioural state. Neuroscience 130(1):165–183

Evans JA et al (2013) Dynamic interactions mediated by nonredundant signaling mechanisms couple circadian clock neurons. Neuron 80(4):973–983

Evans JA et al (2015) Shell neurons of the master circadian clock coordinate the phase of tissue clocks throughout the brain and body. BMC Biol 13:43

Farajnia S et al (2014) Seasonal induction of GABAergic excitation in the central mammalian clock. Proc Natl Acad Sci U S A 111(26):9627–9632

Guido ME et al (1999) Daily rhythm of spontaneous immediate-early gene expression in the rat suprachiasmatic nucleus. J Biol Rhythm 14(4):275–280

Hastings MH (1991) Neuroendocrine rhythms. Pharmacol Ther 50(1):35–71

Hazlerigg DG, Ebling FJ, Johnston JD (2005) Photoperiod differentially regulates gene expression rhythms in the rostral and caudal SCN. Curr Biol 15(12):R449–R450

Hoffmann K, Illnerova H (1986) Photoperiodic effects in the Djungarian hamster. Rate of testicular regression and extension of pineal melatonin pattern depend on the way of change from long to short photoperiods. Neuroendocrinology 43(3):317–321

Illnerová H (1988) Entrainment of mammalian circadian rhythms in melatonin production by light. Pineal Res Rev 6:173–217

Illnerová H, Hoffman K, Vaněček J (1986) Adjustment of the rat pineal N-acetyltransferase rhythm to change from long to short photoperiod depends on the direction of the extension of the dark period. Brain Res 362(2):403–408

Illnerová, H., 1991 The suprachiasmatic nucleus and rhythmic pineal melatonin production, In Suprachiasmatic nucleus: the Mind's clock, D.C. Klein, R.J. Moore, and S.M. Reppert, Editors, Oxford Univ. Press: New York. p. 197–216

Illnerová H, Vaněček J (1980) Pineal rhythm in N-acetyltransferase activity in rats under different artificial photoperiods and in natural daylight in the course of a year. Neuroendocrinology 31(5):321–326

Illnerová H, Vaněček J (1988) Entrainment of the rat pineal rhythm in melatonin production by light. Reprod Nutr Dev 28(2B):515–526

Illnerová H, Vaněček J, Hoffmann K (1989) Different mechanisms of phase delays and phase advances of the circadian rhythm in rat pineal N-acetyltransferase activity. J Biol Rhythm 4 (2):187–200

Illnerová H, Zvolský P, Vaněček J (1985) The circadian rhythm in plasma melatonin concentration of the urbanized man: the effect of summer and winter time. Brain Res 328(1):186–189

Inagaki N et al (2007) Separate oscillating cell groups in mouse suprachiasmatic nucleus couple photoperiodically to the onset and end of daily activity. Proc Natl Acad Sci U S A 104 (18):7664–7669

Jáč M et al (2000) Daily profiles of arginine vasopressin mRNA in the suprachiasmatic, supraoptic and paraventricular nuclei of the rat hypothalamus under various photoperiods. Brain Res 887 (2):472–476

Klein DC, Moore RY (1979) Pineal N-acetyltransferase and hydroxyindole-O- methyltransferase: control by the retinohypothalamic tract and the suprachiasmatic nucleus. Brain Res 174 (2):245–262

Kornhauser JM, Mayo KM, Takahashi JS (1993) Immediate-early gene expression in a mammalian circadian pacemaker: the suprachiasmatic nucleus. In: Young MW (ed) Molecular genetics of biochemical rhythms. Dekker, New York, pp 271–307

Lerner AB et al (1959) Melatonin in peripheral nerve. Nature 183:1821

Meijer JH, Schwartz WJ (2003) In search of the pathways for light-induced pacemaker resetting in the suprachiasmatic nucleus. J Biol Rhythm 18(3):235–249

Messager S et al (2000) Photoperiod differentially regulates the expression of Per1 and ICER in the pars tuberalis and the suprachiasmatic nucleus of the Siberian hamster. Eur J Neurosci 12 (8):2865–2870

Nuesslein-Hildesheim B et al (2000) The circadian cycle of mPER clock gene products in the suprachiasmatic nucleus of the siberian hamster encodes both daily and seasonal time. Eur J Neurosci 12(8):2856–2864

Ohta H, Yamazaki S, McMahon DG (2005) Constant light desynchronizes mammalian clock neurons. Nat Neurosci 8(3):267–269

Pittendrigh CL, Daan S (1976) A functional analysis of circadian pacemakers in nocturnal rodents. V. Pacemaker structure: a clock for all seasons. J Comp Physiol A 106:333–355

Reiter RJ (1974) Influence of pinealectomy on the breeding capability of hamsters maintained under natural photoperiodic and temperature conditions. Neuroendocrinology 13(6):366–370

Reppert SM (2000) Cellular and molecular basis of circadian timing in mammals. Semin Perinatol 24(4):243–246

Schwartz WJ et al (2000) Differential regulation of fos family genes in the ventrolateral and dorsomedial subdivisions of the rat suprachiasmatic nucleus. Neuroscience 98(3):535–547

Sosniyenko S et al (2009) Influence of photoperiod duration and light-dark transitions on entrainment of Per1 and Per2 gene and protein expression in subdivisions of the mouse suprachiasmatic nucleus. Eur J Neurosci 30(9):1802–1814

Steinlechner S et al (2002) Robust circadian rhythmicity of Per1 and Per2 mutant mice in constant light, and dynamics of Per1 and Per2 gene expression under long and short photoperiods. J Biol Rhythm 17(3):202–209

Sumová A, Illnerová H (1996) Endogenous melatonin signal does not mediate the effect of photoperiod on the rat suprachiasmatic nucleus. Brain Res 725(2):281–283

Sumová A, Illnerová H (1998) Photic resetting of intrinsic rhythmicity of the rat suprachiasmatic nucleus under various photoperiods. Am J Phys 274(3 Pt 2):R857–R863

Sumová A, Kováčiková Z, Illnerová H (2007) Dynamics of the adjustment of clock gene expression in the rat suprachiasmatic nucleus to an asymmetrical change from a long to a short photoperiod. J Biol Rhythm 22(3):259–267

Sumová A, Trávníčková Z, Illnerová H (1995a) Memory on long but not on short days is stored in the rat suprachiasmatic nucleus. Neurosci Lett 200(3):191–194

Sumová A, Trávníčková Z, Illnerová H (2000) Spontaneous c-Fos rhythm in the rat suprachiasmatic nucleus: location and effect of photoperiod. Am J Physiol Regul Integr Comp Physiol 279(6): R2262–R2269

Sumová A et al (1995b) The rat suprachiasmatic nucleus is a clock for all seasons. Proc Natl Acad Sci U S A 92(17):7754–7758

Sumová A et al (1998) Spontaneous rhythm in c-Fos immunoreactivity in the dorsomedial part of the rat suprachiasmatic nucleus. Brain Res 801(1–2):254–258

Sumová A et al (2002) The circadian rhythm of Per1 gene product in the rat suprachiasmatic nucleus and its modulation by seasonal changes in daylength. Brain Res 947(2):260–270

Sumová A et al (2003) Clock gene daily profiles and their phase relationship in the rat suprachiasmatic nucleus are affected by photoperiod. J Biol Rhythm 18(2):134–144

Takahashi JS (2017) Transcriptional architecture of the mammalian circadian clock. Nat Rev Genet 18(3):164–179

Takahashi JS et al (2008) The genetics of mammalian circadian order and disorder: implications for physiology and disease. Nat Rev Genet 9(10):764–775

Tournier BB et al (2003) Photoperiod differentially regulates clock genes' expression in the suprachiasmatic nucleus of Syrian hamster. Neuroscience 118(2):317–322

van den Pol AN (1991) The suprachiasmatic nucleus: morphological and cytochemical substrates for cellular interaction. In: Klein DC, Moore RJ, Reppert SM (eds) Suprachiasmatic nucleus: the Mind's clock. Oxford Univ. Press, New York, pp 17–50

VanderLeest HT et al (2007) Seasonal encoding by the circadian pacemaker of the SCN. Curr Biol 17(5):468–473

Vondrašová D, Hájek I, Illnerová H (1997) Exposure to long summer days affects the human melatonin and cortisol rhythms. Brain Res 759(1):166–170

Vuillez P et al (1996) In Syrian and European hamsters, the duration of sensitive phase to light of the suprachiasmatic nuclei depends on the photoperiod. Neurosci Lett 208(1):37–40

Welsh DK, Takahashi JS, Kay SA (2010) Suprachiasmatic nucleus: cell autonomy and network properties. Annu Rev Physiol 72:551–577

Welsh DK et al (1995) Individual neurons dissociated from rat suprachiasmatic nucleus express independently phased circadian firing rhythms. Neuron 14(4):697–706

Yoshikawa T et al (2017) Localization of photoperiod responsive circadian oscillators in the mouse suprachiasmatic nucleus. Sci Rep 7(1):8210

Zelinski EL et al (2013) Persistent impairments in hippocampal, dorsal striatal, and prefrontal cortical function following repeated photoperiod shifts in rats. Exp Brain Res 224(1):125–139

Further Recommended Reading

Tackenberg MC, McMahon DG (2018 Jan 9) *Photoperiodic Programming of the SCN and Its Role in Photoperiodic Output.* Neural Plast. 2018:8217345. https://doi.org/10.1155/2018/8217345 This review represents a comprehensive overview of research on the SCN as a coordinator of photoperiodic responses, the intercellular coupling changes that accompany that coordination, as well as the SCN's role in a putative brain network controlling photoperiodic input and output.

Porcu A, Riddle M, Dulcis D, Welsh DK Photoperiod-Induced *Neuroplasticity in the Circadian System.* Neural Plasticity 2018:5147585. https://doi.org/10.1155/2018/5147585 The review summarizes data proposing that the SCN may be an essential mediator of the effects of seasonal changes of day length on mental health. The authors explore various forms of neuroplasticity that occur in the SCN and other brain regions to facilitate seasonal adaptation, particularly altered phase distribution of cellular circadian oscillators in the SCN and changes in hypothalamic neurotransmitter expression.

Coomans CP, Ramkisoensing A, Meijer JH (2015) *The suprachiasmatic nuclei as a seasonal clock.* Frontiers in Neuroendocrinology 37:29–42 https://doi.org/10.1016/j.yfrne.2014.11.002

The review provides an overview on seasonal SCN modulation, including relevance to human physiology.

Dardente H, Wyse CA, Lincoln GA, Wagner GC, Hazlerigg DG, Dardente H et al (2016 Jul 26) *Effects of Photoperiod Extension on Clock Gene and Neuropeptide RNA Expression in the SCN of the Soay Sheep.* PLoS One. 11(7):e0159201. https://doi.org/10.1371/journal.pone.0159201
Overall, these data demonstrate that synchronizing effects of light on SCN circadian organization proceed similarly in diurnal ungulates and in nocturnal rodents, despite differences in neuro-peptide gene expression.

Circadian Timekeeping in the Suprachiasmatic Nucleus: Genes, Neurotransmitters, Neurons, and Astrocytes

11

Michael H. Hastings and Marco Brancaccio

Abstract

The nocturnal secretion of melatonin by the pineal gland drives photoperiodic seasonal rhythms in mammals. In turn, the pineal is controlled by daily cues generated intrinsically by the circadian (circa- approximately, −*diem* a day) clock of the hypothalamic suprachiasmatic nucleus (SCN). Photic cues from the retina both synchronize the SCN and also acutely suppress melatonin synthesis. As a result, the duration of the nocturnal secretion of melatonin encodes the length of the night and hence season. This chapter will consider recent developments in understanding how the SCN generates an internal representation of solar time and thereby functions as a clock and calendar. The first level of timekeeping pivots around intracellular transcriptional and translational feedback loops (TTFLs) that constitute cell-autonomous circadian timers. These mechanisms are common to many, if not all, mammalian tissues, but three properties beyond its TTFLs make the SCN the principal pacemaker. First, it is the sole component of the mammalian circadian system to receive retinal input and is therefore directly entrained to the cycle of day and night. The TTFLs of SCN cells are therefore a high-fidelity, internal proxy of solar time. Second, its neural connections to the hypothalamus and beyond enable the SCN to direct rhythmic endocrine (including melatonin) and autonomic and behavioral rhythms that in turn coordinate the innumerable cellular and tissue-based clocks distributed across the body. Third, the

M. H. Hastings (✉)
MRC Laboratory of Molecular Biology, Cambridge, UK
e-mail: mha@mrc-lmb.cam.ac.uk

M. Brancaccio
Department of Brain Sciences, UK Dementia Research Institute at Imperial College London, London, UK
e-mail: m.brancaccio@imperial.ac.uk

F. J. P. Ebling, H. D. Piggins (eds.), *Neuroendocrine Clocks and Calendars*, Masterclass in Neuroendocrinology 10, https://doi.org/10.1007/978-3-030-55643-3_11

timekeeping power that enables the SCN to sustain this internal coordination is derived from the circuit-level integration of the ~20,000 neurons into a robust and resilient circuit-level pacemaker. Activity across the cellular TTFLs is tightly synchronized but not simultaneous, as cells peak in activity in different phases. Importantly, this network-level pattern of activity is plastic, the long days of summer increasing the phase dispersal between cells. This response of the SCN to daylength causes a reciprocal widening or narrowing of the dependent melatonin profile. The daily clock thereby generates an internal representation of season. The intercellular mechanisms that underpin network integration are twofold. First, neuropeptidergic cues released from various populations of SCN neurons act in a slow paracrine manner, over circadian time and SCN circuit space, to synchronize and amplify the individual intracellular TTFLs. Second, it has recently become clear that astrocytes play an important role in network function, as they are able to initiate SCN neuronal oscillations and behavioral circadian rhythms and impose their own cell-autonomous period. Analysis of the network-level interactions between neurons and astrocytes will therefore advance understanding of how both circadian and seasonal information is encoded and distributed by the SCN.

Keywords

Circadian · Period · Cryptochrome · Melatonin · Astrocytes · Melanopsin · OPN4

11.1   Introduction: Clocks and Calendars

The cycles of day and night and winter and summer offer particular opportunities and present specific environmental challenges to organisms on a regular, predictable basis. Evolution has therefore favored the development of internal timing mechanisms that allow organisms to anticipate, and thereby prepare for, these events. In vertebrates, the cycle of sleep and wakefulness, which allows adaptive daily alternation between engagement with, and withdrawal from, the world, also imposes a strict temporal order to other systems such as feeding and social engagement. Equally, seasonal rhythms of physiology (fertility), metabolism (adiposity), and behavior (migration) allow species in temperate and polar regions to adapt to their periodically harsh environments, marshaling precious resources to best effect. Such seasonal rhythms are cued by two types of timers, the first is a circannual clock with self-sustained rhythms of approximately 1 year that are entrained (synchronized) by environmental stimuli such as daylength, food availability, and temperature (see chapters by Helm and by West et al. in this issue). When organisms with such a timer are held in experimental isolation, their circannual clocks continue to mark time autonomously and thereby maintain overt seasonal rhythms in the absence of external timing cues. The second mechanism does not involve a circannual oscillator: it responds in an obligate way directly to changes in daylength (photoperiod) to cue seasonal phenotypes. Typically, therefore, when daylength is experimentally held constant, the organism remains in one or other seasonal state and it does not repeatedly alternate between winter and summer phenotypes. In some larger, long-lived species that are primarily photoperiodic in their seasonality, spontaneous switches between seasonal phenotypes may occur, but they lack the precision of cycles controlled by bona fide circannual oscillators.

In mammals, the location and mechanism of the circannual clock(s) are poorly understood. In contrast, it is very clear that the principal circadian clock (circa-approximately -*diem* day) of the hypothalamic suprachiasmatic nucleus (SCN) plays a pivotal role in photoperiodic time measurement. It does this by controlling the secretion of melatonin by the pineal gland: the long nights of winter are internally represented in the accompanying prolonged nocturnal melatonin profile, whereas in summer, the melatonin profile is truncated. In pinealectomized animals, photoperiodic seasonality is curtailed, but it can be restored by daily delivery of exogenous melatonin with an appropriate winter- or summer-like duration (Bartness et al. 1993). The SCN controls the pineal in two ways, involving both serial and parallel, polysynaptic neural pathways that ultimately regulate the autonomic activation of the secretory pinealocytes. First, it is the conduit for retinally derived signals that acutely curtail the ongoing biosynthesis of melatonin: light at dawn and dusk prevents melatonin synthesis and release. Second, the SCN generates intrinsic circadian signals that initiate (anticipated evening) and terminate (anticipated morning) melatonin synthesis. Thus, when animals are held in continuous darkness, they exhibit a well-defined circadian rhythm of nocturnal melatonin secretion (SCN-dependent), whereas experimental exposure to continuous light suppresses the melatonin signal in a retinally dependent manner. The relative contributions of the acute photic effect and the more sustained circadian control in sculpting the melatonin profile vary between species, with ungulates emphasizing the former and rodents and primates the latter (Lincoln et al. 1985; Stokkan et al. 2007; Maywood et al. 1993; Zawilska et al. 2009). It is nevertheless the case that, by entrainment to the prevailing light/dark cycle, the SCN acts as both a daily clock and a photoperiodic calendar (see the chapter by Sumova and Illnerova), mediating the effects of experienced or anticipated daylight on the neuroendocrine axis (see chapter by Hannibal). Downstream of the pineal, the duration of the melatonin profile is transduced into a seasonal neuroendocrine phenotype both directly and indirectly by melatonin-sensitive cells in the pituitary and hypothalamus (see chapters by Barrett and Morgan; Wood; Dufourny and Franceschini; Stevenson). Although typically thought of in terms of "vegetative" neuroendocrinology, under extreme conditions, these subliminal effects of light, the clock, and melatonin can breakthrough to influence human mood and mental state (see the chapter by Partonen). Given its central role in timekeeping, the purpose of this review is to consider recent developments in understanding how the SCN acts as a central circadian clock, because without it, there would be no photoperiodic calendar in mammals.

11.2   Cell-Autonomous Circadian Timekeeping in Mammals: TTFLs

Before considering the SCN in particular, it is important to review the remarkable discoveries from the past 20 years or so concerning the molecular genetic and cellular bases of circadian timekeeping in mammals. These discoveries came from initial work on *Drosophila melanogaster* and the subsequent tracing of genetic homologies to mammals (Rosbash et al. 2007; Reppert and Weaver 2000), as well as by decoding directly the circadian effects of spontaneous and induced de novo mutations in rodents and more recently in human pedigrees (Takahashi 2016). This body of work has revealed that the circadian clock of mammals is a cell-autonomous mechanism involving intracellular transcriptional/ translational feedback loops (TTFLs). At the heart of the canonical TTFL lies a pair of transcription factors, Clock and Bmal1 (Fig. 11.1). These proteins heterodimerize through their Per-Arnt-Sim (PAS) dimerization domains (two in each protein, PAS-A and PAS-B) and bind to target DNA sequences that contain E-box (Enhancer) regulatory elements via their basic helix-loop-helix DNA-binding motifs. There, the heterodimers recruit the general transcriptional apparatus to drive expression of their target genes, which include *Period* (*Per1 and Per2*) and *Cryptochrome* (*Cry1 and Cry2*). Importantly, these genes encode proteins that also heterodimerize, forming Per/Cry complexes that enter the nucleus and recruit the generic inhibitory machinery to suppress Clock/Bmal1-dependent transcription. After a delay of ~12 h, the Per/Cry complexes have therefore closed a negative feedback loop. De novo Clock/Bmal1-dependent gene expression can only start again once the existing Per and Cry proteins have been degraded, and this in turn takes ~12 h. The delayed negative feedback by Per/Cry is therefore the source of TTFL oscillation, which can be readily monitored by real-time imaging of bioluminescent and fluorescent reporters of Per and Cry transcription and protein abundance (Hastings et al. 2005) (Fig. 11.1).

The aggregate period of the TTFL (~ 24 h) is determined by a suite of factors that incorporates the rates of Clock/Bmal1-dependent transcription, the intracellular dynamics of nuclear transfer, and the stability/degradation of Per and Cry proteins (Reppert and Weaver 2002). Many of these processes are in turn regulated by posttranslational modifications of the various positive- and negative-regulatory proteins. As a result, the period of the cell-autonomous clock can be shortened or lengthened by spontaneous or induced mutations of regulatory enzymes such as protein kinases and ubiquitin ligases that affect the stability of the proteins, or mutations of the core clock proteins themselves that alter their transcriptional activity and/or their susceptibility to such regulation (Hirano et al. 2016; Hastings et al. 2018). Equally, the cell-autonomous clock can be accelerated, slowed down or even stopped by pharmacological targeting of the clock proteins or their regulatory enzymes. In rare human pedigrees, mutations affecting the core clock proteins are associated with inherited sleep disturbances (Jones et al. 2013), whilst the natural range of "lark" and "owl" behavioral phenotypes ("chronotype") seen in human populations is likely a result of multigenic inheritance of several circadian alleles, each of small effect (Roenneberg and Merrow 2016). It is important to note,

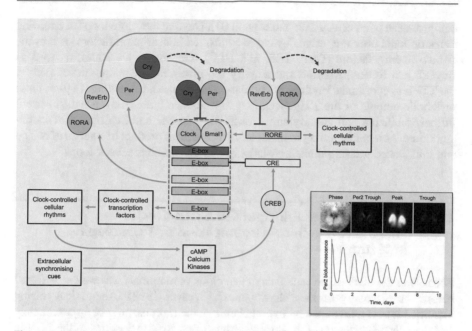

Fig. 11.1 Schematic representation of the interlocked feedback loops of the mammalian circadian clock. At the heart of the circadian oscillator is the control of transcription by the positive regulators Clock and Bmal1, which act via E-box enhancer sequences (dotted line). Genes encoding Per and Cry are activated by Clock/Bmal1, and their protein products in turn oppose the action of Clock/Bmal1 heterodimers, establishing an oscillatory delayed negative feedback loop (the TTFL). Degradation of Per/Cry complexes relieves this negative regulation to initiate a new circadian cycle. The loop is stabilized further by E-box-mediated expression of RevErb and RORA, coregulators of Bmal1 expression, so that TTFL output becomes an input. The circadian signal generated by the TTFL directs cellular functions via a cascade of E-box- and RORE-regulated circadian output genes, with many of them being transcription factors. Additional feedback to the TTFL is provided by cellular cycles of cAMP, calcium and its dependent kinases impinging on CREB, which in turns controls Per expression via calcium/cAMP-regulatory elements (CREs). This pathway is also important for synchronization of the TTFL by extracellular cues. INSET: Upper panel shows phase and bioluminescence images of SCN slice from a Per2::Luciferase mouse, held in static organotypic culture. Bioluminescence images, acquired using a CCD camera, illustrate two serial troughs and one peak of Per2 expression. Lower panel shows aggregate intensity of Per2 bioluminescence signal from the slice recorded over 10 days, exhibiting robust and precise circadian oscillation reflecting the ongoing timekeeping of the TTFL (n.b. declining peak height arises from utilization of luciferin substrate, not attenuation of TFL oscillation) (Hastings, unpublished data)

however, that even though the Per/Cry loop is thought of as the "core" mechanism, it is also sustained by additional accessory feedback loops revolving both around E-boxes and other transcriptional enhancers (e.g. D-Box and CRE-box) (Fig. 11.1). For example, the nuclear hormone receptors RevErbα, RevErβ, and RORA are expressed on a circadian basis via their E-boxes and serve to amplify the core oscillation by controlling the expression of Bmal1 through its RORE regulatory sequences (Preitner et al. 2002) and in their absence, circadian behavior is compromised (Cho et al. 2012; Yin et al. 2007). Beyond the "core loop", a circadian transcriptional program, driven by clock-controlled transcription factors such as the D-box-binding factors (DBP, TEF, and HLF) (Gachon et al. 2006), as well as RevErb and RORA, transmit and amplify the proxy for solar time developed by the TTFL to coordinate rhythms of cellular metabolism and signaling. In turn, these metabolic outputs of the TTFL feedback to modulate the clock mechanism itself, further stabilizing and amplifying the oscillation (Asher and Schibler 2011). Cell-autonomous circadian timing in mammals is therefore a product of a series of nested and interlocked transcriptional/translational and metabolic feedback loops.

11.3 The SCN as the Principal Circadian Clock and the Hierarchical Organization of Timekeeping in Mammals

The role of the SCN as the central circadian clock of mammals was well established before the discovery of the "clock genes" (Weaver 1998). Anatomical tracing identified it as a retinorecipient hypothalamic nucleus, consisting of approximately 10,000 cells on each side of the third ventricle (Text Box 1). Lesions of the SCN in experimental animals curtailed circadian rhythms of behavior and physiology (including melatonin), identifying it as a necessary component of the circadian system. Equally, compression of the SCN by pituitary tumors in human patients disrupts sleep/wake cycles. Lesions also curtail photoperiodic rhythms in seasonal species as a result of compromised melatonin synthesis. Importantly, when isolated in slice culture, the SCN can exhibit autonomous circadian rhythms of neuronal electrical activity and the dependent release of neurotransmitters and neuropeptides: it is, therefore, a self-sustained "clock in a dish". Moreover, grafting of neonatal SCN to arrhythmic SCN-ablated recipient animals can restore circadian patterning to behavior with a period determined by the intrinsic period of the grafted tissue (Ralph et al. 1990). The SCN is therefore necessary and sufficient for circadian organization of behavior. These observations placed the SCN at a privileged position as one of the three mammalian tissues known to contain autonomous circadian clocks, with the others being the retina and perinatal pineal gland (Patton and Hastings 2018), but the SCN uniquely is able to control circadian behavior and physiology.

Text Box 1: Intrinsically Photoreceptive Retinal Ganglion Cells, Melanopsin, and Circadian Entrainment by Light
In contrast to lower vertebrates, where circadian entrainment to light can be mediated by extra-retinal photoreceptors in the brain and pineal complex, in mammals, the retina is the sole route for photic entrainment of daily and photoperiodic seasonal rhythms (Patton and Hastings 2018). The conventional cone and rod photoreceptors of the outer retina mediate perceptual vision,

(continued)

Text Box 1 (continued)

being hyperpolarized by light of appropriate wavelength and intensity. This leads in turn, via changes in bipolar and amacrine interneuronal signaling, to increased firing of retinal ganglion cells (RGCs) of the inner retina, the axons of which project to the visual relay stations of the brain, including the SCN via the retinohypothalamic tract (RHT). The experimental genetic ablation of rods and cones together renders mice perceptually blind. Such animals can, however, still entrain to cycles of light and darkness: the circadian clock of the SCN does not free run as it would under continuous darkness or following ablation of the eye or the RHT. Assuming the genetic ablations were complete and no residual population of rods and/or cones remained, this observation pointed toward a noncone and nonrod circadian photoreceptor (Freedman et al. 1999). Such receptors also mediate pupillary responses and, of relevance to photoperiodism, suppression of melatonin production by the pineal (Lucas et al. 1999), presumably employing an unknown photopigment. A candidate photopigment, melanopsin (OPN4), was first identified in a screen of G-protein-like receptors from frog skin, which also led to the cloning of melatonin receptors. Mammalian homologues for both receptors were rapidly identified: melatonin receptors being expressed in the SCN and pars tuberalis (Reppert et al. 1994) and hOPN4 in RGCs of the inner retina (Provencio et al. 2000). Did OPN4 mark the unknown photoreceptors of the inner retina, and, if so, was it the photopigment responsible for their responses? Direct evidence to answer the first question was obtained in two ways. First, electrophysiological recordings showed that OPN4-expressing RGCs that project to the SCN are intrinsically photoreceptive (Hattar et al. 2002). Second, calcium imaging of the responses to light of wild-type and rod/cone-deficient retinae in culture revealed an extensive network of light-activated RGCs across the inner retina. These cells exhibited a range of intensity-dependent, sustained, transient, and repetitive responses to light pulses in the absence of rods and cones and expressed OPN4 (Sekaran et al. 2003). The functional necessity of OPN4 for circadian entrainment was demonstrated by triple-mutant mice, lacking rod, cone, and OPN4-mediated phototransduction (Hattar et al. 2003; Panda et al. 2003), which were unable to entrain to lighting cycles, exhibit pupillary responses and suppression of melatonin secretion.

Thus, subliminal, i.e., nonvisual, processing of light information is mediated by a newly discovered class of retinal photoreceptors: intrinsically photoreceptive retinal ganglion cells (iPRGCs) (Lucas 2013). In the case of circadian entrainment, a molecularly defined subpopulation of iPRGCs projects directly to the SCN and alone is sufficient to mediate daily and photoperiodic entrainment (Fernandez et al. 2016). Genetic ablation of these iPRGCs removes nonimage forming vision but leaves intact image formation, which is mediated in parallel via RGCs with input from conventional rods and

(continued)

Text Box 1 (continued)

cones (Guler et al. 2008). Under natural conditions, however, it is likely that circadian entrainment can be mediated by signaling through OPN4 in combination with rod and cone opsins, rendering OPN4 (but not the iPRGCs expressing it) partially redundant (Van Gelder and Buhr 2016). In contrast to the fast and spatially sharp responses of the conventional rod and cone photoreceptors that mediate conscious vision, the intrinsic responses to light of iPRGCs are characteristically slow, sustained, and spatially diffuse (Schmidt et al. 2011). These properties are better suited to integrate the daily and seasonal changes in daylight, which are relevant to the clock and calendrical functions of the SCN. They are dependent on the cell-autonomous properties of the iPRGCs and also their extensive dendritic morphology but sparse retinal distribution, which allows them to "harvest" photons and so obtain and integrate information on general lighting intensity across visual space.

The discovery of such a novel cell population in the extensively studied retina was remarkable, but equally exciting was the revelation that OPN4 is the molecule that confers photoreceptivity because OPN4 is an invertebrate-like blue-light photopigment. In contrast to rod and cone opsins, which signal via an inhibitory Gi-protein signaling cascade to hyperpolarize the photoreceptor cell, OPN4 acts via a Gq-protein cascade to depolarize the iPRGC and so increase firing rate (Lucas 2013). This mechanism of action of OPN4 is consistent with its structural similarity to invertebrate opsins that signal in a similar way. Thus, light can activate iPRGC firing rate and thereby stimulate the SCN either by the intrinsically induced depolarization or by serial disinhibition conferred by the cone/rod, bipolar cell cascade. Beyond the SCN, it is now also clear that the iPRGCs, through their influence over various subcortical brain area projections to which they connect, can exert a powerful effect on mood and likely cognition (Lazzerini Ospri et al. 2017). Thus, the discovery of the melanopsin-expressing iPRGCs not only revealed a novel anatomical and functional substrate for the subliminal perception and anticipation of light/dark cycles by the circadian system but also highlighted a key pathway connecting seasonal changes to mood control (Fig. 11.2).

This settled view of circadian organization in mammals, with the SCN as the "driving oscillator" causing daily behavioral and physiological rhythms, was, however, radically challenged by the discovery of clock genes, which showed that SCN cells were not the only ones expressing the intracellular timing clockwork. Rather, clock genes are expressed widely across the body, supporting the possibility that other, perhaps many, cells and tissues also contain genetically competent, cell-autonomous circadian oscillators. This was first tested in cell culture using biochemical measures of clock gene expression and then more extensively by developing bioluminescent and fluorescent reporters for long-term real-time imaging of isolated

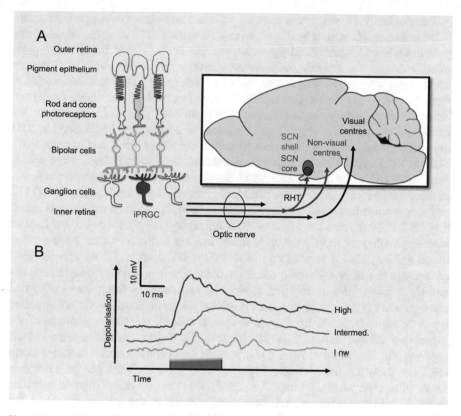

Fig. 11.2 (**a**) Schematic view of the mammalian retina showing location of conventional photoreceptors (rods and cones) in the outer layer connected by bipolar neurons to the retinal ganglion cells (RGCs) of the inner retina. Some of the RGCs (red) express melanopsin/OPN4 and are intrinsically photoreceptive (iPRGCs). RGC axons project to various centers in the brain, the visual centers receiving information from rods and cones. A subpopulation of iPRGCs projects to the SCN core via the retinohypothalamic tract (RHT) to mediate daily and seasonal entrainment and to nonvisual centers to mediate other subliminal responses to light. (**b**) Schematic view of cell-autonomous depolarizing responses of pharmacologically isolated OPN4-positive, iPRGC, to brief light pulses of progressively higher intensity. Note slow, progressive, and sustained, intensity-dependent depolarizing responses. Redrawn from (Berson et al. 2002)

tissues and cell cultures (Nagoshi et al. 2005; Stokkan et al. 2001; Yoo et al. 2004). The resulting discoveries were astonishing: most, if not all, tissues tested were able to express autonomous circadian rhythms of TTFL activity when isolated in culture. There is not a single clock of the SCN: there are numerous clocks active in all major organ systems, all of them pivoted around variants of the intracellular feedback loops driven by Clock/Bmal1, Per/Cry, and associated factors. In turn, these local clocks drive local cellular functions, via the transcriptional cascades and clock-controlled genes noted above, which ultimately determine the behavioral, metabolic, and physiological cycles that adapt mammals to the solar world.

Paradoxically, however, this discovery did not undermine the importance of the SCN; rather, it enhanced it because it revealed that the SCN was not a simple driving pacemaker to which peripheral organs respond passively. Rather, the SCN is capable of orchestrating the intrinsic circadian programs of this astoundingly sophisticated multi-organ system (Hastings et al. 2018) by integrating both the environmental input from the light/dark cycles and the internal feedback by peripheral oscillators. This ensures an accurate representation of internal body time and its corresponding iterations of optimally adapted daily cycles of physiology and behavior. This integration is achieved by daily cues under the control of the neural outputs of the SCN to local hypothalamic nuclei, the brainstem and beyond. These cues, arising from sleep and wakefulness, eating and fasting, and the associated autonomic and neuroendocrine activation, directly and indirectly amplify local tissue-based TTFLs and synchronize them into a coherent whole (Reppert and Weaver 2002; Hastings et al. 2003). In the absence of the SCN, cellular rhythms do not cease, but they do lose amplitude and rapidly desynchronize, leading to the arrhythmia observed at tissue and organismal levels (Yoo et al. 2004; Welsh et al. 2004). The cardinal property of the SCN within this circadian hierarchy is that it can generate autonomously a powerful and coherent rhythm of spontaneous firing rate (SFR) that conveys a set of time cues that are extremely precise and stable (circadian period typically varies by <1% from cycle to cycle). Indeed, real-time recordings of the expression of Per and Cry at the transcriptional and protein levels in SCN organotypic slice cultures, revealed by various genetically encoded bioluminescent reporters, show that the ensemble TTFL function of the SCN can persist in isolation for months, even years (Hastings et al. 2014). It is this power and robustness (allied to the facts that it is the sole retinorecipient element of the system and that it has suitable efferent pathways to effect internal synchronization), which make the SCN the principal circadian clock.

11.4   The Importance of Neural Circuit-Level Interactions in Circadian Timekeeping by the SCN

When its circuit is intact, either in vivo or as an organotypic slice in culture, the circadian TTFLs of individual SCN cells oscillate with high amplitude and synchronized activity with a shared ensemble period (Fig. 11.1). Peak expression of Per occurs in mid-to-late circadian day, lagging a few hours behind the peak of membrane depolarization and spontaneous electrical firing (Yamaguchi et al. 2003; Brancaccio et al. 2013; Noguchi et al. 2017). In contrast, when circuit-level interactions are compromised, for example, by cellular dissociation, pharmacological blockade of neural activity, or genetic compromise of intercellular signaling, the disconnected cells become sloppy, low amplitude oscillators, losing regularity, definition, and synchrony as they start to oscillate with their cell-intrinsic period. The individual SCN cell in isolation is therefore no more effective as an autonomous oscillator than peripheral cells, such as fibroblasts (Noguchi et al. 2017). The powerful and robust tissue-level oscillation of the SCN is a product of cellular interactions and is therefore an emergent property of the circuit, which is conferred by intercellular signaling pathways (Hastings et al. 2018). What are the synchronizing cues? Neurons of the SCN all utilize the inhibitory neurotransmitter GABA, but pharmacological blockade of GABA has little effect on the ensemble circadian oscillation of the SCN (but see below in the context of seasonal timing), indicating a minimal role for GABA signaling in determining the emergent properties of the circuit. SCN neurons also express a variety of neuropeptide transmitters, including vasoactive intestinal polypeptide (VIP) and gastrin-releasing peptide (GRP) in the retinorecipient region of the "core" SCN (Text Box 1, Fig. 11.2). The surrounding "shell" of the SCN has limited direct retinal innervation, and cells therein express other neuropeptides, including arginine vasopressin (AVP), prokineticin 2 (Prok2), and their cognate G-protein-coupled receptors (GPCRs) (AVPR1a and 1b, Prokr2) as well as GPCRs for VIP (VPAC2) and GRP (BB2). In terms of circuit coherence, loss of Prok2 or Prokr2 in rodents has little effect on the SCN, but it does compromise circadian behavior, disorganizing evening activity patterns (Prosser et al. 2007). This highlights a role for Prok2 signaling in mediating SCN output. Joint loss of the 1a and 1b receptors for AVP again does not compromise ongoing molecular (TTFL) oscillation and circadian behavior, but in mice lacking these two GPCRs, cellular synchrony across the SCN slice is more readily disorganized by pharmacological perturbations and the circadian behavior of mice is reset much more rapidly by experimentally advancing or delaying the lighting cycle (Yamaguchi et al. 2013). These effects have been interpreted as a role for AVPR1a/1b signaling in binding together the individual clock cells of the SCN shell: it is not necessary for ensemble oscillation to occur, but it does contribute to circuit coherence.

By far, the most dramatic effect of the loss of neuropeptidergic signaling, however, is seen in the case of VIP and its receptor, VPAC2 (Harmar et al. 2002; Colwell et al. 2003). Mice lacking either gene exhibit disorganized circadian behavior, often with elements of very short period, and in slice culture, the SCN rapidly loses ensemble molecular rhythms, as the individual cellular TTFLs damp in amplitude and desynchronize (Maywood et al. 2006). Application of exogenous VIP to a VIP-null SCN acutely resets TTFL amplitude and synchrony, but this is not sustained. When a wild-type SCN is grafted onto a VIP-null slice, however, the graft is able to initiate and sustain very clear TTFL cycles in the mutant "host" SCN (Maywood et al. 2011). Moreover, the period of the cycles is determined by the period of the graft, confirming the graft as the origin of the driving circadian signal. This signal is paracrine: it does not require synaptic contact between host and graft SCN because it can function between slices separated by a porous membrane with a molecular weight cutoff that allows VIP and other small neuropeptides to move through it. Paracrine signaling may be ideally suited to the prolonged timeframe of the circadian cycle and the requirement for cells distributed across the three-dimensional space of the SCN to be smoothly synchronized. Such properties are very different from rapid and locally restricted synaptic signaling. In this paracrine system, the VIP/VPAC2 axis is predominant but not exclusive: in the absence of the VPAC2 receptor, pharmacological blockade reveals additional contributions by

AVP- and GRP-dependent graft-to-host signaling. Furthermore, recent single-cell analyses of peptide and receptor expression suggest that additional neuropeptidergic axes may form an important topological element of SCN circuitry (Park et al. 2016).

Thus, a diversity of neuropeptidergic signals binds together the individual clock cells of the SCN and their TTFLs amplified and synchronized to make the circuit a far more powerful timekeeper than would be the sum of its cellular parts. The likely mechanism underlying this synergy by neuropeptidergic signaling is via GPCR-mediated production of cAMP and mobilization of calcium ($[Ca^{2+}]_i$) from intracellular stores, triggering kinase-dependent transcription of Per genes, via calcium/cAMP-responsive elements (CREs) (Fig. 11.1). Bioluminescence imaging of CRE-dependent transcription has indeed shown CRE-driven transcription in the SCN to be under tight circadian control, peaking in mid-circadian day (CT06, where CT00 is the start of subjective day) (Brancaccio et al. 2013), which coincides with the peaks of cAMP and $[Ca^{2+}]_i$ in the SCN and is suitably a few hours in advance of dependent Per expression, which peaks between CT09-CT12 (Hastings et al. 2014). In addition, rhythms in CRE-mediated transcription are lost in VIP-null SCN, but can be restored by a wild-type SCN graft, consistent with their paracrine regulation, whilst direct chemogenetic activation of the synthesis of cAMP or mobilization of $[Ca^{2+}]_I$, or treatment with exogenous VIP itself, activates CRE-dependent transcription (Brancaccio et al. 2013; Hamnett et al. 2019). Furthermore, pharmacological inhibition of adenylyl cyclase (AC) compromises TTFL function completely, whilst reducing the rate of AC activity slows down SCN circadian period (O'Neill et al. 2008). Complex interactions between intercellular (secreted) cues and intracellular signaling pathways are therefore critical regulators of the core TTFL in the SCN.

The sophistication of this neuropeptide-dependent synchronization is evident from simultaneous imaging of cellular Per expression and $[Ca^{2+}]_i$ levels, both of which are highly circadian and phase-locked (with $[Ca^{2+}]_I$ advanced) on a cell-by-cell basis (Brancaccio et al. 2014). Furthermore, across the SCN, both rhythms show regionally specific phasing, evident as spatiotemporal waves that progress over circadian time from the dorsomedial to the ventrolateral SCN. Although synchronized, the TTFLs of local populations of SCN cells are not, therefore, simultaneously active from region to region; rather, they exhibit stereotypical phase dispersal, with some regions phase-leading others (Fig. 11.3). This generates a spatiotemporal wave that is comparable from slice to slice and independent of overall ensemble period, but its function is not clear (Patton et al. 2016). Theoretical modeling indicates that an oscillatory population is more resilient if phases of synchronized activity are not simultaneous, whilst a biological function may be related to differently phased cells of the SCN conveying temporally distinct cues to their particular targets in the hypothalamus and beyond. Finally, it has been suggested that the phase wave is a mechanism of photoperiodic encoding by the SCN (see below), which raises the question of how light cues from the retina control the cell-autonomous and circuit-level emergent circadian properties of the SCN.

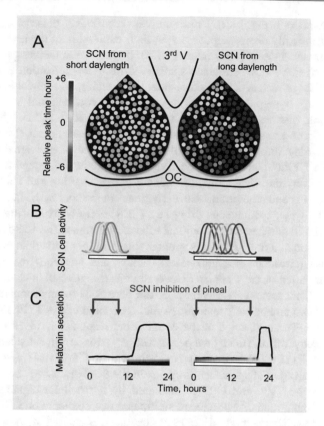

Fig. 11.3 Seasonal (photoperiodic) encoding by phase dispersal of SCN neurons determines profile of nocturnal melatonin secretion. (**a**) Schematic representation of the relative phase distributions of neurons recorded across SCN slices taken from mice previously exposed to a short daylength (12 L::12D, left) or an extremely long day (20 L::4D, right). Circadian phase of each cell is color-coded, dark blue is early and dark red is late. The phase dispersal is much greater in the long daylength and is anatomically explicit with an earlier core and a later shell SCN (based on data presented in (Evans et al. 2013)). (**b**) The photoperiodic phase dispersal distributes active SCN neurons across the circadian daytime, with greater dispersal in long daylengths. (**c**) Under short photoperiods, the compressed phase clustering of SCN inhibitory signaling allows nocturnal pineal melatonin secretion to persist for longer, whereas dispersed SCN cellular activity in summer-like days compresses the melatonin profile. Such changes in the duration of the melatonin profile are the key internal cue driving photoperiodic seasonal rhythms in mammals. OC, optic chiasm, V, ventricle

11.5   Daily and Seasonal Entrainment of the SCN Pacemaker

Entrainment of the SCN is mediated by the light-evoked release of glutamate by terminals of the RHT (Abrahamson and Moore 2001), which are the projections of an anatomically and neurochemically distinct population of retinal ganglion cells

(RGCs) (Text Box 1, Fig. 11.2). Unlike conventional RGCs, those projecting to the SCN are intrinsically photoreceptive due to their expression of the invertebrate-like photopigment melanopsin (Fernandez et al. 2016). Moreover, their responses to light are characterized by slow, sustained spatially diffuse depolarization events, which are better suited to sustain daily and seasonal timekeeping, in contrast to the fast and spatially sharp hyperpolarizing responses of the conventional rod and cone photoreceptors that mediate conscious vision (Schmidt et al. 2011). The VIP cells of the SCN core are the critical gateway for retinal entrainment (Mazuski et al. 2018). By acting through an intracellular, calcium-dependent signaling cascade triggered via NMDA- and AMPA-type ionotropic glutamate receptors, the retinal cues delivered by the RHT terminals activate electrical firing and also induce the expression of Per and other immediate early genes in the core SCN. In the middle of circadian day when spontaneous firing rate (SFR) and Per expression are already high, this stimulation has little additional effect. In contrast, the acute induction of Per transcription at a time when it is spontaneously falling (circadian evening) or is about to rise (circadian morning) resets (delays and advances respectively) the ongoing oscillation of the TTFL in SCN core cells (Shigeyoshi et al. 1997; Herzog et al. 2017). This acute responsiveness of the core SCN to environmental lighting regimes at dawn and/or dusk maintains synchronization of the TTFLs to daily and seasonal time. The next stage of the entrainment response involves second-order effects, whereby VIP and GRP (and perhaps other factors) from activated cells in the core act on cells in the shell that express their cognate GPCRs. As with the circuit-level synchronization of spontaneous cycles in the SCN discussed above, this acute resetting effect of VIP and GRP is mediated by intracellular signaling cascades involving calcium- and cAMP-dependent kinases that converge on CREs to induce Per expression (Hamnett et al. 2019). The same signaling axes are therefore employed both to acutely reset the entire SCN circuit and to sustain its intrinsic coherence and cellular synchrony in the absence of lighting cues.

Under normal conditions, the day-to-day shifts that maintain synchrony of the SCN to environmental light are small, of the order of a few minutes, and thus, they correct the mismatch between the intrinsic circadian period of the animal, which is slightly less than or slightly greater than 24 h, and the exact 24 h period of solar cycles. Experimentally, however, much larger phase shifts of one, even 2 h, can be induced by light pulses presented to mice and hamsters during early or late circadian night (Shigeyoshi et al. 1997; Best et al. 1999). Equally, the SCN slice can be rapidly phase-delayed by 1 h by treatment in vitro with exogenous glutamate (Ding et al. 1994) and VIP (Hamnett et al. 2019) as proxies for activation of the RHT. This sensitivity of the SCN to light at dusk (delays) and dawn (advances) provides the basis not only for daily entrainment but also for photoperiodic encoding by the TTFL. Theoretical considerations have suggested that the SCN circuit incorporates distinct elements that are differentially sensitive to dawn and dusk light, so-called morning (M) and evening (E) oscillators (Daan and Berde 1978), and that as the relative timing of dawn and dusk changes seasonally, then so M and E converge and diverge to create a photoperiodic topology. Whether or not the M and E oscillators are neuroanatomically real and if so, what are their genetic and neurochemical substrates are unresolved questions (Daan et al. 2001; Hastings 2001). Nevertheless, it is clear that photoperiod alters the waveform of ensemble electrical activity in the SCN (Meijer and Michel 2015), and the discovery of clock genes made it possible to ask how TTFL function in the SCN might react to, and thereby encode, daylength (Inagaki et al. 2007). Initial analyses of Per expression integrated across the entire SCN of mice and hamsters revealed that, similar to the SFR electrical rhythm, the peak of expression is extended under long daylengths, filling most of the light phase under entrained conditions (Messager et al. 1999; Nuesslein-Hildesheim et al. 2000). This extension is retained at least for a few cycles under free-running conditions and therefore reflects a photoperiodically dependent plasticity in the circadian waveform of the TTFL (see Sumova et al. this volume) (Fig. 11.3). Importantly, this change in the diurnal SCN signal duration is the inverse of the nocturnal melatonin duration (the arbiter of photoperiodic rhythms), highlighting its potential physiological relevance. Moreover, it should be noted that even in species that do not exhibit clear photoperiodic seasonal metabolic and physiological traits, not least modern humans and laboratory mice, this seasonal encoding within the SCN waveform, and downstream of it in the pineal, is retained: it is a core property of photoperiodism.

The broader TTFL waveform seen under summer lighting schedules could be a cell-autonomous or a circuit-level effect. Fluorescence and bioluminescence imaging of cellular circadian cycles in SCN slices taken from mice previously exposed to long or short daylengths indicates that it is the latter. Specifically, different cell populations can be seen to peak at different times with the result that the aggregate measure of Per expression is broader but that of individual cells is not (Evans et al. 2013; Yoshikawa et al. 2017) (Fig. 11.3). The "fault-line" in this broadening is between the core and the shell SCN. In slices taken from mice exposed to long photoperiods (20 L:4D), the core peaks ~6 h in advance of the shell, whereas in SCN from mice exposed to 12 L:12D, the shell and core exhibit similar phases. The spatiotemporal wave of the SCN circuit is therefore plastic, responsive to daylength and thus able to incorporate seasonal cues into its circadian oscillation. One cause of this may be that the retinorecipient core is acutely responsive to lighting regimes and rapidly tracks them, whereas resetting of the shell SCN, mediated by core-to-shell neuropeptidergic cues, takes longer and may be less complete. Consequently, under summer photoperiods, the two regions segregate in circadian time, with the core behaving as the putative M and the shell as the E oscillator, broadening the aggregate duration of elevated Per expression and expanding the spatiotemporal wave. Pharmacological studies show that once established, the "stretched", long-day condition is sustained by a combination of VIP and GABA signaling (Evans et al. 2013), but on loss of the photic cues, the system "relaxes" back to a more temporally compressed condition, with VIP promoting synchrony and GABA opposing it to maintain a steady state. Thus, circuit-level rather than cell-autonomous mechanisms are at the heart of the ability of the SCN to encode seasonal time via the circadian TTFL and thereby control melatonin secretion and photoperiodic physiology (Fig. 11.3).

11.6   Neurons, the TTFL, and Circadian Timekeeping in the SCN Circuit

The robust circadian rhythm of SFR suggests that it is principally an output of the SCN TTFL clockwork. But neuronal activity is also necessary for SCN function: pharmacological compromise of action potential firing with tetrodotoxin (TTX) causes rapid damping of the cellular TTFLs and cellular desynchrony, with normal circuit functions being progressively restored when TTX is withdrawn (Yamaguchi et al. 2003). The emergent properties of the circuit; robust oscillation, ensemble period and phase, and cellular synchrony with phase dispersal (i.e. the "wave"), are, therefore, resilient and self-organizing (Hastings et al. 2018). Their control mechanisms are embedded within the structure of the circuit and are expressed via neuronal activity. This importance of neuronal electrical activity to TTFL function occurs at two levels. First, at the cell-autonomous level, electrical firing drives changes in $[Ca^{2+}]_i$ that will in turn trigger the expression of Per, via CREs, and thereby amplify the ongoing TTFL cycle (Fig. 11.1). In this way, an output of the molecular clock, circadian changes in neural firing rates, is also an input to the molecular clock: another example of how the circadian system exploits nested loops to enhance stability and amplitude. Second, at the circuit level, electrical activity will drive the release of neuropeptides, which, as described above, will further bind and amplify the individual cellular TTFLs across the SCN. The powerful effects of coupling between neuronal electrical activity and the cell-autonomous TTFL are therefore a critical feature of the SCN, which are not shared by other, less robust tissue clocks.

An alternative way to explore the relationship between neuronal TTFLs and circuit-level timekeeping is provided by genetic complementation. In Cry-deficient (Cry1, Cry2-null) SCN slices and mice, molecular and behavioral circadian rhythms are absent because the core feedback loop of the TTFL is incomplete. Pan-cellular, transgenic expression of Cry1 or Cry2 under their minimal promoter and delivered by adeno-associated viral (AAV) vectors rapidly initiates SCN TTFL rhythms in slice culture and behavioral rhythms in vivo (Edwards et al. 2016; Maywood et al. 2018). Importantly, the period of these rhythms is determined by the isoform of Cry expressed: Cry1 supports long (>26 h) cycles, whereas Cry2 supports short period (~ 22 h) cycles. This confirms that the AAV-expressed Cry protein is the determinant of rhythmicity and not simply a permissive factor for the expression of a cryptic, Cry-independent oscillator. By making expression of the AAV-Cry1 conditional on a Cre recombinase (Cre), it can be targeted selectively to neurons by cotransfection with an AAV expressing Cre under the neuronally specific synapsin 1 promoter. Under these circumstances, TTFL function in slices and behavioral rhythms in mice are, again, rapidly restored (Brancaccio et al. 2019). Indeed, Cry1-dependent negative regulation of the Per2 bioluminescent reporter in SCN slices is evident within 6–12 h, and full TTFL oscillations are established within 24 h. In vivo it requires approximately 1 week for behavioral rhythms to be initiated, although this may in part reflect the slower timecourse for in vivo transduction. These results showed that when SCN neurons are the only cells in the organism with a molecularly competent

TTFL, they are nevertheless sufficient to drive circadian behavior. Given that the behavioral cycles will govern feeding/fasting and core body temperature rhythms, it is likely (but not yet verified) that such mice will also exhibit peripheral metabolic and physiological circadian rhythms. The ability of these animals to cope effectively with changing lighting regimes and thereby encode photoperiodic cues within their circadian waveform, however, is yet to be tested, although such approaches will be an interesting model to study the relevance of input from the (TTFL-deficient) periphery to the SCN in supporting the flexibility and plasticity required within the SCN for seasonal adaptation. Finally, these results demonstrate that developmental specification and specialization of the molecules and circuitry required to sustain a functional SCN clock, and to control behavioral outputs, occur independently of Cry proteins: mice that have never encountered Cry proteins prior to AAV-mediated complementation have the circuit structures in place to immediately sustain TTFL function and control circadian behavior. Significantly, if AVP signaling in the SCN is curtailed by application of a cocktail of AVPR receptor blockers, the initiation of circuit-wide TTFL function is prevented until washout of the blockers (Edwards et al. 2016). Given that AVP expression is regulated by the TTFL, this suggests that as a cell-autonomous target of AAV-Cry1, AVP is necessary to initiate circuit-wide ensemble oscillations, consistent with role of AVP/AVPR in cellular coupling in the SCN (Yamaguchi et al. 2013).

The contribution of neuronal TTFL function in driving circadian behavior has been explored further by using "translational switching" (Text Box 2, Fig. 11.4) (Maywood et al. 2018). This allows the reversible and temporally explicit expression of Cry1 in SCN neurons but only when a noncanonical amino acid (ncAA) is provided via culture medium. Such acute induction of Cry1 in arrhythmic Cry-null SCN slices rapidly (within 24 h) initiated TTFL function, both cell-autonomously and with circuit-level emergent properties (comparable to those observed with recombinase-restricted neuronal expression) (Fig. 11.5) (Maywood et al. 2018). Importantly, the rhythms dissipated equally rapidly (within 24 h) on withdrawal of ncAA, but were reinstated by repeated addition of ncAAs. These novel manipulations of the cell-autonomous and circuit-level mechanisms governing SCN timekeeping can allow a highly dynamic control of the molecular clockwork: the Cry-dependent TTFL requires little priming to be initiated and has no carryover because Cry-independent oscillations stop after Cry1 expression is terminated. Moreover, treatment of SCN slices with different concentrations of ncAA resulted in dose-dependent expression of Cry1 and consequent dose-dependent lengthening of the period of the TTFL. Higher levels of Cry1 prolonged the phase of negative suppression within the TTFL and thus extended its total duration, with the TTFL period being highly tunable. By providing ncAAs in the drinking water of suitably pretreated Cry-null mice, the same rapid, dynamic, and reversible control was seen at the level of circadian behavior, as Cry1 translation in the SCN was alternately supported and terminated across several weeks *on demand* (Maywood et al. 2018) (Fig. 11.5). Again, transitions between circadian competence and disorder were completed within one or two cycles. It is clear, therefore, that the Cry1-dependent TTFL of SCN neurons is tightly interlocked with electrical firing and that it is pivotal

Translational read-through by incorporation of ncAA at ectopic stop
codon allows expression of full length protein: switch on.

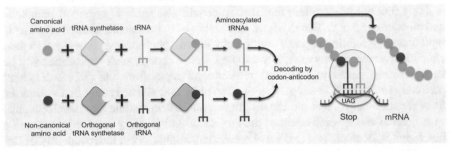

Withdrawal of ncAA allows translational termination: switch off.

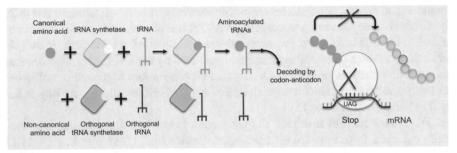

Fig. 11.4 Schematic representation of translational switching by amber suppression. Upper panel: by providing an orthogonal tRNA synthetase to charge an orthogonal tRNA with a noncanonical amino acid (ncAA), an ectopic amber stop codon in the gene of interest can be read through at the ribosome and full-length protein expressed. The protein will incorporate the ncAA at the chosen residue. Lower panel: in the absence of the ncAA, the amber stop codon is free to terminate translation and no full-length protein is expressed (Elements of figure redrawn from (Chin 2017))

in controlling circuit-level and animal-level circadian rhythms, but not in specifying the SCN circuits and extra-SCN neural circuits within which the TTFL and its timing signal operate.

Text Box 2: Amber Suppression for Translational Switching of Protein Expression

The translation of genetic information embedded in mRNA into protein at the ribosome is a central property of living organisms. The unit of translation is the nucleotide triplet codon, which is engaged by a cognate tRNA previously charged with one of the 20 canonical amino acids (AA) used by living organisms. Sequentially, AAs are added to the growing polypeptide chain as specified by the mRNA codon sequence. Translation is terminated when one of the 3 stop codons, which lack a cognate tRNA, is engaged at the ribosome

(continued)

Text Box 2 (continued)

and recognized by a release factor that facilitates ribosomal disassembly. Genetic code expansion is a means for synthetic biology to increase the diversity of amino acids available for protein production by incorporating noncanonical amino acids (ncAA) (Chin 2017). One way to achieve this is to repurpose the mRNA amber stop codon (UAG) to code for ncAA. Artificially engineering amber into a cDNA and thence mRNA encoding a protein of interest provides an avenue for translational incorporation of a ncAA into that protein. This requires the reengineering of a suitable tRNA to recognize amber and be chargeable with the ncAA, alongside a reengineered tRNA synthetase to charge the tRNA with the ncAA (Willis and Chin 2018) (Fig. 11.4).

Suitable orthogonal tRNAs (otRNA) and otRNA synthetases have been developed from prokaryotic factors, and they have been encoded into AAV-based vectors with cell-type specific promoters for use in mouse brain (Ernst et al. 2016). By using synapsin to drive the otRNA synthetase, the potential for translational switching can be restricted to neurons, although access to other cell types is readily achievable (Krogager et al. 2017). To exploit that potential, a second AAV vector is used to deliver the cDNA encoding the protein of interest, bearing an amber stop within the reading frame. Potential expression is again restricted by choice of promoter; in the case of Cry1^{amber}, this is the minimal Cry1 promoter sequence capable of conferring circadian transcription (Maywood et al. 2018). To apply the translational switch, SCN slices or the SCN in vivo are transduced with the AAV vector encoding otRNA with otRNA synthetase, alongside the vector encoding Cry1-Cry1^{amber}, with a second copy of the otRNA.

There is no expression of Cry1 (evidenced by a C-terminal EGFP tag) in the absence of ncAA, in this case alkyne lysine, as the ectopic amber stop codon terminates translation. Provision of ncAA in culture medium or in drinking water rapidly (within hours) induces protein expression via translational read though of the existing mRNA at the amber stop codon. Equally rapid loss of protein expression follows withdrawal of the ncAA. A critically important aspect of amber suppression is that it does not disregulate the proteome of the transduced cell. Potentially, the effectiveness of endogenous amber codons and correct translational termination could be compromised. This does not, however, appear to be the case (Chin 2017), likely because other aspects such as secondary structure and flanking sequences around the native amber codons maintain their effectiveness, whereas the single ectopic amber codon is more accommodating of translational read through. Applying the translational switch to control Cry1 expression in the context of circadian timekeeping provided proof-of-principle of the utility of the method in the mouse brain, both in vitro and in vivo (Fig. 11.5). The reversibility and dose-dependence of

(continued)

11.7 Are there Pacemaker Neurons in the SCN Circuit?

The neuronal heterogeneity of the SCN, evidenced by the diversity of
neuropeptidergic signaling axes noted above (Park et al. 2016), raises the question
of whether some neuronal populations/axes are more important than others. Clearly,
VIP/VPAC2 signaling is critical for the interrelated functions of cellular synchronization and entrainment by lighting cycles, but beyond that is the SCN, a hierarchical
circuit with embedded pacemaker cells, as in the heart for example, or do all cells
contribute equally in the computation of its emergent properties? To answer that
question, it is necessary to be clear about what "pacemaker" means. Is it a group or
"node" of cells that is essential for circuit-wide oscillation to occur or a group that
sets the ensemble period of the circuit (literally "makes" its "pace") or that initiates
and directs the spatiotemporal waves that progress across the SCN? A series of
studies have sought to answer these questions by employing intersectional genetics
to manipulate the cell-autonomous properties of defined neuronal groups in the SCN
and then test the consequences for circuit function and/or circadian behavior
(Hastings et al. 2018). The most extensive test has been of cells expressing
Neuromedin S (NMS), which overlap with both VIP and AVP neurons and constitute ~40% of the SCN across core and shell (Lee et al. 2015). Temporary suspension
of their synaptic transmission by conditional expression of tetanus toxin light chain
reduces the amplitude and cellular synchrony of TTFLs across the SCN slices and
reversibly makes mice behaviorally arrhythmic, highlighting the NMS cells as
determinants of circadian organization. Furthermore, loss of their cell-autonomous
TTFL by conditional deletion of Bmal1 also disrupts circadian behavior, as does
over-expression of Per2. Finally, conditional expression of a mutant version of
Clock (Clock$^{\Delta 19}$), which lengthens cell-autonomous period, causes reversible
lengthening of the period of circadian behavior and the ensemble TTFL of SCN
slices. It is clear, therefore, that by the criteria of sustaining circadian oscillation and
setting ensemble period, NMS cells act as pacemakers within the SCN circuit. Is this
because they have particular distinctive properties?

Paradoxically, the pacemaking roles of NMS cells are not dependent on signaling
by their defining neuropeptide because circadian timekeeping is not perturbed in
mice devoid of NMS (Lee et al. 2015). This result contrasts dramatically with the
role of the VIP/VPAC2 cellular axis in which the neuropeptide and receptor are the

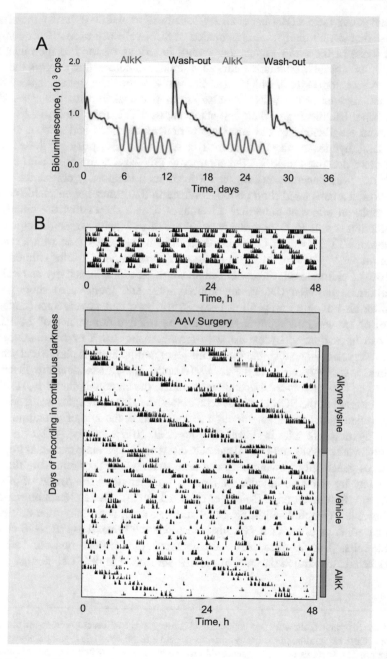

Fig. 11.5 Reversible control of SCN TTFL and behavioral circadian rhythms in Cry-null mice by translational switching of neuronal Cry1 expression. (**a**) Per2::Luc bioluminescence from arrhythmic Cry1,Cry2-null SCN slice transduced with AAVs encoding neuronally specific orthogonal tRNA synthetase, orthogonal tRNA, and Cry1[amber]. Addition of alkyne lysine (AlkK), which will

essential active factors (Harmar et al. 2002; Colwell et al. 2003). It may therefore be the case that any similarly sized population of SCN cells can exert effects comparable to those of the NMS population: circuit functions respond to the quantity of active cells, not their qualitative attributes. Indeed, neurons that express the dopamine 1A receptor (Drd1a), which constitute ~60% of the SCN and also span the core and shell regions of the SCN, can also act as pacemakers (Smyllie et al. 2016). Conditional lengthening of their cell-autonomous TTFL from 20 h to 24 h causes equivalent lengthening of the ensemble period of the SCN and also of circadian behavioral rhythms in mice (Fig. 11.6). This is perhaps unsurprising if these cells are viewed as a dominant majority, but contrary to this expectation, their period-setting role is not fully penetrant insofar as ~30% of such temporally chimeric SCN and mice exhibit an unaltered short period, confirming that control of ensemble period is not simply an effect of numerical advantage. It also shows that the circuit-wide computation is able to incorporate populations of cells with widely divergent cell-autonomous TTFL periods (20 h and 24 h) into a coherent whole with a common ensemble period (20 h or 24 h). In addition, approximately 10% of chimeric SCN and 10% of chimeric mice show circadian rhythms of TTFL activity and behavior that alternate between (Drd1a-determined) long and (nonDrd1a) short periods, revealing an ongoing competition between the two cell populations (nodes) for control of the ensemble period. Moreover, the relative dominance of 24 h Drd1a cells can be redirected by exposure to (antagonistic) 20 h or (facilitative) 24 h lighting regimes, indicating that the circuit-level computation is plastic and sensitive to retinal inputs mediated via the core VIP cells. Notwithstanding this fascinating insight into how circuit-level operations underlie the emergent plasticity, resilience, and robustness of the SCN clock, as with NMS, the Drd1a receptor is not necessary for circadian function per se, although in its absence, the rate of re-entrainment to altered lighting schedules is slower (Grippo et al. 2017). Finally, AVP cells (which partially overlap NMS and Drd1a) can also exert an independent pace-making effect, insofar as genetically slowing their cell-autonomous TTFL or removing the TTFL completely by selective deletion of Bmal1, both lengthen the period of circadian behavioral rhythms in mice (Mieda et al. 2015, 2016). These effects on period are not, however, recapitulated in the SCN slice ex vivo, suggesting that any circuit-level pacemaking effect of AVP cells is less powerful than those of NMS cells and Drd1a cells. But it does leave unanswered the critical question are there neurochemically explicit pacemaking nodes embedded in the SCN circuit?

Fig. 11.5 (continued) allow for translational read through of the amber stop codon and thus sustain neuronal Cry1 expression, immediately initiates negative feedback on Per2 and de novo circadian oscillation. The rhythms are rapidly reversible as the translational switch is turned off and on by removal and addition of AlkK. (**b**) Actograms (double-plotted on 48 h time base for clarity) of arrhythmic Cry1 and Cry2-null mouse before (upper) and after (lower) surgical transduction with AAVs, as above. Provision of AlkK via drinking water rapidly initiates de novo circadian behavior, which is reversibly lost and restored by swapping between vehicle and AlkK (Redrawn from (Maywood et al. 2018))

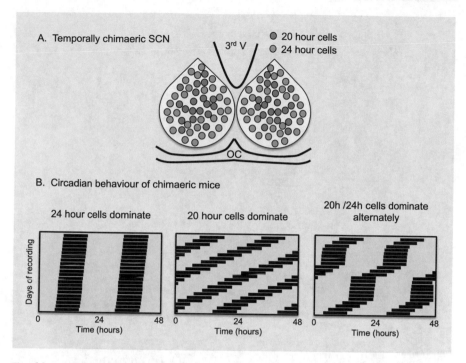

Fig. 11.6 Circadian pacemaking in mice with temporally chimeric SCN reveals network-level interactions between cell groups. (**a**) Schematic representation of temporally chimeric SCN containing cells with cell-autonomous TTFL periods of 24 h or 20 h created by intersectional deletion of the CK1ε^{Tau} alleles in cells expressing Drd1a-driven Cre recombinase. (**b**) Schematic actograms (double-plotted on 48 h time-base for clarity) of mice with temporally chimeric SCN. In the majority of mice (60%), the long period cells predominate (left), but in ca. 30% of mice, the short period cells are pacemakers, whilst in 10% of mice, the two populations control behavioral period alternately (Redrawn from (Smyllie et al. 2016)). OC, optic chiasm; third V, third ventricle

11.8   Neurons Are Not the Only Pacemakers in the SCN Circuit: The Contribution of Astrocytes

Although analysis of SCN timekeeping has focused on neurons, some attention has been paid to their neighboring cells, such as astrocytes, especially in the context of retinal innervation of the SCN. SCN astrocytes strongly express the marker glial fibrillary acidic protein (GFAP), a component of intermediate filaments of the cytoskeleton. Notably, the distribution of GFAP in the SCN is rhythmic, becoming more extensive during circadian daytime and contracting in circadian night (Serviere and Lavialle 1996; Santos et al. 2005). This has been interpreted in the context of astrocytic modulation of retinal innervation to the SCN (closing or allowing access of RHT terminals to SCN core neurons) and/or circadian changes in the metabolic support demanded of astrocytes by neurons, as neuronal electrical firing rates rise

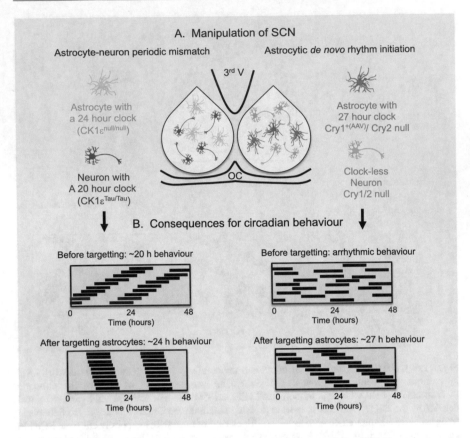

Fig. 11.7 Control of circadian behavior by the cell-autonomous clock of SCN astrocytes. (**a**) Schematic view of intersectional genetic manipulations of SCN neurons and astrocytes. Left: neurons homozygous for $CK1\varepsilon^{Tau}$ have a 20 h cell-intrinsic period, whereas GFAP-dependent deletion of $CK1\varepsilon^{Tau}$ in astrocytes creates an ~ 24 h cell-intrinsic period. Right: in the absence of Cry proteins, SCN neurons lack a functional circadian TTFL, whereas GFAP-dependent expression of Cry1 initiates a long-period oscillation in astrocytes. (**b**) Schematic views of the circadian behavior, under constant darkness, of (left) short period $CK1\varepsilon^{Tau/Tau}$ and (right) arrhythmic Cry1 and Cry2-null mice, before and after AAV-mediated, GFAP-dependent targeting of SCN astrocytes

and fall in circadian time. More recently, a more direct influence of astrocytes on SCN timekeeping has been revealed by conditional manipulation of the astrocytic cell-autonomous TTFL in the SCN. The *Tau* mutant version of casein kinase 1 accelerates the TTFL from 24 to 22 (heterozygous) or 20 h (homozygous). In short-period mutant mice, Cre-mediated deletion of the Tau allele(s) from SCN neurons (and Drd1a neurons, see above) returns behavioral period to wild-type-like 24 h, as would be expected given the central role of SCN neurons in driving behavior. Remarkably, deletion of the mutant allele from SCN astrocytes (targeted by AAV in which the GFAP promoter drives Cre) also causes homozygous mice to change from a 20 h to a 24 h behavioral rhythm (Brancaccio et al. 2017) (Fig. 11.7).

The cell-autonomous TTFL of SCN astrocytes can therefore impose its intrinsic period on the daily behavior of the animal, an effect also seen in heterozygous mice with a period of 22 h that reverts to 24 h when astrocytes are targeted with a different astrocytically specific promoter, Aldh1l1 (Tso et al. 2017). Strikingly, data from this "astrocytic neuronal periodic mismatch" protocol therefore showed that astrocytes of the SCN can function as circadian pacemakers, eliciting circadian patterns of locomotor activity, which are indistinguishable from analogous neuronal manipulations. To test whether or not the astrocytic clock may also be sufficient to initiate de novo SCN and behavioral rhythms, SCN slices from Cry-null mice were cotransduced with AAVs encoding Cre, restricted to neurons, or astrocytes, together with a Cre-dependent Cry1. This protocol of de novo rhythm initiation would reveal the sufficiency of astrocytes in establishing circadian activity. Moreover, because of the absence of competing rhythms in the cell type, which has not undergone the genetic manipulation, it would also allow an easier comparison and contrast of the circadian properties of the newly established rhythms, driven by neurons versus astrocytes. As anticipated, expression of Cry1 in Cry-null SCN neurons initiated circadian TTFL and neuronal $[Ca^{2+}]_i$ rhythms, with a Cry1-definitive long period. Equally, selective expression of Cry1 in astrocytes of Cry-null SCN also initiated TTFL and neuronal $[Ca^{2+}]_i$ rhythms with a Cry1-definitive long period (Brancaccio et al. 2019) (Fig. 11.7). The potency of this control by astrocytes was emphasized further by in vivo studies, in which Cry1 was expressed conditionally in neurons or astrocytes in the SCN of arrhythmic Cry-null mice, which confirmed that Cry1 expression in astrocytes alone was sufficient to both initiate and support long-term daily patterns of locomotor behavior (Brancaccio et al. 2019). Importantly, although the rhythms of the newly generated oscillations were always longer than 24 h, as expected for a Cry1 rescue, astrocytic Cry1 encoded for periodicities that were consistently shorter than those supported by neuronal rescue. Thus, this protocol revealed for the first time that cell-autonomous circadian properties imparted by the astrocytic TTFL clock could be distinguished from those imparted by neurons. Given that astrocytes do not have direct access to behavioral control centers, this also raised the question of how the genetic manipulation of astrocytes could be translated into a motor output, which, although distinguishable in period, was no less robust than the one generated by neurons. Astrocytic Cry1 rescue was capable of reinitiating regular circadian patterns of neuronal $[Ca^{2+}]_i$ in SCN slices showing that the astrocytic TTFL can generate circadian signals able to control cellular circadian function in SCN neurons, which in turn may engage brain centers controlling arousal and locomotion. The possibility to distinguish a cell-autonomous clock in neurons and astrocytes was confirmed by the conditional expression of a bioluminescent transcriptional reporter for Cry1, showing that the TTFLs of neurons and astrocytes are indeed differentially phased, with Cry1 peaking at CT11 in neurons and about 6 h later in astrocytes (Brancaccio et al. 2019). This time-of-day-dependent dichotomy in astrocytic and neuronal activities was confirmed by detecting antiphasic $[Ca^{2+}]_i$ rhythms in astrocytes and neurons in wild type SCN slices, which raised the possibility that astrocytes of the SCN would release a signal capable of directly or indirectly inhibiting neuronal activities at nighttime.

11.9   Astrocytically Released Glutamate Synchronizes Activity of SCN Neurons

What type of signal is provided by astrocytes to drive the surrounding neurons? The first indication of such a signal came from real-time recording of extra-cellular levels of glutamate ($[Glu^-]_e$) in SCN slices. By using a genetically encoded fluorescent reporter (iGluSnFR) delivered by AAV vectors, it was possible to show that $[Glu^-]_e$ varied on a pronounced circadian basis, peaking in circadian night in register with astrocytic $[Ca^{2+}]_i$, a phase of neuronal quiescence (Brancaccio et al. 2017). These $[Glu^-]_e$ oscillations were abolished in SCN slices from Cry-null mice, but emerged when Cry1 was expressed in astrocytes. Furthermore, blockers of the astrocytically restricted Cx43 hemichannels (Abudara et al. 2014; Sengiku et al. 2018), which mediate release of glutamate and other "gliotransmitters" into the extracellular space, impaired such newly generated rhythms and also damped rhythms of clock gene expression in wild type SCN. Inhibition of glutamate transporters caused a large rise in $[Glu^-]_e$ as clearance by neurons and astrocytes was curtailed and flattened its circadian pattern. It is even more surprising that this was accompanied by damping and desynchrony of the cellular TTFLs and neuronal $[Ca^{2+}]_i$ rhythms of the SCN, suggesting that the circadian cycle of $[Glu^-]_e$ is important in circuit-level coordination. The regulation of glutamate by astrocytic Cx43 and transporters showed that glutamate is essential to keep circadian oscillations in SCN slices. In this configuration, retinal innervation is absent, and so any spurious effects from glutamatergic RHT stimulation can be ruled out. In the exclusively GABA-ergic and neuropeptidergic SCN circuit, astrocytes may therefore control neuronal activation by releasing gliotransmitters, such as glutamate, to regulate synaptic function (Savtchouk and Volterra 2018). Glutamate can act via metabotropic and ionotropic receptors, with the latter including NMDA- and AMPA-type groups. However, broad-spectrum blockers of NMDARs or AMPARs alone or jointly had no effect on the disruption of SCN timekeeping caused by elevated $[Glu^-]_e$, arguing against an action of glutamate via these molecules. NMDARs are heteromers of NR1 and various NR2 subunits, and NMDARs containing NR1, NR2A, and NR2B mediate the effects of glutamatergic retinal innervation in the core SCN. These variants are sensitive to the broad-spectrum, open channel NMDAR-blocker MK801, but a third NMDA subunit, NR2C, is also expressed in the SCN and NR2C and NR1/NR2C heteromers are not sensitive to MK801. Furthermore, NR2C is expressed in the dorsal SCN shell, not the retinorecipient core, raising the possibility that glutamate acting via NR2C-containing NMDARs may play a previously unrecognized role in SCN timekeeping. Consistent with this idea, treatment of SCN slices with a blocker of NR2C/NR2D complexes caused rapid and reversible damping and period lengthening of the ensemble TTFL. This damping arose from phase-dispersal of the neurons in the NR2C-expressing region of the dorsal SCN and was reflected in the consequent distortion of the spatiotemporal phase wave across the circuit. Given that NR2D is not expressed in the SCN, this effect highlights a role for the NR2C subunits in circuit synchronization. Further evidence comes from electrophysiological studies, showing that NR2C blockade in circadian day (when $[Glu^-]_e$ is minimal) has no effect on neuronal firing rate or membrane potential, whereas treatment in circadian night, in an environment of high $[Glu^-]_e$ and when SCN neurons are electrically silent, caused an acute and reversible increase in resting membrane potential (depolarization by ~2 mV) and firing rates. These effects were accompanied by an increase in presynaptic $[Ca^{2+}]_i$ levels and decrease in (postsynaptic) cytosolic $[Ca^{2+}]_i$ levels, suggesting that elevated glutamate acts nocturnally on presynaptic NR2C-containing NMDARs to increase the likelihood of GABA release and thereby maintain a suppressive GABAergic tone across the SCN circuit. Removal of this suppressive tone at the beginning of circadian day, when $[Glu^-]_e$ falls as astrocytes become less active, will enable the SCN neurons to increase their spontaneous firing rate and thereby drive their TTFLs at a high amplitude and stable period. How neurons in turn regulate the TTFL of astrocytes is not at all clear, but the working hypothesis is that SCN circuit-level timekeeping arises from interdependent and mutually supportive astrocytic-neuronal signaling. Thus, the "secrets" that make the SCN such a powerful pacemaker are as follows: first, the intracellular linkage between the TTFL and neural electrical activity; second, the intercellular linkage mediated by neuropeptidergic signaling; and third, the mutually supportive antiphasic activities of neuronal and astrocytic TTFLs.

11.10 Perspectives

The SCN is the circadian clock that underpins photoperiodic time measurement in mammals. Understanding of the cell autonomous basis of circadian timekeeping in the SCN has benefited from advances made in elucidating the composition of the TTFL of other cell types, including cell lines. A new challenge is to understand how this generic TTFL interfaces with the particular electrical and metabolic activity of the SCN neuron and how those neurons are networked together to generate the emergent properties that confer such stability and robustness on the SCN. Calcium-responsive elements have been identified as an access point into the TTFL for cellular signaling pathways, although they are most obvious in Per1, and the mechanisms by which other TTFL factors respond to changes in firing rate and/or intercellular signaling await clarification. For example, retinal activation leads to the rapid induction of immediate early genes and their protein products (cFos, Egr1, etc.) in the SCN core. On the other hand, the shell exhibits a low level but sustained circadian oscillation of cFos expression. These acute and tonic changes may in turn direct TTFL gene expression via their AP-1 target sequences. Thus, the conduits for electrical/signaling activation into the TTFL may differ between cell types, for example, between the rapidly resetting core and the slower shell and also between different neuropeptidergic populations. They may also differ between signals that maintain the synchrony of ongoing TTFL oscillations and those that direct phase resetting in response to environmental inputs: are there privileged signaling inputs to the TTFL? Given that TTFLs are active in many other brain regions, lessons learned from the SCN may also be applicable to understand how, for example, cell-autonomous neuronal clocks are integrated and synchronized across the neocortex or within the hippocampus. Circadian disruption carries a heavy cost for cognition, and loss of local cellular circadian synchrony may be one cause of this.

The nature of the intercellular signals that "bind" the SCN circuit also remains unclear. Notwithstanding the power of neuropeptidergic pathways, the role of GABA transmission in the SCN remains an enigma. It has been suggested that peptidergic and GABAergic cues act in tandem by defining the operational range of membrane potential within which SCN neurons can function (Herzog et al. 2017), an idea prompted by the observation that blockade of GABA signaling can rescue the compromised TTFL of VIP-null SCN, even though it is without effect in wild-type SCN. Thus, the balance between pathways may be as important as the activity in any one particular pathway. In addition, a paradox of the SCN as a GABAergic circuit has been its ability to increase spontaneous firing rate on a circadian basis. Increased firing would increase GABAergic tone across the SCN and thereby hyperpolarize the cells and suppress firing, and so how could peak firing be initiated and sustained for several hours in the middle of circadian day? One possibility is that circadian changes in the reversal potential of the GABAR channels may "toggle" them between inhibitory and excitatory states (Pennartz et al. 2002). Alternatively, the model that astrocytes control GABAergic tone independent of neuronal firing rate, via glutamatergic presynaptic depolarization, resolves the paradox because control of GABAergic tone is now devolved from neurons to astrocytes. Is it the circadian change in astrocytic activity that ultimately directs GABAergic tone and thereby determines neuronal firing rate?

The importance of circuit-level signaling to SCN function raises further questions, such as do some populations of neurons influence the circuit more than others, what is the nature of the neuronal computations performed by the circuit, and what is the logic of its topology as a network? Clearly, the answers to these questions will be mutually informative. Some progress (noted above) has been made in searching for pacemaking cells, but the formal circuit topology of the SCN is not understood. Preliminary data have been used to infer a small-world network (Abel et al. 2016), in which hubs consisting of well connected nodes (cells) are located in the central SCN, whereas the cells in the shell are sparsely connected. The challenge is to determine the biological embodiment of these functionally defined structures. Are the hubs characterized by a particular complement of neurotransmitters, do they have greater influence over ensemble properties, and are there systematic differences in synaptic connectivity between nodes and hubs, should they exist? It is also very likely that the network topology is multiplexed, incorporating levels that operate at different temporal and spatial scales. Whereas the small-world may reflect rapid and local GABAergic synaptic linkages, additional neuropeptidergic paracrine and astrocytic modules may operate orthogonally, at a greater spatial scale, and across a longer time domain.

Calendrical function in the SCN is mediated by temporal (phase) rearrangements between cells, rather than any change intrinsic to the cell-autonomous TTFLs. The identity of the SCN cell populations that encode daylength and the neural pathways by which they direct the pineal gland to generate a photoperiodically appropriate melatonin signal are unknown. Improved understanding of SCN circuit topology will better inform this problem, but until recently, photoperiodism was envisioned in the context of neurons. The discovery of the circadian role of astrocytes affords new perspectives: could astrocyte-neuronal interactions contribute to the SCN calendar? At a mechanistic level, the ensheathing of RHT synapses by astrocytes seems to change according to time of the day, and so this aspect of the behavior of astrocytes in the SCN core may also change seasonally, tracking daylength. But the more powerful circadian role of astrocytes appears to be in the dorsal SCN, raising the possibility that the roughly defined core-shell schism caused by long photoperiods may be modulated by and/or may involve localized changes in astrocytic functions. For example, once SCN neuronal populations are locked into their long-day state by retinal cues, are astrocytes important for maintaining it?

A final consideration is how the duration of the melatonin signal is read by target cells in the pituitary and hypothalamus. It is clear that the SCN does not make a significant contribution to this process, but that does not mean that circadian factors are not involved. Indeed, the expression of Per1 in the pars tuberalis (PT), a central target of melatonin in all photoperiodic mammals, is dependent on pineal melatonin (Messager et al. 2001) and the amplitude of the peak expression of Per1 mRNA phased to lights on is higher in hamsters held under shorter photoperiods (Messager et al. 1999). A more extensive characterization of circadian gene expression and season in sheep (Lincoln et al. 2002) not only confirmed the broadening of Per expression in the SCN under summer daylengths but also showed that *Cry2* is expressed in the PT at the start of the dark phase. Consequently, its melatonin-dependent phase relationship to the morning-locked Per peak is photoperiodically sensitive, narrowing on winter photoschedules. The downstream mechanisms by which these melatonin-dependent photoperiodic changes in expression of clock genes in the PT generate seasonal phenotypes are poorly mapped. The PT is thought to control prolactin secretion from the anterior pituitary by secreting a yet-to-be-identified releasing factor, whereas seasonal fertility is thought to be controlled by PT-derived TSH acting in the mediobasal hypothalamus to alter local thyroid hormone activity. Given that a large number of genes are photoperiodically regulated in the PT (Dupre et al. 2010), it may be that the cell-autonomous circadian mechanism is not relevant and all the critical timing machinery involves melatonin (Lu et al. 2010). If so, this would extend the functions of canonical clock genes beyond the oscillatory clock and toward a molecular photoperiodic "egg-timer".

Acknowledgements MH was supported by the Medical Research Council, U.K. MC_U105170643. MB was supported by the UK Dementia Research Institute which receives its funding from UK DRI Ltd, funded by the UK Medical Research Council, Alzheimer's Society and Alzheimer's Research UK.

References

Abel JH, Meeker K, Granados-Fuentes D, St. John PC, Wang TJ, Bales BB, Doyle FJ, Herzog ED, Petzold LR (2016) Functional network inference of the suprachiasmatic nucleus. Proc Natl Acad Sci U S A 113:4512–4517

Abrahamson EE, Moore RY (2001) Suprachiasmatic nucleus in the mouse: retinal innervation, intrinsic organization and efferent projections. Brain Res 916:172–191

Abudara V, Bechberger J, Freitas-Andrade M, de Bock M, Wang N, Bultynck G, Naus CC, Leybaert L, Giaume C (2014) The connexin43 mimetic peptide Gap19 inhibits hemichannels without altering gap junctional communication in astrocytes. Front Cell Neurosci 8:306

Asher G, Schibler U (2011) Crosstalk between components of circadian and metabolic cycles in mammals. Cell Metab 13:125–137

Bartness TJ, Powers JB, Hastings MH, Bittman EL, Goldman BD (1993) The timed infusion paradigm for melatonin delivery: what has it taught us about the melatonin signal, its reception and the photoperiodic control of seasonal responses. J Pineal Res 15:161–190

Berson DM, Felice FA, Takao M (2002) Phototransduction by retinal ganglion cells that reset the circadian clock. Science 295:1070–1073

Best JD, Maywood ES, Smith KL, Hastings MH (1999) Rapid resetting of the mammalian circadian clock. J Neurosci 19:828–835

Brancaccio M, Edwards MD, Patton AP, Smyllie NJ, Chesham JE, Maywood ES, Hastings MH (2019) Cell-autonomous clock of astrocytes drives circadian behavior in mammals. Science 363:187–192

Brancaccio M, Enoki R, Mazuski CN, Jones J, Evans JA, Azzi A (2014) Network-mediated encoding of circadian time: the suprachiasmatic nucleus (SCN) from genes to neurons to circuits, and back. J Neurosci 34:15192–15199

Brancaccio M, Maywood ES, Chesham JE, Loudon AS, Hastings MH (2013) A Gq-Ca(2+) axis controls circuit-level encoding of circadian time in the suprachiasmatic nucleus. Neuron 78:714–728

Brancaccio M, Patton AP, Chesham JE, Maywood ES, Hastings MH (2017) Astrocytes control circadian timekeeping in the Suprachiasmatic nucleus via Glutamatergic signaling. Neuron 93 (1420–1435):e5

Chin JW (2017) Expanding and reprogramming the genetic code. Nature 550:53–60

Cho H, Zhao X, Hatori M, Yu RT, Barish GD, Lam MT, Chong LW, Ditacchio L, Atkins AR, Glass CK, Liddle C, Auwerx J, Downes M, Panda S, Evans RM (2012) Regulation of circadian behaviour and metabolism by REV-ERB-alpha and REV-ERB-beta. Nature 485:123–127

Colwell CS, Michel S, Itri J, Rodriguez W, Tam J, Lelievre V, Hu Z, Liu X, Waschek JA (2003) Disrupted circadian rhythms in VIP- and PHI-deficient mice. Am J Phys Regul Integr Comp Phys 285:R939–R949

Daan S, Albrecht U, Van der Horst GT, Illnerova H, Roenneberg T, Wehr TA, Schwartz WJ (2001) Assembling a clock for all seasons: are there M and E oscillators in the genes? J Biol Rhythm 16:105–116

Daan S, Berde C (1978) Two coupled oscillators: simulations of the circadian pacemaker in mammalian activity rhythms. J Theor Biol 70:297–313

Ding JM, Chen D, Weber ET, Faiman LE, Rea MA, Gillette MU (1994) Resetting the biological clock: mediation of nocturnal circadian shifts by glutamate and NO. Science 266:1713–1717

Dupre SM, Miedzinska K, Duval CV, Yu L, Goodman RL, Lincoln GA, Davis JR, Mcneilly AS, Burt DD, Loudon AS (2010) Identification of Eya3 and TAC1 as long-day signals in the sheep pituitary. Curr Biol 20:829–835

Edwards MD, Brancaccio M, Chesham JE, Maywood ES, Hastings MH (2016) Rhythmic expression of cryptochrome induces the circadian clock of arrhythmic suprachiasmatic nuclei through arginine vasopressin signaling. Proc Natl Acad Sci U S A 113:2732–2737

Ernst RJ, Krogager TP, Maywood ES, Zanchi R, Beranek V, Elliott TS, Barry NP, Hastings MH, Chin JW (2016) Genetic code expansion in the mouse brain. Nat Chem Biol 12:776–778

Evans JA, Leise TL, Castanon-Cervantes O, Davidson AJ (2013) Dynamic interactions mediated by nonredundant signaling mechanisms couple circadian clock neurons. Neuron 80:973–983

Fernandez DC, Chang YT, Hattar S, Chen SK (2016) Architecture of retinal projections to the central circadian pacemaker. Proc Natl Acad Sci U S A 113:6047–6052

Freedman MS, Lucas RJ, Soni B, Von Schantz M, Munoz M, David-Gray Z, Foster R (1999) Regulation of mammalian circadian behavior by non-rod, non-cone, ocular photoreceptors. Science 284:502–504

Gachon F, Olela FF, Schaad O, Descombes P, Schibler U (2006) The circadian PAR-domain basic leucine zipper transcription factors DBP, TEF, and HLF modulate basal and inducible xenobiotic detoxification. Cell Metab 4:25–36

Grippo RM, Purohit AM, Zhang Q, Zweifel LS, Guler AD (2017) Direct midbrain dopamine input to the Suprachiasmatic nucleus accelerates circadian entrainment. Curr Biol 27(2465–2475):e3

Guler AD, Ecker JL, Lall GS, Haq S, Altimus CM, Liao HW, Barnard AR, Cahill H, Badea TC, Zhao H, Hankins MW, Berson DM, Lucas RJ, Yau KW, Hattar S (2008) Melanopsin cells are the principal conduits for rod-cone input to non-image-forming vision. Nature 453:102–105

Hamnett R, Crosby P, Chesham JE, Hastings MH (2019) Vasoactive intestinal peptide controls the suprachiasmatic circadian clock network via ERK1/2 and DUSP4 signalling. Nat Commun 10:542

Harmar AJ, Marston HM, Shen S, Spratt C, West KM, Sheward WJ, Morrison CF, Dorin JR, Piggins HD, Reubi JC, Kelly JS, Maywood ES, Hastings MH (2002) The VPAC(2) receptor is essential for circadian function in the mouse suprachiasmatic nuclei. Cell 109:497–508

Hastings M (2001) Modeling the molecular calendar. J Biol Rhythm 16:117–123. Discussion 124

Hastings MH, Brancaccio M, Maywood ES (2014) Circadian pacemaking in cells and circuits of the suprachiasmatic nucleus. J Neuroendocrinol 26:2–10

Hastings MH, Maywood ES, Brancaccio M (2018) Generation of circadian rhythms in the suprachiasmatic nucleus. Nat Rev Neurosci 19:453–469

Hastings MH, Reddy AB, Maywood ES (2003) A clockwork web: circadian timing in brain and periphery, in health and disease. Nat Rev Neurosci 4:649–661

Hastings MH, Reddy AB, Mcmahon DG, Maywood ES (2005) Analysis of circadian mechanisms in the suprachiasmatic nucleus by transgenesis and biolistic transfection. Methods Enzymol 393:579–592

Hattar S, Liao HW, Takao M, Berson DM, Yau KW (2002) Melanopsin-containing retinal ganglion cells: architecture, projections, and intrinsic photosensitivity. Science 295:1065–1070

Hattar S, Lucas RJ, Mrosovsky N, Thompson S, Douglas RH, Hankins MW, LEM J, Biel M, Hofmann F, Foster RG, Yau KW (2003) Melanopsin and rod-cone photoreceptive systems account for all major accessory visual functions in mice. Nature 424:76–81

Herzog ED, Hermanstyne T, Smyllie NJ, Hastings MH (2017) Regulating the Suprachiasmatic nucleus (SCN) circadian clockwork: interplay between cell-autonomous and circuit-level mechanisms. Cold Spring Harb Perspect Biol 9

Hirano A, Fu YH, Ptacek LJ (2016) The intricate dance of post-translational modifications in the rhythm of life. Nat Struct Mol Biol 23:1053–1060

Inagaki N, Honma S, Ono D, Tanahashi Y, Honma K (2007) Separate oscillating cell groups in mouse suprachiasmatic nucleus couple photoperiodically to the onset and end of daily activity. Proc Natl Acad Sci U S A 104:7664–7669

Jones CR, Huang AL, Ptacek LJ, Fu YH (2013) Genetic basis of human circadian rhythm disorders. Exp Neurol 243:28–33

Krogager TP, Ernst RJ, Elliott TS, Calo L, Beranek V, Ciabatti E, Spillantini MG, Tripodi M, Hastings MH, Chin JW (2017) Labeling and identifying cell-specific proteomes in the mouse brain. Nat Biotechnol

Lazzerini Ospri L, Prusky G, Hattar S (2017) Mood, the circadian system, and Melanopsin retinal ganglion cells. Annu Rev Neurosci 40:539–556

Lee IT, Chang AS, Manandhar M, Shan Y, Fan J, Izumo M, Ikeda Y, Motoike T, Dixon S, Seinfeld JE, Takahashi JS, Yanagisawa M (2015) Neuromedin s-producing neurons act as essential pacemakers in the suprachiasmatic nucleus to couple clock neurons and dictate circadian rhythms. Neuron 85:1086–1102

Lincoln GA, Ebling FJP, Almeida OFX (1985) Generation of melatonin rhythms. In: Evered D, Clark S (eds) Photoperiodism, melatonin and the pineal gland. Pitman, London

Lincoln G, Messager S, Andersson H, Hazlerigg D (2002) Temporal expression of seven clock genes in the suprachiasmatic nucleus and the pars tuberalis of the sheep: evidence for an internal coincidence timer. Proc Natl Acad Sci U S A 99:13890–13895

Lu W, Meng QJ, Tyler NJ, Stokkan KA, Loudon AS (2010) A circadian clock is not required in an arctic mammal. Curr Biol 20:533–537

Lucas RJ (2013) Mammalian inner retinal photoreception. Curr Biol 23:R125–R133

Lucas RJ, Freedman MS, Munoz M, Garcia-Fernandez JM, Foster RG (1999) Regulation of the mammalian pineal by non-rod, non-cone, ocular photoreceptors. Science 284:505–507

Maywood ES, Chesham JE, O'brien JA, Hastings MH (2011) A diversity of paracrine signals sustains molecular circadian cycling in suprachiasmatic nucleus circuits. Proc Natl Acad Sci U S A 108:14306–14311

Maywood ES, Elliott TS, Patton AP, Krogager TP, Chesham JE, Ernst RJ, Beranek V, Brancaccio M, Chin JW, Hastings MH (2018) Translational switching of Cry1 protein expression confers reversible control of circadian behavior in arrhythmic cry-deficient mice. Proc Natl Acad Sci U S A 115:E12388–E12397

Maywood ES, Hastings MH, Max M, Ampleford E, Menaker M, Loudon AS (1993) Circadian and daily rhythms of melatonin in the blood and pineal gland of free-running and entrained Syrian hamsters. J Endocrinol 136:65–73

Maywood ES, Reddy AB, Wong GK, O'neill JS, O'brien JA, Mcmahon DG, Harmar AJ, Okamura H, Hastings MH (2006) Synchronization and maintenance of timekeeping in suprachiasmatic circadian clock cells by neuropeptidergic signaling. Curr Biol 16:599–605

Mazuski C, Abel JH, Chen SP, Hermanstyne TO, Jones JR, Simon T, Doyle FJ, Herzog ED (2018) Entrainment of circadian rhythms depends on firing rates and neuropeptide release of VIP SCN neurons. Neuron 99(555–563):e5

Meijer JH, Michel S (2015) Neurophysiological analysis of the suprachiasmatic nucleus: a challenge at multiple levels. Methods Enzymol 552:75–102

Messager S, Garabette ML, Hastings MH, Hazlerigg DG (2001) Tissue-specific abolition of Per1 expression in the pars tuberalis by pinealectomy in the Syrian hamster. Neuroreport 12:579–582

Messager S, Ross AW, Barrett P, Morgan PJ (1999) Decoding photoperiodic time through Per1 and ICER gene amplitude. Proc Natl Acad Sci U S A 96:9938–9943

Mieda M, Okamoto H, Sakurai T (2016) Manipulating the cellular circadian period of arginine vasopressin neurons alters the behavioral circadian period. Curr Biol 26:2535–2542

Mieda M, Ono D, Hasegawa E, Okamoto H, Honma K, Honma S, Sakurai T (2015) Cellular clocks in AVP neurons of the SCN are critical for Interneuronal coupling regulating circadian behavior rhythm. Neuron 85:1103–1116

Nagoshi E, Brown SA, Dibner C, Kornmann B, Schibler U (2005) Circadian gene expression in cultured cells. Methods Enzymol 393:543–557

Noguchi T, Leise TL, Kingsbury NJ, Diemer T, Wang LL, Henson MA, Welsh DK (2017) Calcium circadian rhythmicity in the Suprachiasmatic nucleus: cell autonomy and network modulation. eNeuro 4

Nuesslein-Hildesheim B, O'brien JA, Ebling FJ, Maywood ES, Hastings MH (2000) The circadian cycle of mPER clock gene products in the suprachiasmatic nucleus of the siberian hamster encodes both daily and seasonal time. Eur J Neurosci 12:2856–2864

O'Neill JS, Maywood ES, Chesham JE, Takahashi JS, Hastings MH (2008) cAMP-dependent signaling as a core component of the mammalian circadian pacemaker. Science 320:949–953

Panda S, Provencio I, Tu DC, Pires SS, Rollag MD, Castrucci AM, Pletcher MT, Sato TK, Wiltshire T, Andahazy M, Kay SA, Van Gelder RN, Hogenesch JB (2003) Melanopsin is required for non-image-forming photic responses in blind mice. Science 301:525–527

Park J, Zhu H, O'Sullivan S, Ogunnaike BA, Weaver DR, Schwaber JS, Vadigepalli R (2016) Single-cell transcriptional analysis reveals novel neuronal phenotypes and interaction networks involved in the central circadian clock. Front Neurosci 10:481

Patton AP, Chesham JE, Hastings MH (2016) Combined pharmacological and genetic manipulations unlock unprecedented temporal elasticity and reveal phase-specific modulation of the molecular circadian clock of the mouse Suprachiasmatic nucleus. J Neurosci 36:9326–9341

Patton AP, Hastings MH (2018) The suprachiasmatic nucleus. Curr Biol 28:R816–R822

Pennartz CM, De Jeu MT, Bos NP, Schaap J, Geurtsen AM (2002) Diurnal modulation of pacemaker potentials and calcium current in the mammalian circadian clock. Nature 416:286–290

Preitner N, Damiola F, Lopez-Molina L, Zakany J, Duboule D, Albrecht U, Schibler U (2002) The orphan nuclear receptor REV-ERBalpha controls circadian transcription within the positive limb of the mammalian circadian oscillator. Cell 110:251–260

Prosser HM, Bradley A, Chesham JE, Ebling FJ, Hastings MH, Maywood ES (2007) Prokineticin receptor 2 (Prokr2) is essential for the regulation of circadian behavior by the suprachiasmatic nuclei. Proc Natl Acad Sci U S A 104:648–653

Provencio I, Rodriguez IR, Jiang G, Hayes WP, Moreira EF, Rollag MD (2000) A novel human opsin in the inner retina. J Neurosci 20:600–605

Ralph MR, Foster RG, Davis FC, Menaker M (1990) Transplanted suprachiasmatic nucleus determines circadian period. Science 283:693–695

Reppert SM, Weaver DR (2000) Comparing clockworks: mouse versus fly. J Biol Rhythm 15:357–364

Reppert SM, Weaver DR (2002) Coordination of circadian timing in mammals. Nature 418:935–941

Reppert SM, Weaver DR, Ebisawa T (1994) Cloning and characterization of a mammalian melatonin receptor that mediates reproductive and circadian responses. Neuron 13:1177–1185

Roenneberg T, Merrow M (2016) The circadian clock and human health. Curr Biol 26:R432–R443

Rosbash M, Bradley S, Kadener S, Li Y, Luo W, Menet JS, Nagoshi E, Palm K, Schoer R, Shang Y, Tang CH (2007) Transcriptional feedback and definition of the circadian pacemaker in drosophila and animals. Cold Spring Harb Symp Quant Biol 72:75–83

Santos JWQ, Araujo JF, Cunha MJB, Costa SO, Barbosa ALC, Mesquita IB, Costa MSMO (2005) Circadian variation in GFAP immunoreactivity in the mouse suprachiasmatic nucleus. Biol Rhythm Res 36:141–150

Savtchouk I, Volterra A (2018) Gliotransmission: beyond black-and-white. J Neurosci 38:14–25

Schmidt TM, Do MT, Dacey D, Lucas R, Hattar S, Matynia A (2011) Melanopsin-positive intrinsically photosensitive retinal ganglion cells: from form to function. J Neurosci 31:16094–16101

Sekaran S, Foster RG, Lucas RJ, Hankins MW (2003) Calcium imaging reveals a network of intrinsically light-sensitive inner-retinal neurons. Curr Biol 13:1290–1298

Sengiku A, Ueda M, Kono J, Sano T, Nishikawa N, Kunisue S, Tsujihana K, Liou LS, Kanematsu A, Shimba S, Doi M, Okamura H, Ogawa O, Negoro H (2018) Circadian coordination of ATP release in the urothelium via connexin43 hemichannels. Sci Rep 8:1996

Serviere J, Lavialle M (1996) Astrocytes in the mammalian circadian clock: putative roles. Prog Brain Res 111:57–73

Shigeyoshi Y, Taguchi K, Yamamoto S, Takekida S, Yan L, Tei H, Moriya T, Shibata S, Loros JJ, Dunlap J, Okamura H (1997) Light-induced resetting of a mammalian circadian clock is associated with rapid induction of the mPer1 transcript. Cell 91:1043–1053

Smyllie NJ, Chesham JE, Hamnett R, Maywood ES, Hastings MH (2016) Temporally chimeric mice reveal flexibility of circadian period-setting in the suprachiasmatic nucleus. Proc Natl Acad Sci U S A

Stokkan KA, Van Oort BE, Tyler NJ, Loudon AS (2007) Adaptations for life in the Arctic: evidence that melatonin rhythms in reindeer are not driven by a circadian oscillator but remain acutely sensitive to environmental photoperiod. J Pineal Res 43:289–293

Stokkan KA, Yamazaki S, Tei H, Sakaki Y, Menaker M (2001) Entrainment of the circadian clock in the liver by feeding. Science 291:490–493

Takahashi JS (2016) Molecular architecture of the circadian clock in mammals. In: Sassone-Corsi, P. & Christen, Y. (eds.) A time for metabolism and hormones. Cham (CH)

Tso CF, Simon T, Greenlaw AC, Puri T, Mieda M, Herzog ED (2017) Astrocytes regulate daily rhythms in the Suprachiasmatic nucleus and behavior. Curr Biol 27:1055–1061

Van Gelder RN, Buhr ED (2016) Ocular photoreception for circadian rhythm entrainment in mammals. Annu Rev Vis Sci 2:153–169

Weaver DR (1998) The suprachiasmatic nucleus: a 25-year retrospective. J Biol Rhythm 13:100–112

Welsh DK, Yoo SH, Liu AC, Takahashi JS, Kay SA (2004) Bioluminescence imaging of individual fibroblasts reveals persistent, independently phased circadian rhythms of clock gene expression. Curr Biol 14:2289–2295

Willis JCW, Chin JW (2018) Mutually orthogonal pyrrolysyl-tRNA synthetase/tRNA pairs. Nat Chem 10:831–837

Yamaguchi S, Isejima H, Matsuo T, Okura R, Yagita K, Kobayashi M, Okamura H (2003) Synchronization of cellular clocks in the suprachiasmatic nucleus. Science 302:1408–1412

Yamaguchi Y, Suzuki T, Mizoro Y, Kori H, Okada K, Chen Y, Fustin JM, Yamazaki F, Mizuguchi N, Zhang J, Dong X, Tsujimoto G, Okuno Y, Doi M, Okamura H (2013) Mice genetically deficient in vasopressin V1a and V1b receptors are resistant to jet lag. Science 342:85–90

Yin L, Wu N, Curtin JC, Qatanani M, Szwergold NR, Reid RA, Waitt GM, Parks DJ, Pearce KH, Wisely GB, Lazar MA (2007) Rev-erbalpha, a heme sensor that coordinates metabolic and circadian pathways. Science 318:1786–1789

Yoo SH, Yamazaki S, Lowrey PL, Shimomura K, Ko CH, Buhr ED, Siepka SM, Hong HK, Oh WJ, Yoo OJ, Menaker M, Takahashi JS (2004) PERIOD2::LUCIFERASE real-time reporting of circadian dynamics reveals persistent circadian oscillations in mouse peripheral tissues. Proc Natl Acad Sci U S A 101:5339–5346

Yoshikawa T, Inagaki NF, Takagi S, Kuroda S, Yamasaki M, Watanabe M, Honma S, Honma KI (2017) Localization of photoperiod responsive circadian oscillators in the mouse suprachiasmatic nucleus. Sci Rep 7:8210

Zawilska JB, Skene DJ, Arendt J (2009) Physiology and pharmacology of melatonin in relation to biological rhythms. Pharmacol Rep 61:383–410

Glossary

Arcuate nucleus a bilateral cluster of neurons in the mediobasal hypothalamus adjacent to the ventral region of the third ventricle. The presence of fenestrated capillaries in this region gives cells in this structure a more permeable blood–brain barrier than most other regions, so enhancing its capacity to monitor peripheral concentrations of hormones and metabolites.

Astrocyte a type of glial cell, those in the suprachiasmatic nucleus contribute to circadian rhythm generation and regulate neuronal activity.

Blood–brain barrier (BBB) the concept of a selectively permeable barrier between blood in capillaries in the brain and the extracellular fluid that bathes neurons and glia. Tight junctions between endothelial cells restrict the passive transport of substances into the brain.

Bmal "clock" gene encoding Brain and Muscle ARNT-Like 1 (BMAL), a "clock" protein, i.e., a transcription factor involved in intracellular feedback loops that constitute a circadian oscillator. ARNT is Aryl hydrocarbon receptor nuclear translocator-like protein 1.

β thyroid-stimulating hormone (βTSH) a specific β subunit that dimerizes with a common α subunit (αGSU) in thyrotrophs in the anterior pituitary gland. The dimer was initially identified as the pituitary hormone regulating thyroid hormone production, but this specific β subunit can also bind to TSH-R expressed by tanycytes in the hypothalamus to regulate gene expression.

Circadian rhythm a spontaneous cycle in a physiological variable or behavior that can be demonstrated to persist experimentally when organisms are maintained in constant environmental conditions with a periodicity of approximately 24 hours (a day).

Circannual rhythm a long-term spontaneous cycle in a physiological variable or behavior that can be demonstrated to persist when organisms are maintained in constant environmental conditions, in particular a fixed photoperiod. The approximate periodicity is a year, though under experimental conditions the period is usually shorter than 12 months, typically 10.5 months.

Cry1, Cry2 "clock" genes encoding transcription factors (Cryptochrome proteins: CRY1, CRY2) that are involved in intracellular feedback loops that constitute a circadian oscillator.

F. J. P. Ebling, H. D. Piggins (eds.), *Neuroendocrine Clocks and Calendars*, Masterclass in Neuroendocrinology 10, https://doi.org/10.1007/978-3-030-55643-3

Deiodinase a family of enzymes that remove iodine atoms from thyroid hormone, thus regulating bioactivity in target tissues. Whereas deiodinase 1 is widely expressed in the periphery, deiodinase 2 and 3 are expressed in the brain. Deiodinase 2 increases bioactivity by converting thyroxine (T4) to tri-iodothyronine (T3) via removal of an iodine atom from the outer ring, whereas deiodinase 3 reduces bioactivity by converting thyroxine to reverse T3 and by converting tri-iodothyronine to T2 by removal of iodine from the inner ring.

Ependymocyte a glial cell that forms the barrier surrounding the ventricular system in the brain.

Fisher 344 rat a laboratory strain of *Rattus norvegicus* that retains some photoperiodic traits during juvenile development. European strains of Fisher 344 rats are reported to be more photoperiodic that the US strains.

Folliculostellate cells cells in the *pars tuberalis* and *pars distalis* (anterior pituitary) that have a complex morphology with extended cytoplasmic projections. They do not contain secretory granules and so are not classical hormone-producing cells, but may produce factors that exert paracrine regulation. In addition to facilitating local communication, they have an immunomodulatory function.

Free running rhythm a rhythm that is not entrained, so revealing the true innate periodicity.

Hypothalamus part of the basal forebrain (diencephalon) that is a major regulatory center in the vertebrate brain integrating the function of the endocrine, autonomic, and limbic functions. It directly regulates pituitary function.

Long day a photoperiod where the length of the light phase exceeds the length of the dark phase, often abbreviated as LD or LP.

Median eminence a relatively cell-free structure in the mediobasal hypothalamus containing neurosecretory terminals that deliver peptides and amines into portal capillaries that flow to the adjacent anterior pituitary gland.

Melatonin an indoleamine hormone synthesized primarily in the pineal gland in mammals by acetylation and methylation of serotonin. Its production is under the control of the circadian system (suprachiasmatic nucleus) via the sympathetic nervous system, such that secretion occurs during the dark phase.

***Pars tuberalis* (PT)** part of the pituitary stalk that sits at the interface between the median eminence of the hypothalamus and the anterior pituitary gland (*pars distalis*). It primarily comprises thyrotrophs that produce βTSH and folliculostellate cells.

Period the cycle length of a rhythm, the time interval between two successive oscillations.

Per1, Per2 "clock" genes encoding transcription factors (period proteins: PER1, PER2) that are involved in intracellular feedback loops that constitute a circadian oscillator. Period genes were discovered in the 1970s by Ron Konopka in mutant fruit flies (*Drosophila melanogaster*) displaying abnormal circadian periodicities.

Phase the position of a specific point in the cycle of one rhythm relative to an external time reference point or to a specific point in the cycle of another rhythm.

Photoperiodic time measurement (PTM) the pathways, mechanisms, and cellular processes by which annual changes in day length are perceived by an organism.

Phodopus sungorus a species of dwarf Russian hamster often referred to as a "Djungarian" or "Siberian" hamster. This species is widely used in studies of mechanisms underlying rhythmicity because in laboratory conditions it retains seasonality and photoperiodic responses including reproduction, molting, fattening, appetite, and thermoregulation.

Photorefractoriness a phenomenon observed in experimental studies where an initial physiological or behavioral response to a change in photoperiod spontaneously reverts back to the initial state despite the photoperiod being unchanged.

Seasonal affective disorder (SAD) a syndrome in which depression occurs usually during the autumn or winter and remits the following spring or summer, for at least two successive years.

Short day a photoperiod where the length of the dark phase exceeds the length of the light phase, often abbreviated as SD or SP.

Tanycyte a glial cell whose cell body is in the ependymal layer lining the ventral third ventricle, with a cytoplasmic projection that protrudes through the surrounding mediobasal hypothalamus. The end-feet of these tanycytic projections may contact capillaries or ensheath axonal terminals in the median eminence, and a subset of end-feet may contact cells in the surrounding *pars tuberalis*.

TTFLs Intracellular Transcriptional and Translational Feedback loops that constitute cell-autonomous circadian timers

Tuberalin a hormonal factor produced by the *pars tuberalis* that elicits prolactin secretion by lactotrophs in the *pars distalis*. The chemical identity of tuberalin is not known, but several candidates have been proposed including tachykinins and endocannabinoids.

Zeitgeber a photic (light) or non-photic environmental cue that can synchronize or entrain an innate biological rhythm. The term is German for "time-giver".

Index

© The Editor(s) (if applicable) and The Author(s), under exclusive license to
Springer Nature Switzerland AG 2020
F. J. P. Ebling, H. D. Piggins (eds.), *Neuroendocrine Clocks and Calendars*,
Masterclass in Neuroendocrinology 10, https://doi.org/10.1007/978-3-030-55643-3

Printed in the United States
by Baker & Taylor Publisher Services